# Hospital Privileges and Specialty Medicine

## 2nd Edition

# Hospital Privileges
# and Specialty Medicine
# 2nd Edition

Donald G. Langsley, M.D. and
Beauregard Stubblefield, M.B.A.
*Editors*

Foreword by
J. Lee Dockery, M.D.

Published by
the American Board of Medical Specialties
in collaboration with the
Division of Medical Affairs
American Hospital Association

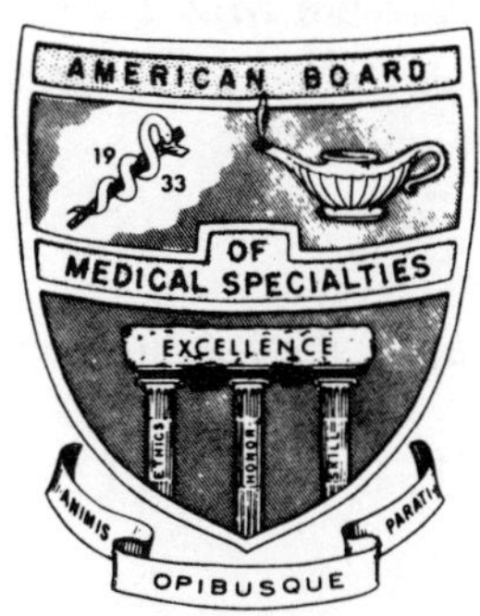


## American Board of Medical Specialties
Evanston, Illinois
1992

ISBN: 0-934277-17-6

Library of Congress Number: 92-073099




Design/Typesetting: North Coast Associates.
Printed in the United States of America.

# Contents



**v**

## SECTION II — Previously Published Papers

See following list of 28 previously published papers

**Chapter**

**Chapter**

**Chapter**

# Contributors of Original Papers

**John R. Ball, MD, JD** is Executive Vice President, American College of Physicians, Philadelphia, PA.

**Philip Bashook, EdD** is Director of Evaluation & Education, American Board of Medical Specialties, Evanston, IL.

**J. Lee Dockery, MD** is Executive Vice President, American Board of Medical Specialties, Evanston, IL.

**Donna D. Fraiche, JD** is a Shareholder in the firm of Locke Purnell Rain Harrell, New Orleans, LA.

**William F. Jessee, MD** is Vice President for Quality Management, Humana, Inc., Louisville, KY.

**Donald G. Langsley, MD** is Executive Vice President Emeritus, American Board of Medical Specialties, Professor of Psychiatry, Northwestern University Medical School and Chief, Psychiatry Service, VA Lakeside Medical Center, Chicago, IL.

**James S. Roberts, MD** is Senior Vice President, Joint Commission on Accreditation of Healthcare Organizations, Oakbrook Terrace, IL.

**Beauregard Stubblefield, MBA** is Program Director, Division of Medical Affairs, American Hospital Association, Chicago, IL.

# Foreword

J. Lee Dockery, MD
Executive Vice President
American Board of Medical Specialties

Credentialing and the declination of hospital staff privileges continue to be issues of primary importance to hospitals and the respective physician applicant for privileges, but ultimately to the public which both entities serve. Through a variety of influences, board certification has become a reference standard as a component of credentialing requirements and privilege delineation for hospital based or affiliated practice. It must be emphasized, however, that documentation of certification is only one of several valid and important criteria for the declination of staff privileges.

The American Board of Medical Specialties (ABMS) and the American Hospital Association (AHA) have a long- standing cooperative relationship. This relationship led to the first joint conference on Hospitals Privileges and Specialty Medicine in September of 1985, and the publication of the first edition of a book by the same title, both designed to enhance the partnerships between physicians and hospital management. These collaborative activities have fostered discussion and the development of compatible mechanisms to deal with credentialing and the delineation of privileges, to the benefit of each constituency and with the outcome of improved patient care.

The first edition of *Hospital Privileges and Specialty Medicine* proved to be a very popular and a useful publication to the over 7,000 hospitals which have the burden and responsibility for defining and verifying the credentials of physicians and awarding the privileges for practice in a respective hospital. The award of privileges must be commensurate with both the resources and the capabilities of the hospital and the skill and capability of the physician compatible with the education, training and demonstrated ability as judged by examination for licensure and certification by boards recognized and approved by ABMS. These credentialing functions, along with peer evaluation and monitoring of practice outcomes, are delegated responsibilities to the medical staff by the governing board of the hospital which require careful evaluation, documentation and decision with shared responsibility. The smoothness with which the credentialing and award of privilege decision are made, predicts the degree of conflict and tension between the hospital and the physician., The second edition of *Hospital Privileges and Specialty Medicine* is another joint project between the ABMS and the AHA reflective of the continued strong relationships and the interest in credentialing and delineation of staff privileges. The new edition is completely revised with a new selection of important articles on credentialing and the delineation of hospital privileges published during the past five years. Seven new original chapters have been added, dealing with the process of credentialing and its relationships to verification of qualifications, practice monitoring, legal aspects of credentialing, Joint Commission on Accreditation of Healthcare Organizations (JCAHO) requirements and influence of continuing medical education on initial privileges, continued privileges and expanded privileges. The reader is informed that none of the reprinted articles or the position statements of any of the authors of these chapters represent the official position of the ABMS or the AHA. It is anticipated that this new revision of the book will be useful to hospitals, medical staff organizations and other organizations involved in credentialing and defining access to institutions by physicians for practice. A strong credentialing system accepted by the hospital and the medical staff is the foundation for the provision of quality health care in any institution. This publication will facilitate and complement any effort in the development of such a system and process.

# Original Papers

**PART**

# 1

# Credentialing, Privileging and Performance: View from the 90s

John R. Ball, MD, JD

The decade of the 80s brought a heightened awareness of the need to deal with health care issues of quality, access, and cost. These issues, along with other changes in the structure of divided responsibility between hospital medical staffs and their governing boards, influenced the processes of credentialing and privileging physicians, but the major motivating factor turned out to be economic rather than either quality or access. The 1990s are even less likely to see a reduction in the focus on cost, but there are encouraging—and disturbing—signs that a number of other important issues will be taken into account. Renewed emphasis by payors on the quality of the "product" may stimulate hospitals to develop and disseminate data on the credentials of the medical staff, their medical outcomes, and their quality assurance processes. Interest in enhancing access to care for the underserved, in the context of cost containment, has prompted proposals for more "managed care," and may catalyze further consolidation of group practices, integrated with hospitals. The newly rediscovered principles of "continuous quality improvement" suggest changes in the way credentialing and de-credentialing may occur. And the ever-present legal system, from the requirements of the National Practitioner Data Bank to changing standards in malpractice cases, will continue to force more data from the health system. These issues will continue to affect the balance of power that has existed between physicians and hospitals for several decades.

*Credentialing* is the process of determining whether a physician may be admitted to membership in the organized medical staff of a hospital.

**3**

Although non-physician health care professionals may also be admitted and granted privileges, this chapter will focus on physicians and only cite issues associated with non-physicians. To be considered for membership in a medical staff, a physician must present evidence of having met very basic qualifications, such as graduation from an acceptable medical school, post-graduate training, possession of a license to practice medicine, and testimony that the applicant has acceptable moral and professional qualities.

*Privileging* is the process of granting the right to perform certain activities within the institution. It presupposes that the physician has become a member of the medical staff. Although it has long been technically and legally the responsibility of the hospital's governing board to grant staff membership and staff privileges, historically the role of the medical staff was much more important and its recommendations were almost automatically accepted by the board. The balance of power in the past was tilted toward physicians, and hospital privilege delineation was centered around staff needs. Moreover, the era of cost reimbursement was one in which cost pressures were not intense, and hospitals had little economic incentive to question medical staff recommendations. Legal changes concerning the hospital's responsibility for quality of care and the presence of a physician manpower surplus have been factors in the recent shift of the balance of power toward hospitals. In addition to the physician surplus, there has been a major increase in non-physician providers who have been able to obtain (frequently via legislation) an expanded role, moving into areas of practice formerly reserved to physicians. The trend toward subspecialization and the consequent competition for privileges between subspecialists and generalists has also influenced privilege delineation. In the economic sphere of prospective payment, hospitals have two basic choices—increase revenues or decrease expenses. The hospital's economic incentive to avoid the sicker patients, whose treatment is more costly, also plays into an economic rationale for granting or withholding privileges.

Privileging is both symbolically and practically important, because it occurs at precisely that junction where professional ethics, the self-interest of the physician, and the complex interests of the institution intersect. Clinical privileges are just that—privileges rather than rights. Licensure conveys the *legal right* to practice but does not mandate a *duty* on behalf of the hospital to permit a licensed physician to practice the broad areas permitted by the license. Privileges define the services the practitioner may perform and are granted by the hospital on the basis of established criteria, applied in each individual case.

Privilege delineation is a two-step process, the initial decision being admission to the medical staff and the second, the privilege to perform certain services within the hospital. For admission to the medical staff, information is provided on education and training, experience, reference regarding competence and character, possession of a current license, professional memberships, and other relevant information about prior negative professional history (e.g., malpractice actions, license revocation, or loss of privileges elsewhere). The Health Care Quality Improvement Act, which established the National Practitioner Data Bank, has added an important dimension to this initial step. Under the act, hospitals are required both to provide information to the Data Bank when there has been a significant reduction in a physician's privileges and to access the Data Bank when admitting a physician to the medical staff or granting privileges. Although the implementation of the National Practioner Data Bank has been fraught with problems, the concept is worthy, and the data potentially critical for responsible credentialing and privileging to occur. The granting of specific privileges usually requires that the applicant give evidence of competence in the management of disease or performance of procedures. The evidence may be in the form of board certification or successful completion of an accredited residency, other types of specific training, case reports or letters from prior supervisors.

 Though other chapters in this book will deal with specific techniques of credentialing and privileging, this one will review the broad areas of health policy and the varied objectives of those in government, other groups with interest in health care, and the health professions concerning these issues. As noted in the first chapter of a prior edition of this book, the environment of health care is changing. Unless both health professionals and health care institutions change, we may not survive, and the people, whose health care is in our charge, will suffer. All of us need to accept the responsibilities associated with our roles. We should accept the theses that:

a) The health professions must undertake the responsibility of providing hospital medical staffs objective standards and information on which to base recommendations for clinical privileges.

b) Hospitals must defer to medical staff judgment on medical qualifications, but strengthen their roles in making independent business decisions.

c) Courts must grant substantial leeway to hospitals in making economic judgments and to the health professions in making medical judgments.

d) Policy-makers must recognize the long term effects on health care caused by short-term decisions driven by cost considerations.


## The Environment

The environment of health care may be considered under three headings: economic, legal and political. The dominant force, at present, of course, is economic, with the practice of health care, the law relating to it, and the politics of health care all shaped by economics. Physician and hospital practice patterns are changing dramatically because of economics. The frontier of the law of health care is antitrust law, deeply rooted in free-market economic theory. And the political choices in health care are driven almost solely by cost considerations. The environment is shaped largely by forces outside the direct control of health professionals.

By way of introduction, the following points should be made:

a) Economic pressures form a two-edged sword for professionals:
1) the opportunity to reassert professionalism, to develop standards and to be willing to be measured by them.
2) the danger of the loss of professionalism, of allowing economic self-interest to usurp the primacy of the patient's best interest.
b) Antitrust law, in which competition is always the primary value, and at times the only value, does not mean that standards cannot be established by health professionals; it does mean that those standards must be established and applied in ways that do not contravene other societal values.
c) In politics, public mistrust of the motives of physicians, coupled with the medical profession's negative political strategy, has resulted in the legitimate concerns of the profession lacking a sympathetic audience and resulting in an unprecedented vulnerability of the profession to political change that does not account for legitimate clinical concerns.

## Economics

Health care costs are like a balloon: squeeze down at one point and another expands. The moderation of Medicare expenditures for hospitals following the institution of prospective payment in 1983 was accompanied by a predictable increase in outpatient expenditures. Health care costs continue to consume an ever-increasing portion of the Gross National Product. And all parties, from the politician to the payor, from the physician and "provider" to the patient, understand that *something* must be done about costs.

Perceptions about economics become political reality. But before turning to the Washington political perspective, consider an anecdote on how not too long ago, physicians perceived medical economics. It is instructive about how far we have come.

Lewis Thomas, in his delightful book of essays, *The Medusa and the Snail*, reflects on the nature of change:

I had forgotten what things were like in the good old days of medicine, and how different. I knew, of course, that the science and technology have undergone changes of great magnitude, and how doctors now can accomplish such cures and relief of disability as were beyond the imagination when I was young. But there is another difference, and I had forgotten about this.

Thomas then goes on to report on a survey, done in his 1937 Harvard Medical School yearbook, of Harvard medical alumni from the classes of 1907, 1917, and 1927. Of greatest interest, both to Thomas and perhaps to us today, were the findings concerning net incomes, incomes that by comparison were significantly higher than those of the average physician of 1937. The median net income was between $5,000 and $10,000 a year, only five alumni making over $20,000. Commented one alumnus in the survey: "I am satisfied with medicine as a life's work. However, I should recommend it only for the man who has plenty of money back of him. Many men never make much in medicine."

In today's world of an affluent medical career, we, like Lewis Thomas, on occasion forget what things were like in the "good old days," and only by pausing can we begin to digest the degree of change and the rapidity with which it has occurred.

On occasion, though, we physicians, unwilling to accept the demythologizing of medicine, do wish to go back to the "good old days"— that brief period perhaps in the 1950s or 1960s, when incomes and control and satisfaction were high, and regulation and other constraints low. It is that occasional, though strong, wistfulness for the past that comes into conflict with today's pervasive perception that something must be done about costs.

## Cost

Concern about health care costs is not new. Almost sixty years ago, a group calling itself the Committee on the Costs of Medical Care published a number of surveys on health care costs. In the late 1930s, the modern debate on "socialized medicine" was begun in this country, a debate that has seen periodic revivals of proposals for national health insurance, some as recent as 1991. The difference, however, between this rather long history and the present debate is that most earlier criticisms of the existing health care system and proposals for its restructuring were based not so much on the view that *costs* in general were high, but that *access* to care should be enhanced. Indeed, that old rationale has returned, as we have become pointedly aware that a large percentage of our population has inadequate access to basic, appropriate health care. However, the juxtaposition of two competing policy ends—enhancing access and controlling costs—makes finding a good solution all the more problematic. There is, nevertheless, a consensus among almost all segments of society that health care costs are unacceptably high and that something must be done about it.

American business is increasingly feeling the pressures brought on by the almost geometric increases in costs. More recently, workers have been affected in a number of ways, from having to pay higher premiums, copayments and deductibles to being unable to change jobs due to the insurers' practice of excluding pre-existing medical conditions in any new employee. Nevertheless, nowhere is the pressure felt more acutely than in government, at the federal level with Medicare, and at the state level with Medicaid, where that single program consumes 15 percent of the average budget. The federal government, especially, is under pressure as voters become frustrated with the lack of leadership and as politicians remain hamstrung by the decade-old mantra "no new taxes." The economic message is a powerful one:

Health care costs are rising at rates far in excess of the increase of other sectors of the economy. Even during the recent times of 5 percent inflation, health care costs were rising at over 15 percent—at times more than three times the rate of inflation. Physician fees continue to be a prominent component of the CPI.

Outlays for Medicare since 1970 have been increasing at an average rate of over 17 percent per year. Medicare outlays have grown from $3.5 billion in 1965 to $35 billion in 1980 to $118 billion in 1991.

In 1992, total annual health expenditures for the nation will be $817 billion. In the past several years we have watched these health care expenditures increase as a percent of our gross national product from 8.9 percent of GNP to the projection for 1992 of 14 percent.

For those concerned with questions of quality and access and the day-to-day practice of medicine or the day-to-day administration of hospital facilities these are the kinds of seemingly dry numbers that make the eyes glaze. But increasingly, these are the kind of numbers that matter to those in Washington charged with the management of the public purse.

Coupled with the economic facts of life of the health care system are another set of economic facts—those relating to the present state of the nation at large. This second set of statistics and economic concepts is even more removed from the day-to-day world of those within the health care sector, and yet in many senses it is more traditional macroeconomic elements that are responsible for imbuing policy makers with a dramatic sense of urgency, even as they remain paralyzed by a lack of consensus, of leadership, and of a solution with which anyone has confidence.

Finding a solution to the problem of \$300+ billion deficits is viewed by economists, businesspeople and others, from all points on the political spectrum, as essential to the continued economic well-being of the nation. This concern is perceived and shared by the Congress. More importantly, it is widely shared by members of Congress irrespective of political ideology or party affiliation. Standard wisdom is that a massive deficit with its appetite for capital consumption crowds out other investment opportunities in the market place. Money that could be devoted to industrial development gets used instead by the federal government in the financing of the federal debt.

But the annual deficit of \$300+ billion is only a part of the story; it is adding to a cumulative national debt quickly approaching \$5 *trillion*. Again, what is so important here is the trend in the rate of growth of that underlying debt: in January of 1981, the debt was \$940.5 billion. For fiscal year 1993, it is projected to be \$4.5 trillion. The cost of feeding this debt—interest—was roughly \$75 billion in 1980. It will approach \$317 billion in 1993. In short, Congress must find a way to curb the rate at which the debt is being increased. Perhaps even more importantly, and less often discussed, debt of this magnitude is providing opportunities for unprecedented levels of foreign capital to enter the American system. This in itself raises important questions far beyond the scope of this paper, but serves parenthetically as a reminder that in our role as health care providers (in all senses of the term), we cannot lose sight of our larger responsibilities as citizens.

What then, do these national economic concerns, including the need to reduce federal expenditures, have to do with any of us who care about the delivery of health care in this country? The importance of the linkage is twofold. First, because of the size of the federal contribution to health care, any attempt to address the overall federal budget must focus at least some attention on the health care segment of that budget. The budget of the Department of Health and Human Services constitutes over a third of the total federal budget. Of that budget nearly 96 percent goes to entitlements including Social Security and Medicare. Given our present societal commitment to the preservation of Social Security, even more budgetary attention is focused on the Medicare and Medicaid expenditures.

Secondly, it signals once and for all the transition from an era in which the provision of health care services was the sole province of physicians, hospitals, and insurers, to an era in which the government must and will be a key, if not the principal, determinant of policy approaches.

Now these fiscal and economic realities are considered in the context of a set of powerful *political* realities:

A societal consensus that health care costs are unacceptably high.

A consensual analysis that third-party retrospective reimbursement is at the root of the cost problem by enhancing incentives to provide services—to spend—and by eliminating most incentives to be parsimonious.

The widespread view that governmental programs of cost containment from Medicare coverage policies, PRO review, health planning, and UCR reimbursement were inadequate, at least in part because of providers' attitudes.

The widespread view that private sector provider-dominated programs, such as the Voluntary Effort of the late 1970s were failures.

An increasing frustration at all levels of government with the opposition of providers to every governmentally proposed program of cost containment, including PRO, health planning, the cost containment/capital expenditure cap proposals and even prospective payment.

A further frustration, particularly in Congress, that highly touted proposals for resolving the cost problem have so far appeared to be without substance.

A whetting of the appetite for reform secondary to the apparent success (in economic terms) of the prospective payment system.

A general view that something must be done, especially during a presidential campaign when much attention is being given to health care reform.

This focus is on Washington because there the broad brush of public policy is played out and the cost issue—since government pays 40 percent of health care costs—is most acute.

The actions of government on the economics of health care predictably, though belatedly, have had spillover effects onto the private sector. Rooted in concepts of "social justice" that grew in the 1950s and 1960s, the idea of a "right" to at least some level of medical care led to two elemental governmental activities: (1) decreasing barriers to access, both economic (through Medicare and Medicaid) and geographic (community health centers and regional health programs), and (2) increasing supply, primarily through small, albeit successful, capitation grants to medical schools. The result was increased access by the poor; a fostering of a sense of "entitlement" by the elderly; and a doubling of medical school outputs.

When, however, costs began to increase without apparent commensurate benefits, government turned to what it knew best: regulation. Regulation proceeded on two fronts: supply and payment. For example, since its inception, Medicare has focused single-mindedly on the mechanics of payment rather than the goals of payment. Only with the 1982 TEFRA legislation did legislation or regulation directly attack the economic incentives that in part determine hospital behavior. Strangely the federal government never fully utilized the economic clout that comes with its 40 percent share of the inpatient market; rather than becoming a prudent purchaser, it was content to remain an increasingly "picky payor."

The consequence of racheting down reimbursement levels for the provider was that providers increasingly began to meet their obligations to public payers through funding from the private sector: cost-shifting. Thus, care of the undercompensated, financing of graduate medical education, innovation, and other activities for which government was unwilling to compensate fully was shifted to others—private payors, business, the large insurers. The same global economic pressures beginning to be felt by government are felt by business, however, and that sector has quickly become unwilling to pay for activities in health care that appear unrelated directly to the services received by patients for whom they are responsible.

As an indication of the linkage of apparently disparate economic elements, consider the harvest we now reap of the position of this country in world economic markets following World War II, a position of domination. In such a position, this country's businesses could and did pay a premium to its labor force, not only in terms of wages but most acutely in terms of fringe benefits. Since fringes have been selectively immune from taxation, they have grown at ratios faster than wages, and they have become subject to separate attack by government and industry. Symbolic of the attack by government is the periodic proposal to limit the tax deductibility of health insurance, a proposal that presently lacks enough political clout to pass, and proposals attacking the newer pension arrangements. Business, however, seeking ways to become more competitive in an increasingly competitive international market, has moved in two directions—politically towards protectionism, and internally towards limiting health insurance costs through a variety of steps: self-insurance and tough utilization review; mandatory second surgical opinions; lower cost providers; tougher negotiating stances with insurers and the newer practice plans—HMOs, IPAs, PPOs. However, business, like government, has thus far moved primarily on the *how* of payment and still leaves, for the most part, the *what* of payment (*what service* is provided) to the provider. This is to a certain extent appropriate, but we cannot expect it to continue for long. Business is sophisticated to know (even if government does not) that price *and* quality are the two components of any service, and I believe, that business will soon involve itself, not merely with the price it is willing to pay, but also in the quality of services it buys.

ond, there is concern among gerontologists and among those who treat a high proportion of the poor that hospital pressure to shorten length of stay put both their patients and them at a disadvantage because of the greater-than-average resource utilization such patients generally require. And third, there is some concern that a variety of pressures will force the acute care hospitals into subspecialization and intensive care and potentially away from meeting full community needs. Whether this last trend is bad or good is debatable, but it suggests an increasing likelihood of the hospital to grant privileges to the subspecialist and intensivist to the detriment of the generalist.

The message is that there is change in health care, driven not by quality concerns or access considerations, but driven overwhelmingly by economics. Those changes have not plateaued, but are accelerating. Systems that fail to respond constructively to them will not survive. At meetings of physicians throughout the country, there are many individual and small group practitioners who acutely feel change—an eroding practice base, decreasing income, lack of confidence in for-profit institutions, and fear of exclusionary PPOs and major employer groups. Change is here, but how to meet it constructively!

One can make the case for a new strategy, not merely a new political strategy, but one that would reaffirm the role of physicians as a profession, placing the interests of the patient primary and self-interest subordinate, and a strategy that would require medicine to accept the responsibility for standard-setting. We can no longer demand the sole authority to set standards. While opposing the actions of others in standard-setting, we can no longer refuse to accept the responsibility to set standards *and* be willing to be measured by them. Those who hope that the government will get out of the health care regulation business will be disappointed, especially if we, the medical profession, fail to act responsibly.

The history of organized medicine's involvement in politics in the 1980s is one of opposition—opposition to all governmental attempts to introduce cost consciousness. The opposition may have had some short-term effectiveness, but it had longer-term detriment, both in terms of political credibility and of programmatic outcome. Consider the political issues identified by organized medicine as its top priorities in the 1980s:

*Health Planning:* Organized medicine and the Reagan administration strongly favored elimination of health planning, since medical organizations felt it intruded on practice and government decried the cost. The result is that oversupply and maldistribution are worse rather than better.

*Peer Review Standards Organizations (PSRO):* Organized medicine and the Reagan administration favored elimination of the program, with physicians opposing "cookbook medicine," and the administration on the basis of cost. Peer Review Organizations continue, and their nearly sole focus is on the cost, not the quality, of health care.

*Technology Assessment:* Organized medicine and the administration favored elimination of the structured way by which Medicare decides what to pay for, but the activity continues, enhanced by further legislation.

*Federal Trade Commission:* Organized medicine argued that there should be no application of the antitrust laws to professionals. But the US Supreme Court upheld FTC authority to review the business of medicine, the Executive Branch opposed legislative change, and Congress refused to eliminate FTC authority.

*Mandatory assignment/Medicare fee freeze:* Organized medicine opposed both but Congress passed a fee freeze and defeated mandatory assignment in name only.

*Expenditure Targets:* Organized medicine opposed any cap on overall expenditures, arguing that the proposal would hurt patients. Consumer groups disagreed, and medicine meekly accepted the re-named "Voluntary Performance Standards."

What do these examples tell us? Though it was hoped that a conservative administration would be sympathetic to the private sector and the medical profession, the health policy issues identified by organized medicine as those of highest priority were all decided against the position favored. This suggests that the strategy of fighting absolutely every presumed incursion by government is bankrupt. It also suggests that by focussing on the economic battles, the profession has overlooked a more important issue, the erosion of clinical autonomy. As medicine fought for the privilege of the practitioner to bill without restriction, it forgot to fight for the right of the physician to make appropriate clinical decisions, informed by the data.

A strategy based on what professionals are supposed to be most concerned with—quality—will be best for the patients we serve, for the continuation of professionalism, and for positioning in the marketplace. For too long we used "quality" as a response to explain away legitimate concerns of society about variations in process, differences in outcomes, and costs. Yet we have refused to define what we mean by quality and have held the proposition that controls on input (licensure, accreditation, etc.) and to some extent process (medical audits, "peer review") are the only acceptable controls. We have acted as a medieval guild, admitting the craftsmen, controlling their apprenticeship, and after they have run the gauntlet, rarely questioning what they then do. We have refused to respond to the legitimate questions of an increasingly sophisticated population of the connection between those inputs and health outcomes.

It is time to dispel the notion that anything any practitioner wishes to do is legitimate. It is time for our profession to set reasonable limits to practice, to establish standards rather than allowing the exception to rule.

There is heartening evidence that the old ways are changing. The work of the American College of Physicians over the last fifteen years in the development of guidelines for clinical practice, the more recent work of the American Medical Association (AMA), with specialty groups, on "practice parameters" indicate a real willingness on the part of the profession to lead. Recent leadership changes within the AMA have set a new direction, one that at least on its surface professes to work cooperatively with government and with the payers of health care. The power of these positive signals to the individual practioner should not be underestimated. The idea that the profession as a whole should set the standards of practice, and the concept that an inter-connected health system requires cooperation among all its participants is, strangely, revolutionary. But the direction is as potentially productive as it is right.

How might all this play out in privilege delineation? It is time for the medical profession to determine what the minimum qualifications are—in terms of training, experience, and outcomes—for the performance of medical and surgical services. We should not be afraid of cookbooks; we use them all the time. What we need, simply, is a better cookbook—one based on the best data and the best current professional consensus, and one that is flexible enough to allow legitimate variation and innovation. How to accomplish this?

Step 1: Convene panels, broadly based, in each of the subspecialty areas represented in clinical practice (not necessarily subspecialties, but for convenience of grouping, subspecialty areas). Make the panels broadly based, by including representatives of all who perform and wish to perform services in the subspecialty area. Include non-clinicians and intelligent observers.

Step 2: Identify all the major services in the subspecialty area. "Major" may be subject to debate, but a useful starting point and would include those whose number or cost is significant, and whose potential for benefit or risk is great.

Step 3: Identify the literature applicable to each service, with attention to two basic aspects: a) its effectiveness, risks, indications, and costs; and b) the degree of experience necessary to perform the service with optimal outcomes, both initially and to maintain competence.

Step 4: Derive, through a structured group process, the minimal qualifications necessary to perform each service. It has been shown that surgeons, rather quickly in a structured process, can come to consensus on the relative complexity of surgical procedures. The difficulty in reaching consensus is not that it is not possible; it is the conceptual difficulty of converting unwritten subjectivity to written objectivity, of being comfortable that the process is inherently imperfect, and understanding that self-interest can be overcome and unanimity is not the only valid consensus.

Step 5: Validate the standards, based on external review, much as is now done by the JCAHO in its standards and survey process and by the federal government in regulations writing.

Step 6: Revise the standards, based on outside review, to balance the goal of standards based on hard data with the need that they be acceptable practically.

Step 7: Place an official imprimatur on the standards by some decision maker.

Step 8: Allow for variation. Legitimate local circumstances do differ. But do not allow the variation or exception to be the rule; require that variations be justified.

Step 9: Periodically re-evaluate the standards, as practice and technology change, as training changes, and as data fail to confirm the original standard.

What would be the result of such a performance-based standard for privilege delineation?

1. Most importantly would be its conceptual purpose. It would, in its best sense, demonstrate the responsibility of the profession to set standards and to be willing to be measured by them. It would further demonstrate a willingness to respond to legitimate societal questions of the relation between health outcomes and medical processes, and would enhance one of the central components of professionalism—the responsibility of serious self-regulation.
2. Such a step would respond to the immense practical need of hospitals and medical staffs for data-based objective criteria, based on medical considerations, for the delineation of privileges.
3. Consequently, hospitals and their staffs would more likely be protected from the unproductive litigation now surrounding privilege delineation.
4. Finally, the process would allow for the enhancement of *efficient* medical care, for the truly best medical care is the most cost-effective care.

In summary, I hope to have provoked discussion by laying out the economic perspective which now drives decision makers, and by challenging the medical profession to be what it is: a profession in the best interest of patients, rather than a trade in its own self-interest; and to further that challenge, to propose a process for data-based performance-based privilege delineation.

# Assessing, Monitoring, and Improving Medical Practice In the Hospital

William F. Jessee, MD

There is perhaps no single responsibility of the hospital medical staff which is of greater gravity than that of assessing, monitoring and continuously improving the quality of care provided in the hospital. Over the last two decades, these responsibilities have been substantially expanded, both through judicial decisions of various state and federal courts, and by the changes which have taken place in the relationship between hospitals and their medical staffs. The continuing evolution of hospital-medical staff relationships, coupled with changes in the accreditation standards of the Joint Commission on Accreditation of Healthcare Organizations, has required that physicians assume new roles in the process of continuous quality improvement in the delivery of health care. Accordingly, it is now critical that every hospital have in place effective mechanisms for the ongoing monitoring and assessment of both processes and outcomes of care as tools for identifying opportunities for process improvement, as well as for triggering peer review mechanisms.

The responsibility for the quality of care provided in any hospital ultimately rests with its governing body. A major component of the mission of the hospital Board of Trustees is to maintain and constantly improve the quality of care and service provided.[1] While maintaining financial viability is often viewed as an equally important component of trustee responsibility, no institution can long survive if it is unable to provide quality care. In the increasingly competitive world of hospitals and health care, a hospital which does not have in place effective mechanisms to measure

**19**

and continually improve both clinical and service quality is unlikely to be successful in serving its community or remaining as a viable institution. Good quality health care includes four primary components: 1) optimal achievable process and outcomes of care; 2) efficient use of resources; 3) minimal risk of patient injury or illness associated with care; and 4) patient satisfaction with care. While quality is complex and multidimensional, each of the above four components can be measured and information obtained from that measurement can be used as a tool for continuous improvement in quality. It is important to note that measurements of each of these four components of quality may yield differing results. For example, care which has led to a favorable outcome is not always efficient or satisfactory to the patient. Conversely, patients may not achieve desirable outcomes despite a process of care that was entirely consistent with professional standards, efficient, low risk,and entirely satisfactory to the patient or family. Quality is not easily reduced to a single global index, but each of the four components of quality noted above is a critical part of the medical staff's responsibility for measurement and self-improvement.

To accomplish the objective of maintaining high quality care, hospital trustees must be able to maintain a system of accountability over four areas of hospital operations: 1) credentialing and privilege delineation, 2) the quality assessment and improvement program, 3) risk management, and 4) employee performance evaluation. Unfortunately, lay trustees are often insecure in their ability to deal with quality of care issues. While most are familiar with financial management and are quite comfortable with those aspects of trusteeship related to their role as financial fiduciaries, they are much less comfortable with their role in maintaining quality care. Accordingly, the trustees look to the hospital's organized medical staff to serve as their agents in accomplishing their quality improvement objectives, while recognizing that ultimate responsibility continues to rest with the board. It is important that the hospital board establish effective mechanisms to assure accountability between the board and medical staff in the conduct of these responsibilities. An organized approach to maintaining such a system of accountability has been outlined elsewhere and will not be discussed further in this chapter.[1]

Concepts of continuous quality improvement recognize that the care received by patients in the modern hospital is a consequence of the interaction of large numbers of individuals, organized into multiple organizational units, through which patients pass. While the conventional wisdom has, for many years, held the attending physician primarily responsible for the quality of care provided, the reality of practice in today's hospital is that the physician is but one member of a complex care team involved in attempting to provide the coordinated services necessary to good quality patient care. Conventional quality assurance programs have, in the past, focused on identifying errors in care and attempting to attribute those errors to individuals. Contemporary concepts of continuous improvement by contrast recognize that hospital care is an extremely complex process and that when processes, outcomes, efficiency, or satisfaction are less than expected, evaluation of the processes involved is much more likely to be productive than are efforts to affix blame for the result.[2,3] For example, a care process consisting of only one step, which step is correctly performed 95% of the time, has a probability of favorable results of 0.95. When the complexity of the care process increases to ten steps, with each step still being performed correctly 95% of the time, the probability of a favorable outcome from the process declines to $0.95^{10}$ or 0.599. A forty-step process, a level of complexity common in many hospital processes such as medication administration, has a probability of favorable outcome of $0.95^{40}$ or less than 13%, when each step is performed correctly 95% of the time. Accordingly, attention to understanding care processes which cut across disciplinary and departmental lines in the hospital, and to simplifying those processes, is a key to improvement in the quality of health care.

Nonetheless, the performance of individuals involved in care processes remains critical. In the example cited above, if the frequency of correct performance of a single step should fall to 50%, it lowers the probability of a favorable outcome by almost half. Accordingly, attention to individual performance of medical staff members, as well as of hospital employees, is an important part of quality improvement efforts. This should, however, be a by-product of the overall quality assessment and improvement effort rather than its central focus. It is only by refocusing quality improvement efforts on process improvement, and away from traditional punitive efforts to affix blame, that we will be able to move forward to the next stage of our efforts to improve health care quality in the American hospital.

Responsibility for assuring that the physicians involved in the provision of medical care are competent and that their performance meets acceptable standards is delegated by the Board of Trustees to the medical staff. This delegation of responsibility encompasses peer assessment and monitoring of professional competence, clinical performance, and judgment in the delivery of care. It is important that a clear distinction be made between those issues involved in assessing and monitoring medical practice which relate to quality, and those issues which relate primarily to the business aspects of hospital management. The organized medical staff must play a key role in evaluating quality issues, but must carefully avoid becoming involved in business issues which may be construed as having the objective of restraining competition. The growth of antitrust litigation, perhaps most cogently exemplified by the *Patrick* case in Oregon,[4] has made it imperative that the medical staff studiously avoid any *appearance* that decisions or recommendations made on hospital privileges are based on attempts by potential competitors to control or eliminate competition. Such naive statements as "we already have too many cardiologists" may offer a potential litigant valuable ammunition in arguing that an adverse decision on credentials or privileges was based primarily on economic grounds, rather than on quality of care.

In carrying out its delegated responsibilities for assessing and improving the quality of care, the medical staff has five specific roles to play:

1. Initial assessment of applicants for privileges.
2. Ongoing monitoring of the performance of medical staff members.
3. Periodic reevaluation and renewal of privileges.
4. Specific delineation of clinical privileges.
5. Assessing and monitoring compliance with privileges.

Each of these five areas of responsibility is discussed in detail below.

1. *Initial Assessment*—The most important structural control which the medical staff has over the quality of care provided by its members is in the careful review of the credentials, experience, character, and performance of each physician or other individual who may make application for staff membership or for clinical privileges. The medical staff's ability to influence its composition in a way that will favorably affect patient care quality is at its greatest at the time of initial application. Accordingly, it is essential that there be a comprehensive in-depth evaluation of the background of each applicant to assure the validity of the credentials presented, and to assure that the applicant's performance historically has demonstrated acceptable professional competence and clinical judgment.

The major issues which should be considered in this process are summarized in Table 1. Validation of the educational background and residency training of the individual is critical. Reliance should not be placed upon copies of documents as evidence of completion of either medical education or residency training. Rather, inquiries should be made directly to the medical school and residency program involved. These inquiries are most useful if they ask for specific information on such attributes as fund of clinical knowledge, basic science knowledge, diagnostic acumen, skill in patient management, surgical skills, clinical judgment etc. Both requirements of the Joint Commission on Accreditation of Healthcare Organizations[5] and a large volume of case law make clear that verification of this information with original sources, wherever feasible, is essential. A study of the credentials presented by applicants for staff positions in a large ambulatory care program demonstrated that as many as five percent of the applicants misstated their educational credentials.[6] For this reason, verification of such information is absolutely essential.

In addition to verification of training, inquiries should also be made specifically regarding the types of procedures the resident was trained to perform and the types of patients cared for during the residency program. This has become increasingly important as the scope of residency programs has become more varied. While each specialty board has made a significant effort to define the scope of practice for that specialty, full reliance cannot be placed upon those definitions in the case of individual residents. For example, residents in surgical training programs may have significant experience with gastrointestinal endoscopy in some cases and much more limited in experience in others depending upon the nature of the program and the types of patients they have seen during their residency experience. It is important before granting clinical privileges to recognize where each individual's training may be strong or weak, since that will have substantial implications for the privileges granted and for the subsequent monitoring of that individual's practice.

Board eligibility or certification also should be carefully examined. Increasingly, both hospitals and specialty boards have discouraged use of the term "eligibility" since grants of privileges made on this basis are difficult to revoke in the event that the applicant subsequently is unable to successfully pass the certification examination. In lieu of the eligibility requirement, many hospitals now require board certification, but will accept

---

**Table 1. Quality of Care Considerations in Credentialing & Privilege Delineation**

- Education
- Residency Training
- Numbers of Procedures Performed and Results
- Medical Specialty Board Eligibility/Certification
- Professional Liability Experience
- Peer Relationships, Peer Evaluations
- Ability to Work with Staff
- Availability to Provide Patient Care
- Process and Outcomes of Care, Clinical Competence, Professional Judgment

completion of an approved residency program in lieu of such certification for a limited time period. If the applicant is unable to successfully complete the certification process by the end of that period, clinical privileges are not necessarily withdrawn, but may be modified to permit the practitioner to care only for less seriously ill patients. Such an approach protects both the public and the institution, while still permitting the physician to practice in the hospital.

Quality of care considerations must also include the individual's professional liability experience. A physician who has been involved as a defendant in a professional liability action is not necessarily one who is practicing poor medicine. However, any instance of liability litigation should be a flag which triggers a more careful review of the circumstances and of the patient management evidenced by the facts. Whenever there have been multiple instances of professional liability, particularly if they involved similar diagnoses or patient care circumstances, questions should be raised concerning the quality of care provided by the practitioner. Often it may be necessary to request medical records or to ask for a complete explanation of the facts of the case from the physician concerned. Information on professional liability actions is in the public domain once a lawsuit has been filed. Generally, such information can be obtained from the physician's liability insurance carrier with a signed release from the physician applicant. In some instances, however, carriers will not release such information under any circumstances. In such an event, it may necessary to request information from public records.

The institution of the National Practitioner Data Bank has facilitated inquiry into the professional liability experience of the individual physician. This data bank, established by Federal law, contains information on any malpractice settlement or judgment made involving an individual physician. It also contains a record of any disciplinary action which may have been taken by a hospital or state licensing board. Accordingly, a critical part of the credentialing process is inquiry of the data bank concerning any information that they may have available concerning the applicant. Here, too, the existence of information in the data bank does not in and of itself indicate problems of competence. It should, however, lead to a more careful examination of the circumstances in each case. Such careful review by the credentials committee will permit an informed judgment to be made concerning the applicant's performance in that case and the implications of the case for his future competence to practice in the hospital.

Peer relationships and peer evaluations are also important quality of care issues, as is the ability to work with the non-physician staff in the hospital. Providing patient care in a modern hospital is a team effort.

Accordingly, the ability to work as part of a team, and to maintain a harmonious relationship with colleagues and with nurses and other non-physician staff, is a legitimate concern in evaluating the ability of an individual to qualify for staff membership. However, care must be taken to assure that any action taken on an applicant for privileges is directly linked to the quality of care provided. In the the case of *Miller v. Eisenhower Medical Center*,[7] the California supreme court has held that personality per se may not be used as the exclusive grounds for denial of privileges unless a clear relationship can be drawn to the quality of services likely to be provided.

Availability to provide patient care may also be a quality of care consideration. For instance, some hospitals utilize a criterion which states that an applicant for staff privileges must be able to reach the hospital from residence or office within a certain number of minutes, or must be physically located within a certain number of miles. However, such rules need to be flexible. For example, "availability" for an anesthesiologist or obstetrician is substantially different than "availability" for a dermatologist. Accordingly, this criterion, if used, should recognize the differences between specialties and make appropriate allowances.

Finally, the processes and outcomes of patient care provided (clinical competence and professional judgment), are the key criteria for staff membership. If any questions arise in the examination of an applicant's credentials concerning the quality of care which may be provided, it is entirely appropriate and, in fact, increasingly expected, that the applicant be looked to for additional evidence about his care of patients. An examination of patient records from the applicant's current hospital may be a valuable tool in assessing competence for privileges. The burden of proving competence rests with the applicant. Accordingly, if any questions arise, the hospital should request that the applicant provide copies of the medical records of patients for whom care was provided in order to allow those records to be reviewed in the same fashion as are the hospital's own records of patients cared for by current staff members. The burden of proving competence is on the applicant only prior to the granting of privileges. Once this grant has been made, the burden then shifts to the institution, which must prove that the practitioner no longer is competent or that his or her judgment is no longer sound in order to remove or modify those privileges.

2. *Ongoing Monitoring*—Responsibilities for ongoing monitoring of members of the medical staff apply to two categories of staff members: first, new staff members in their provisional membership period, and secondly, full active staff members whose performance must be monitored to assure that it remains appropriate. It is essential that each new member of the staff pass through a period of close observation in order to assure

that the initial decision concerning staff membership and the clinical privileges granted was, in fact, correct. The monitoring program devised for each new staff member should be tailored to that individual's background and qualifications, as well as to the nature of their practice in the hospital. For example, the initial proctoring program for a new staff member who had recently completed residency training would be somewhat different than that for one who has had a long and distinguished career. For surgical specialties, monitoring may include a period of direct observation in the operating room, or, in some cases, scrub supervision by the assigned proctor. For other applicants, including those in nonsurgical specialties, the period of initial monitoring may involve retrospective review of selected patient records. In any event, it is critical that the nature of the monitoring process, including the assignment of responsibility for proctoring to one or more members of the medical staff, be specified at the time that privileges are granted in order to avoid later misunderstandings.

For individuals who are already full members of the medical staff, either with active staff privileges or with courtesy or consulting privileges, the hospital's quality assessment and improvement program should serve as a means for ongoing monitoring. As outlined earlier, the ongoing monitoring activity conducted in the hospital, whether by medical staff departments or through hospital-wide measurements of clinical processes and outcomes, has its primary objective the identification of opportunities for improvement in care processes. As a by-product, however, information should be profiled by physician in order to serve as an early warning system for potential problems of performance. Joint Commission accreditation standards (MS4.6) specify that the department chairman is responsible for "continuing surveillance of the professional performance of all individuals who have delineated clinical privileges in the department" and "assuring that the quality of patient care provided within the department is monitored and evaluated." In the Quality Assessment and Improvement chapter of the Joint Commission standards, it similarly indicates that relevant results from quality assessment activities "when relevant to the performance of the individual, are used as a component of the evaluation of individual capabilities."[5]

Accordingly, information on patient outcomes, such as mortality, complications, readmission, reoperation, and compliance with process criteria for treatment, as well as other key measures selected by the medical staff, should be profiled by practitioner. These profiles should be regularly fed back to each member of the medical staff as a means of self improvement, as well as used by the department in a periodic process of reappraisal. It is important to note that such profiling should not imply attribution of responsibility to the individual physician. For example, a patient who has undergone a surgical procedure and subsequently dies should not be inferred to be a death attributable to the surgeon. Rather, all physicians involved in that care should simply have recorded in their profile that a patient of theirs experienced an undesirable outcome. If one begins to see that certain physicians have substantially higher rates of poor outcomes than do others, unexplained by differences in patient mix, then it should lead to a closer examination of the pattern of practice of the individual. The statistical data in and of themselves, however, do not permit one to make definitive judgments about professional competence or performance.

3. *Renewal of Privileges*—The ongoing collection, profiling and feedback of individual performance information to members of the medical staff is an important part of medical staff self-governance and self-improvement activities. However, at least every two years, the track record of every member of the staff must be comprehensively reviewed. Joint Commission standard MS2.7 requires that, at least every two years, "information concerning the individual's professional performance, the individual's judgment, and the individual's clinical or technical skills, as indicated in part by the results of quality assessment and improvement activities" be reviewed.[5]

To permit this process to occur, clinical performance data must be collected in an ongoing fashion and accumulated in practitioner-specific performance files. Too often, only negative information is accumulated and that is often not well documented. As a result, these evaluations may be perceived very negatively by staff members, and "performance problems" may be a matter of hearsay rather than a matter of documentation. This situation can be obviated by developing a physician specific "peer review" file kept in the medical staff office or, in larger hospitals, in the departmental office. That file should include the results of the monthly departmental quality reviews, infection control reviews, drug usage reviews, blood utilization reviews, surgical case reviews, incident report data, liability experience information, and other sources of data pertaining to the physician's clinical performance, patient relationships, and professional judgment. Data reflecting both favorable and unfavorable performance should be included to permit a balanced and comprehensive evaluation. In addition, caution should be taken to assure that access to that file is limited by hospital policy to preserve the confidentiality of the information it contains. At the specified interval for renewal, this file should be comprehensively examined by the department chairman, or a committee of the department, in order to ascertain the individual's competence for continued privileges in the institution and to make recommendations back to that staff member for improvement.

4. *Privilege Delineation*—The process of privilege delineation is a mechanism for assuring that each practitioner provides only those services which he or she is qualified to provide and for which their competence has been demonstrated. This process should be carried out by the medical staff departments, rather than by the credentials committee. Interdepartmental conflicts must be resolved either at the credentials committee level or by the medical staff executive committee.

Family practice often presents one of the major challenges in the delineation of clinical privileges. Remember that Joint Commission standards require that all practitioners be held to the same standards of performance, regardless of their background and qualifications.[5] In addition, the performance of each member of the medical staff must be monitored by the department in which the service is provided, rather than by the parent department. For example, a family practitioner providing obstetrical services must meet the same criteria, and have their performance evaluated in the same fashion, as do members of the department of obstetrics and gynecology.

Several alternative approaches to privilege delineation have been described. Unfortunately, none of them is ideal. One alternative is to delineate by specialty. This approach assumes that all adequately trained specialists are qualified for all privileges in that specialty. Most physicians intuitively believe that this is not completely true; however, this may be a starting point for delineation of privileges, if combined with more specific criteria for granting privileges for high risk procedures. In more and more hospitals, a categorical approach is being utilized, particularly for non-surgical specialties. This approach defines categories of privileges by the risk to the patient and by the training required to treat patients in that category.

A third alternative approach is the so called "laundry list." This approach is particularly valuable in surgical specialties, but becomes virtually useless in cognitive specialties such as internal medicine or pediatrics. Whatever approach is utilized, it is essential that there be objective criteria developed by each department for granting privileges and that these criteria be uniformly applied. Table 2 gives an example of the categorical approach to delineation of clinical privileges in pediatrics.

In granting privileges for new procedures, it is important that criteria for making privileging decisions be addressed early in the introduction of new technologies into the hospital. Too often, hospitals have found that new procedures or technologies have been adopted by members of their medical staff without specific privilege delineation. At that point, it is difficult if not impossible to control the proliferation of the procedure in the absence of catastrophic results. It is generally preferable, as a new technology is developed and proposed for introduction, to anticipate that members of the staff will wish to perform that procedure or utilize that technology. Consultation from experts in the field may be sought to determine the type of training which should be required, the technical resources which should be present to support the technology, and the criteria which should be utilized to evaluate applications for privileges. Such criteria should then be developed and enforced, requiring completion of defined training prior to granting privileges to perform the new procedure. If such criteria are

---

**Table 2. Categorical Privilege Delineation for Pediatrics.**

Category I
   Illnesses, injuries, conditions, or procedures which have a low risk to the patient (e.g., routine newborn care; uncomplicated pneumonia).
   Nonspecialists with little or no pediatrics residency training, but with reasonable experience in care of these conditions.

Category II
   Major illnesses, injuries, conditions or procedures, but with no significant risk to life (e.g., undiagnosed anemia; status asthmaticus; LP and ABG, except newborns).
   Significant training or experience in pediatrics; not necessarily board certified.

Category III
   Major illnesses; injuries, conditions or procedures which carry substantial threat to life (e.g., meningitis; drug overdose; erythroblastosis fetalis; neonatal resuscitation).
   Board Certification* in pediatrics or other extensive training and experience in the care of these conditions.

Category IV
   Unusually complex or critical illnesses, injuries, conditions, or procedures which carry a serious threat to life (e.g., leukemia; respiratory failure; nenonatal intensive care; renal dialysis).
   Extensive relevant subspecialty training or experience beyond board certification in pediatrics.

   *Completion of three-year residency training in pediatrics may be acceptable in lieu of board certification for a period not to exceed five years following completion of training.

developed and applied uniformly, many of the conflicts associated with the introduction of new procedures or technologies can be avoided.

5. *Assessing and Monitoring Compliance with Privileges*—As part of the periodic review and renewal of clinical privileges, it is important that each practitioner's compliance with the clinical privileges which have been granted be assessed. For procedure-based specialties, such as surgery, this may be accomplished on a concurrent basis by reviewing operative procedures scheduled against the privileges granted. For non-surgical specialties, such review is best accomplished on a retrospective basis. In any event, it is important for purposes of avoidance of corporate liability to assure that each individual complies with the privileges that have been granted. If an individual exceeds the privileges granted, the hospital may potentially be held liable for negligence in permitting such practice to exist. Where an individual is found to have consistently exceeded the privileges, there may be grounds for disciplinary action to be taken.

## Conclusion

Developing effective systems for assessing, monitoring and improving medical practice is a key to fulfilling both the medical staff's and the board's responsibilities for quality of care. As a hospital medical staff establishes mechanisms such as those described in this chapter, it will be assured of more effective peer regulation of practice in the hospital and of more effective self-governance. Accordingly, the overall quality of care in the institution will be improved. For the governing body, assurances that the medical staff has adopted such procedures, and that reports are being provided to the board on a regular basis documenting the operation of these activities, are important for maintaining fiduciary accountability. Such accountability is a key to the avoidance of corporate liability as well as to the development of better quality hospitals. Through such cooperative action between the board and its medical staff, the community and the patients they both serve will benefit.

## References

1. Jessee, W.F. *Quality of Care Issues for the Hospital Trustee.* Chicago: Hospital Research and Educational Trust, 1984.
2. Berwick, D.M., Godfrey, A.B., and Roessner, J. *Curing Health Care: New Strategies for Quality Improvement.* San Francisco: Jossey-Bass, 1990.
3. Kritchevsky, S.B., and Simmons, B.P. Continuous quality improve

ment: concepts and applications for physician care. *JAMA*, 266:1817-1823, 1991.
4. *Patrick v. Burget*, 800 F. 2d 1498 (9th Cir. 1986), rev'd 108 S.Ct. 1658 (1988).
5. *Accreditation Manual for Hospitals, 1992.* Oakbrook Terrace, Illinois: Joint Commission on Accreditation of Healthcare Organizations, 1991.
6. Schaffer, W.A., Rollo, F.D. and Holt, C.A., Falsification of clinical credentials by physicians applying for ambulatory-staff privileges. *New Eng. J. Med.*, 318:356-358, 1988.
7. *Miller v. Eisenhower Medical Center*, 614 p.2d (Cal. 1980).

# Quality Management Data: Their Use in Credentialing

Beauregard Stubblefield, MBA

## Introduction

Credentialing is used by hospitals and their medical staffs to protect patient safety and enhance patient care quality. Credentialing attempts to ensure that only qualified practitioners are permitted to practice and that they practice within the scope of their expertise and competency and within the capacity of the hospital. Both systems and individuals have an impact on the quality of patient care. The credentialing process primarily addresses individuals, by evaluating the qualifications of all clinicians independently providing and/or directing patient care.[1] In addition to all medical staff members, the credentialing process often covers other clinicians (for example, psychologists, nurse midwives) who may not be medical staff members because of state laws and/or medical staff decisions.[2]

Quality management (QM) activities (quality assessment and improvement, risk management, infection control, and utilization management) address both systems and individuals as they affect patient care. QM activities provide data regarding the provider's current competence to provide high-quality care. QM data are generated by hospital staff, medical staff peer review committees, and from external sources. These data are then used as part of a medical staff's and hospital's continuous effort to improve care and as integral elements of the credentialing process.[3]

This chapter will review the credentialing process (or processes), focusing on privilege delineation. The chapter then examines each QM disci-

**33**

pline in turn, reviewing its background and history, processes and data, and the use of that data in credentialing. The chapter concludes with a summary of findings.

## The Credentialing Process

*Credentialing* is used in this chapter as it is often used in the field, to include three interrelated processes: the verification of credentials, medical staff appointment and reappointment, and the delineation of clinical privileges. Each process will be defined and described briefly. The focus of this chapter is on privilege delineation at intial appointment, and particularly at reappointment.

*Credentials verification* is the process whereby a provider's licensure, education, training, board certification, and other structural elements related to practice are validated.[4] Hospitals are required to query the National Practitioner Data Bank[5] as part of credentials verification for physicians and dentists. Credentials verification occurs prior to appointment or reappointment and/or privilege delineation.

Credentials verification often involves both clinical (department chairmen) and nonclinical staff (medical staff coordinators), but there is generally no governing board involvement. Because clinicians will often speak candidly with their peers by phone, some department heads contact residency program directors and other physicians by phone as well as by letter. Hospitals and their medical staffs must individually determine how to verify credentials.

*Medical staff appointment or reappointment* may confer a variety of rights and responsibilities. Many of these are political (for example, right to run for medical staff office, meeting attendance requirements), but others have important quality implications (for example, obligation to maintain current medical records, continuing medical education requirements, and so forth).

The appointment process generally starts with an application, including clinical privileges requested, completed by the prospective member. (Some hospitals use a preapplication process as well.) Credentials are verified as described above. The department director interviews the applicant, reviews the application and related materials, compares them against preestablished criteria, and makes a recommendation to the credentials committee or medical staff executive committee (MSEC). After its review, the MSEC makes a recommendation to the governing board. The governing board makes the ultimate decision on both membership and privileges. Appeals mechanisms at various levels are specified in the medical staff bylaws. The medical staff office provides substantial support throughout the appointment process.

The initial appointment to the medical staff is generally referred to as a provisional appointment. It is for a specified period of time during which the medical staff may review the practitioner's performance directly. The governing board reviews activities during the provisional period before making a decision on promoting the practitioner to regular status (See credentialing cycles.)

Medical staff membership decisions are affected by federal and state law, Medicare Conditions of Participation for Hospitals, standards of the Joint Commission on Accreditation of Healthcare Organizations (JCAHO), and hospital medical staff bylaws. (For example, certain state laws mandate that podiatrists or others be considered as medical staff members.)[6]

*Privilege delineation* (privileging) involves tailoring the scope of care provided by a particular independently practicing[7] clinician on the basis of capabilities of the individual (through his or her training and experience) and the hospital (through its staff, equipment, and systems).

Privileges, as with medical staff membership, are granted by the governing board following the recommendations of the MSEC, credentials committee and/or department chair. MSEC recommendations follow the review of an individual practitioner's application and qualifications compared to previously defined criteria for awarding privileges. Information and support for privileging are provided by the medical staff office, medical records, and quality management areas.

Privileges are generally granted simultaneously with medical staff membership when both are approved. Privileges can be granted without medical staff membership (for example, to a clinical psychologist), and medical staff membership can be granted without privileges (for example, honorary membership for a retiring physician).

Medical staff membership and independent practice governed by privileges are not synonymous. Psychologists, for example, may have privileges to practice independently through state law, and/or medical staff bylaws, yet not be permitted medical staff membership.[8] Approximately 40 percent of hospital medical staffs surveyed in 1989 changed their bylaw provisions regarding clinical privileges and/or medical staff membership for limited license (nonphysician) practitioners.[9]

Quality management data are most useful in this aspect of credentialing. Although other aspects are addressed, the focus will be on privilege delineation, particularly at reappointment. At reappointment substantial QM data are available, and are used to evaluate clinical competence.

## Privilege Delineation

Privileges define the scope of care that a given practitioner can provide in a specific setting. Privileges are far more specific than credentials. Though they are also affected by state laws, case law, and bylaws, privileges must be tailored specifically to the individual provider and the individual institution.[10] For example, the most competent cardiac surgeon in the world would not be given privileges to perform heart transplants at a hospital that did not have the equipment and staff to support this operation. This surgeon could be welcomed on the medical staff and awarded privileges to perform bypass surgery similar to those granted its other cardiac surgeons. The capabilities of the hospital, as well as the surgeon, must be considered in awarding privileges. In this case, the hospital's limitations were preeminent.

Objective professional criteria form the basis for awarding clinical privileges. Before awarding privileges, objective criteria for these privileges are recommended by the medical staff and approved by the governing board. These criteria "pertain to, at the least, evidence of current licensure, relevant training and/or experience, current competence, and health status."[11] Once these criteria are adopted, they are consistently applied to applicants.[12] The goal of the credentialing process is to protect patient safety and enhance patient care quality. This goal is met through the following objectives related to privilege delineation:

- Describe the scope of care a clinician is authorized to provide in a particular hospital. This must be done prospectively and with high degree of certainty.
- Award *privileges for which the clinician has demonstrated* current appropriate licensure, relevant training and/or experience, current competence, and satisfactory health status that qualify him/her to execute the requested privileges.
- Grant *privileges that the hospital can support* with appropriate facilities and equipment, trained staff, quality evaluation systems, and so forth.
- Ensure the practitioner's *compliance* with granted privileges, so that he or she does not exceed the scope of care authorized by the governing board.
- Ensure that all patients receive the same level of quality of care regardless of the location or clinician involved.[13] (A patient seeking an uncomplicated delivery should expect to receive the same high-quality care from a nurse midwife in the hospital's off-site birthing center, an ob/gyn in her specially designed room, or a family physician in the

sician in the delivery suite.) To maintain this level of quality of care, privileges must be granted only to clinicians who demonstrate their ability to provide such care. As the medical staff and hospital continuously improve the quality of care, clinicians must demonstrate their ability to provide care at the higher standard.

- Maintain a credentialing process based on objective criteria, consistently applied to all applicants for privileges.[14] The process should respect clinicians' differing training and expertise, and patients' rights to choose their own clinician (for example nurse midwife, ob/gyn, family physician). Privileges must be awarded in a consistent manner, motivated by interest in patient care. There is no room for decisions based on economic self-interest or clinician bias.[15]

Each of the above objectives is important and has an impact on the quality of patient care. The following four are particularly dependent on quality management data:

- Assessing current clinician competence
- Assessing current hospital competence (support staff, facilities, and so forth)
- Ensuring compliance with privileges
- Maintaining the same quality of care for all patients


## Credentialing Cycles and Current Clinical Competence

Credentialing has two cycles: (1) the initial appointment to the medical staff, including a provisional period, and (2) reappointment (usually biannually thereafter). This chapter concentrates on reappointment, because only limited QM data are generally available at the time of initial appointment.

The provisional period deserves special attention before focusing on reappointment. During the provisional period, the practitioner applying for privileges is reviewed directly by the medical staff as to his or her clinical competence before a final decision is made regarding privileges and/or medical staff membership. This "hands on" review is an essential complement to the verification of credentials. The nature of the review (also called proctoring, preceptorship, and supervision) is tailored to the individual practitioner: a newly trained resident would not be supervised in the same way as a distinguished clinician recruited to head a department; surgeons and others performing procedures may have a colleague "scrub in" to observe, while retrospective chart review may serve in other situations. Nevertheless, all new members must be reviewed more intensely than those who have completed the provisional period. The nature of the review should be defined in advance, and should use quality management processes extensively. This review during the provisional period allows the medical staff to identify issues or problems undiscovered through credentials verification, and address them before privileges and/or medical staff appointment are finalized. The medical staff may respond to any problems by focused education or other interventions. At the end of the provisional period, the medical staff may recommend the governing board grant privileges as requested, grant more limited privileges, continue the provisional period, or disapprove the application for medical staff membership and/or privileges.

William F. Jesse, M.D., argues that the onus is on a provider to demonstrate his or her qualifications at the time of initial appointment and/or privileging. Once the hospital grants privileges, it must prove that the practitioner is no longer competent to exercise these privileges before removing or modifying them.[16] Again, the provisional period is critical because the medical staff can review the practitioner's care before a final decision is made to grant privileges.

Different standards may apply during the practitioner's regular term of membership than at reappointment. During the term of membership, a change in privileges (adding, deleting, or restricting privileges) would require either the practitioner or the medical staff to request a change. Attorneys Zingman and Long address the topic in the Credentialing and Privileging chapter of *Risk Management Handbook for Health Care Facilities:*

> The medical staff bylaws should establish fair procedures by which privileges may be reduced, suspended or terminated. The medical staff and governing body must then comply with the bylaws requirements to ensure that the adverse decision is both *fair and accurate* . . . . Where the decision of the medical staff and governing body is found to be reasonable and not arbitrary or capricious, the courts generally refrain from interfering and uphold the action taken.[17]

Bylaws provisions regarding reduction, suspension, or termination of privileges generally place the responsibility for demonstrating the need for a change on the medical staff.[18]

At reappointment, the burden may rest with the hospital and its medical staff regarding medical staff membership, which includes political rights (such as the ability to run for medical staff office). However, reappointment generally involves a new application for privileges. Even at reappointment, *the practitioner may be required to demonstrate current clinical competence*[19] to execute the privileges requested. The hospital must grant only those privileges for which the provider has demonstrated competence to its satisfaction.

## Quality Management Data and Privilege Delineation

Quality management (QM) data must be considered at reappointment in evaluating a provider's current clinical competence. This is mandated by Joint Commission on Accreditation of Healthcare Organizations (Joint Commission) standards[20] and court opinions[21] and, more importantly, by common sense. The hospital and its medical staff collect QM data to improve patient care. These data can be used to develop appropriate treatment protocols, improve educational efforts, support the need for new equipment, and modify providers' behavior. Modifying privileges is only one way of modifying practitioner behavior.

Each QM discipline provides its own data and perspective. These data should be used on a concurrent basis by hospital and medical staff departments to improve patient care. *Quality improvement activities must not wait for reappointment.* Rather, reappointment offers an opportunity to review the QM activities that have occurred over the preceding months, and determine if QM data address the provider's current competence, the appropriateness of his/her current privileges, and if further action is needed. This chapter examines the QM disciplines in turn and shows how their data may be used in recredentialing.

## Quality Assessment and Improvement

### Background and History

There are at least as many definitions of health care quality as there are definers. An Institute of Medicine committee adopted the following definition: "Quality of care is the degree to which health services for individuals and populations increase the likelihood of desired health outcomes and are consistent with current professional knowledge."[22] More important than the field's definition of quality per se are the philosophy and process for improving quality, how both the philosophy and process have evolved, and the role of credentialing in quality improvement.

Quality Improvement (QI) encompasses all aspects of service (housekeeping to neurosurgery). QI also evaluates a variety of aspects of quality from patient satisfaction to clinical outcomes. This chapter focuses only on patient care provided by privileged practitioners. QI has evolved to focus largely on systems rather than individuals. Credentialing deals primarily with the individual provider. However, QI and credentialing both deal with the intersection between the individual and the larger hospital system. A QI study involving medication errors and drug reactions might examine the roles of pharmacy and nursing staff as well as the role of ordering physicians.23 Privileging must reflect the competence of the hospital system (staff, facilities, equipment, and so forth) as well as the practitioner. Applying QI data to individual privilege delineation and medical staff appointment decisions is the nexus of these two processes.

The evolution of medical staff QI can be traced back to *The Minimum Standard* (table 1 in appendix)[24] promulgated by the American College of Surgeons in 1918. This document is impressive for its brevity, foresightedness, and applicability to today's medical practice. *Integrated Quality Assessment* (IQA) includes an excellent brief history of QI activities.[25] IQA notes the following:

- Quality assurance dates at least to 1918 when The Minimum Standard stated that the medical staff should "review and analyze at regular intervals their clinical experience in the various departments of the hospital . . . ; the clinical records of patients...to be the basis for such review and analyses."
- In 1951, the Joint Commission on Accreditation of Hospitals (now the Joint Commission on the Accreditaion of Healthcare Organizations) was formed to "analyze, review, evaluate, and, where necessary, improve the quality of clinical practice." The Joint Commission then evaluated hospitals by "measuring their performance against minimum standards that reflected the evolving scope of hospital-based practice."
- In 1965, the federal government enacted Medicare and became the single largest purchaser of health care services. With increasing technology and costs came increased research on quality particularly using Donebedian's model of *structure, process, and outcome.*
- Through the 1970s and 1980s, the Joint Commission and other researchers focused on developing processes to review patient care quality. These included medical audits, occurrence screening, and systematic monitoring and evaluation (M and E).

Two interrelated activities have been increasingly important in health care in the past several years: Continuous Quality Improvement/Total Quality Management (CQI/TQM) and Clinical Practice Guidelines (Practice Parameters). Both are described in Technical Briefings prepared by the American Hospital Association Division of Quality Resources:

- Continuous Quality Improvement/Total Quality Management[26] (CQI/TQM) is an ongoing process that goes beyond traditional QA activities, which are often confined to a program. CQI is a management philosophy that promotes a process of organizational participation and team building. It can be applied to any function or process, including the assessment of clinical patient care. CQI relies heavily on the use of scientific methods and statistical analysis to identify, reduce, or control process variations and has been successfully applied to industrial and manufacturing processes. CQI focuses on systems or processes, rather than individuals. It is a complement to, not a substitute for, other QM activities, peer review, and credentialing.
- Clinical Practice Guidelines (CPGs) or Practice Parameters[27] are, in their most basic form, strategies for the management of patients' clinical care. They are also described as points along a continuum. At one end are schedules for immunization of children against childhood diseases. At the other are detailed pathways for the management of diseases, including specific guidelines for hospital staff, equipment, volume of procedures, length of stay, and other specfics. In between lie such CPGs as prescription drug protocols, indications for c-sections, and so on.

CPGs are actively being developed by medical specialty societies with the endorsement and support of the American Medical Association (AMA). They are also being developed under the auspices of the federal government.

The relationship of CPGs to credentialing is controversial and undecided. The AMA's policymaking House of Delegates has consistently opposed the use of practice parameters (CPGs) in credentialing unless and until they have been demonstrated effective in obtaining desired patient outcomes.[28] John R. Ball, M.D., J.D., of the American College of Physicians argues elsewhere in this text for the use of CPGs to drive "data-based performance-based privilege delineation."[29] AHA encourages hospitals and their medical staffs to systematically evaluate CPGs, modify them as needed to suit local circumstances, implement them in various patient care settings, and utilize them as appropriate in institutional planning, for example, in new service development and technology assessment.[30] AHA has not endorsed the use of CPGs in credentialing. Further, hospitals currently implementing CPGs are not using them in the credentialing process.[31]

The constant within these evolving efforts has been the goal of improving patient care. Interventions including education, process/system improvements, policy revisions, practitioner supervision, equipment changes, privilege modification, and others are means to this end.

## Medical Staff Review Functions

There are six monitoring and evaluation functions described by the Joint Commission as the responsibility of the medical staff:[32]

- Monitoring and evaluation of patient care quality
- Surgical case review
- Drug usage evaluation
- Medical records review
- Blood usage review
- Pharmacy and therapeutics (P & T) review

These functions are often mirrored by medical staff committees; however, this structure is not mandated by the Joint Commission. In departmentalized hospitals, these functions may be carried out by the departments themselves. These committees may implement and/or recommend actions. Much of what they do is produce and analyze data that other groups use. When medical staff committees are used, for example, results must be presented to departments and/or the medical staff for analysis and appropriate action. The goals for all involved are that the review functions be properly executed and their results be used to continually assess and improve patient care.

Data trends must also be observed over time for changes in patterns. Data must also be brought down to an individual practitioner level in at least two ways:

- *Departmental reports*—Antibiotic review by St. Anywhere's Pharmacy and Therapeutics (P & T) Committee showed that third-generation cephalosporins were properly used within the Department of Medicine overall, but a report sorted by provider indicated Dr. A's usage was substantially different from her peers. After further stratification of the data, Dr. A's usage was found to be in patients with more severe conditions. Cases that many of her colleagues chose not to manage alone, she handled directly and through consultation. This finding was reported back to the P & T Committee as well as to the department while maintaining the confidentiality of the individual involved.

- *Physician QM profile*—Physician profiles may be generated and maintained by many groups for varied purposes: HMOs, PROs, and so forth. These profiles are those generated through the Quality Management area and maintained by the medical staff office specifically for credentialing purposes. These QM profiles may include both raw data (for example, unplanned returns to the operating room) and the results of peer review activities and analysis of such data (focused education, privilege changes, and so forth).[33] A physician's QM profile is typically reviewed by several groups at the time of promotion from provisional status and at reappointment. The department chair, Credentials Committee, Medical Staff Executive Committee, and the governing board may review such profiles. The specific contents of these profiles, frequency of updating and review, and the parties who review them vary substantially according to state law, hospital custom, and preference. Nearly all profiles include the six monitors cited above and are reviewed by at least the department chair prior to reappointment.

## Department Quality Review

Departments are the focal point for QI in many hospitals today. Small hospitals' medical staffs often meet as a whole because meeting as individual departments would be inefficient or impossible. A growing number of hospitals are also using QI teams that cross department and disciplinary boundaries. Even these teams often share their findings with individual departments because departmental education and approval are often required for lasting behavior and system changes that improve quality.

A variety of processes can identify both problems and opportunities for improvement:

- Monitoring and evaluation of specific aspects of care
- Review of referred cases
- Evaluation of medical staff review function reports
- Comparing departmental parameters with external data sets: practice parameters, specialty society reports, multihospital system data, research projects (Quality Indicator Project,[34] and so forth)
- Risk management, infection control, and utilization management data from internal and external sources (for example, National Practitioner Data Bank, Federation of State Medical Boards Data Bank, Centers for Disease Control, PRO, Blue Cross/Blue Shield, other payers, and so forth)

Departmental review of individual episodes of patient care frequently will find appropriate high-quality care in the vast majority of cases (one QM professional estimates 85 percent),[35] and will not identify problems or opportunities for improvement. *This important information (review found no problems) should be recorded in each affected practitioner's profile and credential file.* These documents are intended to provide a fair and realistic portrait of the practitioner's care. This can be done only if positive, as well as negative, findings are included.

In reviewing entire systems or processes of care (for example, management of congestive heart failure) through a CQI effort, opportunities to improve the process will always be found. There is no contradiction between these statements. Rather there is a shift in focus or emphasis from individuals to systems. A constant balance must be made between the two since both are important to continuously improving patient care.

When problems and opportunities for improvement are found, they should be dealt with expeditiously. The speed and intensity of the corrective action[36] will be determined by the potential impact on patient care: A surgeon discovered to have arrived at the operating room inebriated might require immediate action, perhaps a summary suspension of privileges to permit an appropriate investigation while protecting patient safety.[37] An internist found to have prematurely discharged a patient because he missed a slightly elevated temperature might have this item recorded and monitored over time for possible patterns. In some situations there would be further investigation to determine the reasons for the discharge. The individual result, and the findings of any investigation, would be recorded in the physician's QA profile. Should a pattern of premature discharges emerge, the department would be expected to take corrective action—perhaps focused education. Should the pattern continue, a counseling session with the department chair and/or a required second opinion prior to discharge could be used.

Each department is responsible to the medical staff executive committee, the board, and, most importantly, the patients involved, to see that *effective* corrective action resolves the problem. Corrective action should not wait until reappointment.

Implementing corrective action, particularly when it is an adverse action such as a summary suspension, is a thankless but essential job. Who is required to, or authorized to, take adverse actions? These questions should be clearly answered in the medical staff bylaws and be consistent with relevant laws, court decisions, and Joint Commission standards.

Reappointment offers another chance for corrective action, however. A profile that shows a pattern of repeated premature discharges by Dr. C, but no corrective action by the Department of Medicine, is presented to the Medical Staff Executive Committee (MSEC). The MSEC may ask the department chair for an explanation, and also recommend restriction of privileges and/or other corrective action. The reappointment period adds two year's worth of data and the knowledge that the board will ultimately review and act on the recommendations of the department and the MSEC.

Five points are worth repeating:

1. There is a balance between problems and opportunities attributable to individuals and those attributed to processes and systems. Both are important. Investigation is required to distinguish between them.
2. Most reviews of individual episodes of patient care will find high-quality care with no significant problems or opportunities for improvement.
3. Any process or system can be improved. Organizations will prioritize their QI efforts based on the needs of their patients and other customers.
4. When problems or opportunities are found, effective and appropriate corrective action should be taken expeditiously. The speed and intensity of the corrective action is determined by the threat to patient safety. Again much corrective action will not be directed toward individuals. Education may be the first and only corrective step required to assist a practitioner in improving care.
5. Reappointment time is often too late to institute effective corrective action. If corrective action has not been implemented prior to reappointment, however, each body involved in reappointment has an obligation to recommend and/or take effective corrective action.

## Risk Management

### Background and History

Risk management (RM) has been defined as "the discipline of identifying and managing potential liability situations in the care and treatment of patients."[38] The same authors state: "Effective risk management prevents injury or loss, provides for a safer hospital environment, and contributes to improving the quality of patient care."[39]

Risk management is a relatively new discipline: "The impetus to establish risk management in hospitals came from the insurance crisis in the mid-1970s, when the number of malpractice claims against hospitals and physicians rose dramatically and the amount required seemed to skyrocket." Insurers and self-insured hospitals "perceived that risk management programs were the answer to bringing the cost of malpractice claims under control."[40]

In less than 20 years, RM has become an integral part of quality management and of health care delivery. The Handbook of Health Care Risk Management[41] describes a four-step generic model for risk management:

1. The identification of risk
2. The analysis of the risks identified
3. The treatment of risk
4. The evaluation of risk treatment strategies

The critical elements involving credentialing are risk identification and risk treatment. Risk identification, through the use of occurrence screens, review of complaints and lawsuits, and so forth, can provide data that may be used directly in the credentialing process. These data may also be referred to a department chair, quality committee, or QM staff. The actions from that referral (for example, a obstetrics department review of a cesarean section delayed by the on-call physician's late arrival) could lead to changes in physician privileges (for example, the obstetrician might be required to relocate closer to the hospital in order to remain on the call schedule.)

Effective credentialing itself is an important risk treatment. Ensuring the competence of credentialed, independent practitioners improves patient safety and quality of care, thereby reducing risk. Conversely, failure to effectively credential such practitioners may place the hospital at increased risk of liability should an adverse incident occur. Patients have successfully charged that negligent credentialing was partially responsible for a practitioner injuring them through substandard care.[42]

This section will focus on how RM data can be used to reduce or minimize risk by strengthening the credentialing process.

## Pre-Appointment RM Data

Risk management uses prospective, concurrent, and retrospective approaches as do the other QM disciplines. Risk managers often emphasize the prospective (or preventive) aspects of their field: They remind nurses and physicians which medications are most strongly correlated with falls, teach patient relations and skills, and stress documentation. These efforts are akin to spreading salt on the sidewalk *before* the snowfall.

Yet *retrospective* RM data are used in a prospective way in the initial credentialing process far more often than other QM data. The major reason is that historic RM data on an individual practitioner are readily available from several sources including the practitioner's application, court records, the National Practitioner Data Bank (NPDB), the Federation of State Medical Boards Action Data Bank, and the American Medical Association Masterfile. Data from these sources can be used as part of the credentialing process at a given hospital.

RM data involve actual or potential liability whether the legal system is involved or not. Data include liability insurance coverage and claims settled or pending. Applicants are commonly asked on medical staff application (and reapplication) to provide proof of liability coverage in a specific minimum amount, and a summary of any pending or settled litigation within a specified time period (for example, five years). These items are requested for two related reasons: (1) Liability insurance protects the hospital's assets, and (2) information on liability cases *may* give some insight into the quality of the physician's care. The fact that a practitioner has been sued at least once does not, per se, say anything about the quality of care provided. The facts of the case(s) involved should be reviewed with the practitioner openly and candidly. The results should then be considered with all other information obtained regarding the applicant.

The establishment of the National Practitioner Data Bank (NPDB) in September 1990 created new opportunities and new requirements for hospitals. As of this writing, all malpractice payments of one dollar or more paid on behalf of physicians, dentists, and other specified practitioners are reported to the NPDB. (There are proposals to establish a "floor" of $30,000 to $50,000, below which payments would not be reported. This is to eliminate the reporting of "nuisance suit" payments, where it is less costly for a practitioner to settle a lawsuit than to successfully defend it.) In addition, hospital actions adversely affecting physician privileges for longer than 30 days, state licensure board actions, and professional society actions are all available through the NPDB.[43] These reports do not provide detailed or conclusive evidence regarding physician conduct or competence. Rather they are red flags, "newspaper headlines" that require further investigation to reveal the full story.

Hospitals are *required* to both report adverse actions to the NPDB, and to query the NPDB at the time of appointment and reappointment, and whenever a practitioner requests additional privileges. (Failure to report and/or query can result in civil penalties up to $10,000 and other problems.) Hospitals (and other specified entities performing peer review) may query the NPDB at any other time.[44] Some have suggested incident-based NPDB queries; for example, if a claim is made, or a significant incident is reported, some hospitals query the NPDB to see if there are any similar occurrences in the practitioner's past.[45]

Much, if not all, of the data available in the NPDB should be provided by the applicant in response to a well-written medical staff membership application. Hospitals and their medical staffs should consider: (1) requiring such information on the application; (2) requiring a new application (or reapplication) to begin the reappointment process; (3) making false statements, by commission or omission, grounds for disciplinary action up to and including revocation of medical staff membership and/or clinical privileges; (4) using the NPDB as one source of information regarding the practitioner, but proceeding with the credentialing process pending the NPDB report, and if the NPDB report provides new information, reviewing the new information together with existing information and taking any appropriate action; and (5) requiring the applicant to notify the medical staff office promptly if any information on the application changes.

### Postappointment RM Data

Once the practitioner has been granted privileges, and is actually using the hospital's facilities, additional RM data become available. In addition to claims made and attorney inquiries (both of which often name the hospital), incident (or occurrence) reports and other early warning systems are invaluable. Such notices often allow a risk manager to proactively work with patients, practitioners, and attorneys to resolve potential liability problems without substantial legal expenses, delays, and other headaches. Examples of incidents reported to RM include patient falls, medication errors, patient injuries, complaints, and so forth. Risk managers also receive final reports and/or case referrals from QM committees and other medical staff and hospital committees. Informal reports of hospital employees, physicians, and others interested in patient care quality are also of value.

RM data are frequently used for educational purposes. A frank discussion of a case recently closed for a substantial settlement can focus a QA Committee or department's attention and make discussion of documentation, preventing patient falls, or effective peer review far more compelling. RM data are also reported in practitioners' QM profiles and accumulated over time to identify trends. When either patterns or similar incidents require further review, appropriate data are referred to the department(s) involved. This referral is often done through the QA/QI area because quality of care is a primary concern and also because QA/QI activities are protected from discovery under many state laws.

As described under Quality Assessment and Improvement, either an individual finding (for example, an inebriated surgeon), a pattern (for example, repeated premature discharges), and the corrective action taken in response to these data (focused education, mandatory second surgical opinion) are each important. One or more of these may result in actions affecting a practitioner's privileges. Risk managers also attempt to use the retrospective data collected to anticipate and prevent similar situations in the future. They use RM data to improve patient care quality.

## Infection Control

### Background and History

Infection control (IC) has been an important issue in public health and hospitals since before the turn of the century.[46] Tremendous strides have been made, for example, in sanitation for public water supplies and in the identification, prevention, and treatment of nosocomial infections. IC, like other QM disciplines, strikes a balance between the impact of systems or processes of care and individual practitioners on patient care.[47] IC's balance is heavily shifted towards the impact of systems, therefore IC has a very limited role in credentialing. IC's focus on systems stems from several sources: (1) large volumes of data are required to perform IC analysis; (2) many infections are not preventable at all, and others cannot be prevented by individual action; (3) there is no currently acceptable risk adjustment method to allow individual clinician comparisons. This section focuses on the evolution of IC into an integrated component of the QM process, and its limited role in credentialing.

IC as an activity is usually the responsibility of the hospital epidemiologist in consultation with the medical staff or hospital Infection Control Committee. There has been an effort in recent years to integrate IC into QM activities to take advantage of overlapping resources (for example, uilization management (UM) coordinators identifying suspected nosocomial infections) and enhance hospitalwide perspective and visibility for the IC function. Whether IC is *structurally* part of the QM Department, as advocated in *Integrated Quality Assurance*,[48] is not critical. The IC function, and the other QM disciplines, benefit from close coordination and integration of efforts.

### Infection Control Process—Identification of Suspected Nosocomial Infections

*Integrated Quality Assurance* states three major ways that suspected or known nosocomial (hospital-acquired) infections may be identified: (1) IC practitioner review of daily admission diagnoses may identify possible nosocomial infections related to previous admissions; (2) IC practitioner review of positive laboratory reports may identify suspected nosocomial infections; (3) QM coordinators may identify suspected nosocomial infections during continued stay reviews as mentioned in the UM section.[49] In addition, other clinicians such as nurses and respiratory therapists may identify suspected nosocomial infections through incident reports, occurrence screens, and oral reports.

All hospital personnel involved in surveillance activities should use ommon definitions, approved by the infection control committee, for the identification of nosocomial infections. The Centers for Disease Control (CDC) definitions for nosocomial infections are the most widely acception definitions. They may be adopted by hospitals for use in their nosocomial infections surveillance programs. Modifications in the CDC definitions may be made where the infection control committee deems appropriate.


### Infection Control Process—Reporting of Nosocomial Infections

Surveillance activities, including the indentification of nosocomial infections in most hospitals, are the responsibility of the IC practitioner in collaboration with the IC committee. Although the IC committee approves the type and scope of surveillance activities, the exact division of these responsibilities varies among hospitals. Methods of reporting findings are largely at the discretion of the individual hospital.

As with other QM disciplines, it is recommended that IC data be compared with reference points and monitored over time. However, the nature of the data and comparisons are different for IC. IC data are often presented in an aggregated form to identify possible trends, patterns, and changes in them. The aggregations are done by type of infection, not individual physician. (For example, rates of ventilator-associated nosocomial pneumonia.) These rates can then be compared with historical rates and national norms, but not on an individual practitioner basis.

The only nosocomial infection that has been found to be preventable by an individual physician is the surgical wound infections (SWI). The 10-year $8 million Study on the Efficacy of Nosocomial Infection Control

(SENIC) found reporting their own surgeon-specific rates to individual surgeons was one major factor in reducing infections. The others are all systemic interventions: one infection control practitioner per 250 beds, intensive surveillance efforts, and a knowledgeable physician in charge of the infection control committee.

Reducing surgical wound infection rates by providing feedback to surgeons on their own rates is valuable, and has been shown to reduce infection rates. This should not be interpreted as a call to immediately include surgeon-specific SWI data on physician profiles used in credentialing. Consider the following reasons:

1. While there may be acceptable ranges within a particular hospital, there are no national norms yet for hospitalwide SWI rates.
2. Comparisons would require huge denominators for reliability, and few surgeons would generate such volumes. Would medical staffs and hospitals evaluate only those few?
3. Educational feedback of their own data to surgeons can be implemented now to help reduce infection rates.

Aggregate IC data should be used as an educational tool in a variety of settings, including the IC Committee, individual departments, and the entire medical staff. Providing individual data on SWIs to physicians may also be useful. At this time, individual IC data should generally not be used in the credentialing process.


## Utilization Management


### Background and History

History Utilization management (UM) focuses on the appropriate and efficient use of hospital resources to provide high-quality patient care. This broad mandate includes concern with under- and overutilization of hospital days and ancillary services; early identification of patients' possible QM problems (for example, infections, falls, premature discharge); providing services in the most appropriate setting (that is, inpatient acute care, subacute or skilled nursing facility, ambulatory care center or physician office, hospice, and so forth); working with external review agencies (for example, PRO, insurers) in evaluating these issues; and collaborating with medical staff and hospital personnel in addressing these challenges.

The role of the UM team has expanded rapidly over the past several years. The traditional role focused on reviewing the necessity for inpatient acute care: prospectively through preadmission review; concurrently through continued stay reviews; and retrospectively through chart reviews and audits. Today UM is used in evaluating ambulatory surgery, ancillary utilization, and managed care contracts; representing the hospital and physicians in appeals of PRO and payer denials and audits; collaborating with discharge planning; and referring cases to other QM staff.

The following factors have fueled expansion to the current state:

- Implementation of the Medicare prospective payment system (PPS) and diagnosis-related groups (DRGs) led to concern that patients were being discharged prematurely ("quicker and sicker").
- Inpatient ancillary utilization increased significantly as physicians tried to discharge patients sooner, but hospitals being paid per case were and are concerned with total expenditures.
- UM staff have frequent patient and/or chart contact on a concurrent basis and may identify QM issues earlier than other staff. This became more important as many hospitals reduced staffing and consolidated functions.
- Ambulatory care has become the growth area of the hospital field. As outpatient expenditures increase, both hospitals and payers are looking to UM to ensure that funds are spent wisely.
- External review agencies including PROs, insurers, utilization management firms, and managed care organizations (HMOs, PPOs, and so forth) have gained increasing control over the practice of medicine inside and outside the hospital by controlling the revenue stream to physicians and hospitals. UM represents hospital and physician interests in putting high-quality patient care first, and receiving adequate reimbursement for services appropriately rendered.

  External agencies always have a financial incentive to minimize reimbursement to providers. UM works with medical staff and other hospital personnel to see that this incentive does not have a detrimental impact on patient care.
- Medical staff and hospital personnel must provide patient care that yields excellent outcomes in a cost-efficient manner. The demand for value by payers, employers, and the public is important today and growing. UM staff and the medical staff's Utilization Management Committee are on the forefront of education and collaboration in improving and demonstrating the value of patient care services.

### Internal and External Data Sources

UM uses internal and external data prospectively, concurrently, and retrospectively to enhance patient care quality. As with RM and other QM disciplines, the retrospective data are most useful in the credentialing process. These UM data are provided directly to credentialing bodies through practitioner QM profiles, and indirectly through referral to QM functions (departmental, medical, committee, and QM staff).

There are several internally generated UM statistics that are frequently used to compare individual practitioners to their peers within a department or medical staff, and with national or regional norms.

Internal data include the following:

- Average length of stay (ALOS)—Overall and by diagnosis, procedure, or DRG
- Ancillary resource utilization
- Practitioner case-mix/severity index—Must be used to adjust the previous two items to allow "apple to apple" comparisons

There are also important external indicators. We will stress repeatedly, however, that external indicators must be confirmed through internal peer review processes before they are used in the credentialing process. Credentialing is primarily an internal hospital function. Credentials verification can largely be subcontracted to an outside group. However, medical staff appointment and privilege delineation cannot be delegated to external agencies. Only the hospital governing board can take these actions after receiving recommendations through the medical staff as stated in the medical staff bylaws.

External data include the following:

- DRG day outlier (may also be generated internally)
- DRG cost outlier (may also be generated internally)
- Admissions/days denied by PROs, Blue Cross/Blue Shield, and other payers
- Quality letters/generic screen violations identified by payers
- Severity of illness/intensity of service (SI/IS) criteria issued by payers and evaluated by the UM committee and/or affected departments

### Identification of QM Data by UM Coordinators

The identification of relevant QM data was an important addition to the UM coordinator's job description. It was added because of the coordinator's concurrent contact with the patient and medical record (see Continued

Stay Review), PROs' adoption of generic screens,[50] and the consolidation of responsibilities within shrinking staffs. Integrated Quality Assessment (IQA),[51] previously cited, gives an excellent summary of the UM coordinator's expanded role in QM.

QM data identifiable by UM coordinators include the following:

- Complications of procedures (especially cardiac arrest, hemorrhage, or death)
- Medication errors
- Slips, falls, or any other injuries
- Suspected nosocomial infections
- Adverse drug reactions
- PRO generic screens
- Cases not meeting other approved occurrence screens

Data identified by UM coordinators are generally routed through the appropriate QM department (QA, RM, IC) for review and appropriate further action. This may include investigation by QM staff, referral to a department chair or QA committee, or merely monitoring the information over time. The appropriate action depends on individual circumstances, particularly the potential impact of the findings on patient care quality.

### The Utilization Management Process—
### Preadmission Review (Prospective)

UM staff members prospectively review the necessity of inpatient admission in certain cases. Cases may be selected for preadmission review based on a random sample, specified diagnoses or procedures, particular payers, particular physicians, or some combination of these.

The following review process is fairly representative, but it is not the only process by any means. We should also note that similar precertification protocols are sometimes used for *selected procedures*, whether performed on an inpatient or outpatient basis.

The physician and/or the physician's staff contact UM staff with the initial diagnosis, estimated length of stay, proposed procedure, if any, and similar relevant data. These are reviewed against preestablished criteria, typically focusing on the patient's severity of illness and the intensity of service proposed (SI/IS criteria). If the case does not meet these criteria, it is referred to the UM physician advisor (PA). After reviewing the case, the PA may approve the admission on the basis of his or her medical judgement, deny the admission, or contact the physician for further information. UM staff members do not make determinations of the medical necessity for admission. The PA makes such decisions on a peer-to-peer basis with the admitting physician. There is an appeals process if the admitting physician disagrees with the PA's decision. Often a second PA, the medical director, or a department chair is called in to resolve the dispute. Professional disagreements are understandable and completely acceptable. Each party must put the patient's best interests first. Physicians and hospitals must first consider the impact of a decision on patient care.

If a decision to admit is made, UM staff or physician office staff will contact any external review agency that requires admission precertification to receive authorization. These agencies also have appeals processes that should be used if the hospital and admitting physician disagree with the initial decision. In guarding the patient's interest, remember the words of one emergency department physician: "Reviewers authorize payment, not treatment."

## The Utilization Management Process—
## Continued Stay Review (Concurrent)

Patients are monitored periodically throughout their inpatient stay to determine their continued need for inpatient acute care. The frequency of monitoring depends on the patient's diagnosis and condition, staffing levels, external review requirements, and other factors. The process will remain relatively stable and include the comparison of the patient's condition with preestablished criteria (SI/IS, appropriateness evaluation protocol). Those that fail to meet criteria are referred to the physician advisor for review as described above. If the PA decides the patient no longer requires acute care, he or she may recommend that the attending physician consider discharge, transfer to a more appropriate facility, reclassification of care provided to subacute[52] (providing lower reimbursement, while allowing the patient to remain in the hospital), or other alternatives. This conversation is again peer-to-peer between the PA and the attending physician. In practice, many UM coordinators have developed good working relationships with attending physicians. The coordinator may discuss a case with the physician, and he or she may decide to change the course of action. Nevertheless, any formal determination of medical necessity is a peer-to-peer decision. As with the preadmission situation, an appeals process is available if the PA and attending disagree regarding the necessity for continuing acute care.

Utilization Management Process—Retrospective Review (Audit)

UM may be thought of as the rapid response area of QM. It is certainly true that decisions on patient admission, discharge, and transfer must often be made under time constraints, and always for the patient's benefit. Decisions are also often under significant conflicting pressure from admitting physicians and external reviewers who disagree over what course of treatment is most appropriate. UM data are also used constructively on a retrospective basis to improve delivery systems, to educate practitioners, to change behavior, and through other QM functions, to influence credentialing decisions.

UM data (including ALOS, ancillary utilization, PRO denials, and so forth) are often included in QM profiles. Referrals from UM to other QM functions and/or committees may also be included. These data are particularly useful when they are adjusted for case mix/severity, external data are reviewed and validated by internal peer review processes, data are compared with reference points (departmental averages, national norms), and they are monitored over time on both an individual and a group basis.

These data are often presented first to a medical staff UM Committee. Other hospitals dispense with this committee and have departmental reviews instead. The UM Committee may also be the group to validate external data. Alternatively, this may be done by departmental QA committees and/or departments to allow specialty-specific peer review. The UM Committee may identify patterns requiring further review on a unit-specific, departmental, individual practitioner, or hospitalwide basis. Data may involve particular diagnoses and/or procedures, and thus tie to specific clinical privileges. The UM Committee often refers the data in question to a specific department for further analysis and corrective action, if required. The department is then expected to report back to the UM Committee, and both groups are held accountable by the Medical Staff Executive Committee. Assistance in investigation is often provided by one or more QM areas, administration, the medical staff office, other hospital departments, and, nearly always, medical records.

The results of investigations based on UM referral are recorded in each affected practitioner's credentials file, as with other QM data. The data will often be used for educational purposes and may change practitioner behavior. They are also available to credentialing bodies to aid their decisions.

## Conclusions and Summary

Credentialing includes the following three interrelated processes:

- Credentials verification
- Medical staff appointment
- Privilege delineation

Credentialing is a major quality tool, because it works to assess and improve the competence of independently privileged practitioners. Credentialing involves multiple individuals and bodies including: the applicant, department chairmen, credentials committee, Medical Staff Executive Committee, and the governing board.

Ultimate responsibility for medical staff appointment and privilege delineation rests with the hospital governing board. The board must be assured that functions delegated to the medical staff, and supported by the administration, are carried out appropriately. This is an essential precursor to the board's actual appointments and privilege delineation.

Quality management (QM) includes the following four interrelated disciplines:

- Quality assessment and improvement
- Risk management
- Infection control
- Utilization management

QM data can and must be used continually to improve patient care without waiting for the reappointment process to begin. Most QM data will document good patient care quality. Where problems or opportunities for improvement are identified, most will be related to systems and processes, not individual practitioners.

Credentialing, particularly privilege delineation, can and should be influenced by QM data. Medical staff appointment may be particularly influenced by QM data during the provisional period of initial appointment. During the provisional period prior to promotion to active status, and at reappointment, the onus of demonstrating current clinical competence rests with the applicant. This applies to competence in general and specifically for the privileges requested.

QM data should be presented and used in both aggregate (for example, departmental and specialty level) and practitioner-specific forms for quality improvement purposes. Practitioner-specific data are essential for credentialing purposes and should be presented to credentialing bodies in QM profiles and to departments and committees as referrals for review and action. The results of department and committee actions should also be presented to credentialing bodies for their use.

The credentialing process is one important tool in medical staff/hospital partnership to improve patient care. The credentialing process itself must be continually improved so that it may help to improve patient care. The integration of quality management data into the credentialing process is an important step in this continuing evolution.

## References

1. Independent practice is patient care provided by "an individual who is permitted by law and who is also permitted by the hospital to provide patient care services without direction or supervision, within the scope of his/her license and in accordance with individually granted clinical privileges." (JCAHO, *Accreditation Manual for Hospitals (AMH)*, footnote, p. 55)

2. State licensure acts specify the scope of practice of physicians, dentists, podiatrists, clinical psychologists, chiropractors, and other practitioners. California, Florida, and others specify that certain practitioners may not be denied medical staff membership as a group.

   Hospital medical staff bylaws specify which categories of practitioner are eligible for membership and/or privileges, and define the application process. They also specify objective criteria for categories of membership and specific privileges. Individuals then apply and are considered for membership and/or privileges on their individual merits. The American Hospital Association (AHA) takes no position regarding membership and/or privileges for any category of practitioners. This decision is made by individual hospitals and their medical staffs. For more information, see AHA statement on the profession of chiropractic and hospitals in the appendix.

3. A *hospital* must have inpatient beds and an organized medical staff, among other characteristics (A. Fox Keiger, ed., *Hospital Administration Terminology*, 2nd ed., Chicago: American Hospital Publishing, Inc., p. 27). Many other types of organizations have medical staffs and award privileges: ambulatory surgery centers, health maintenance organizations, long-term care facilities, ambulatory health care centers, and so forth. This chapter addresses credentialing as a medical staff/hospital partnership. Many, but not all, concepts would apply in other settings.

4. National Association Medical Staff Services, *Principles of Medical Staff Services Science*, pp. 57-72; Zusman, J., *Credentialing and Privileging Systems*, pp. 33-36; JCAHO, AMH 1992, MS.2.4.1.3.1, p. 56.

Note: Community (or centralized) credentials verification services (CCVSs) will query the NPDB, obtain original copies of medical school transcripts, and perform similar mechanical duties that burden physicians and hospital staffs. This may not eliminate the need for individual clinicians to contact their peers during the credentials verification process. That is an individual medical staff/hospital decision.

CCVS programs are offered by a number of medical societies (for example, the American Medical Association's National Credentials Verification Service), private organizations, and hospital associations either alone or in partnership with medical societies (for example, Hospital Council of Southern California, Hospital Association of Greater Des Moines (Iowa), and so forth). McCormick, B., Community credentialing saves time and money, *Trustee*, November, 1989; Koska, M. T., Credentialing service demise a disappointment', *Hospitals*, February 20, 1992.

5. The National Practitioner Data Bank (NPDB) is a federally mandated computer system containing adverse actions lasting over 30 days taken against specified practitioners (presently physicians and dentists) by hospitals, licensing boards, or professional societies. Malpractice payments for a broader variety of practitioners are also included. Hospitals must query prior to appointing or reappointing physicians or dentists to the medical staff, or awarding/revising privileges. Failure to do so voids immunity provisions granted under the Health Care Quality Improvement Act of 1986, allows a plaintiff or his or her attorney access to the practitioner's NPDB record, and could lead to charges of negligent credentialing if there was information contained in the NPDB that the hospital did not obtain.

   For further information on reporting requirements and negligent credentialing, see: *National Practitioner Data Bank Guidebook*, U.S. DHHS, Public Health Service, Health Resources and Services Administration, pp. 3-6; *Elam v. College Park Hospital*, 132 Cal. App. 3d 332, 183 Cal. Rptr. 156 (Cal. App. 4 Dist. 1982); *Johnson v. Misericordia Community Hospital*, 99 Wis. 2d 708, 301 NW 2d 156 (1981), both cited in D. Fraiche, Legal Aspects of Clinical Privilege Delineation, in H*ospital Privileges and Specialty Medicine*, 2nd edition.

6. Medical staff membership decisions are affected by federal and state law, Medicare Conditions of Participation, JCAHO standards, and medical staff bylaws. As examples: The Health Care Quality Improvement Act of 1986 outlines fair hearing process for adverse membership decisions. Guidelines must be followed to gain protection under the HCQIA for peer review activities. California state law specifies

that the rules and regulations of a health facility may not discriminate among MDs., DOs, and DPMs (podiatrists), Cal. Health and Safety Code s. 1316. The same code (s. 1316.5) states that psychologists may be allowed medical staff membership. Other states (for example, Florida) prohibit banning groups of practitioners from hospital medical staffs. JCAHO standards specify that: (1) the medical staff includes licensed physicians and may include independent practitioners from other professions; (2) competence must be considered as part of appointment/reappointment and privilege delineation; and (3) appointment/reappointment must occur biennially, or more frequently. (JCAHO, *AMH92*, MS.1.1.1, p. 55; MS.2.6, p. 57; MS.2.13, p. 58)

Bylaws define which practitioners are eligible for medical staff membership, but must be written to conform with applicable laws and standards.

7. See note 1.
8. Data collected by the American Hospital Association Division of Medical Affairs in 1989 showed that 43.2 percent of hospitals' medical staff bylaws allowed clinical psychologists as medical staff members, while 46.4 percent were granted privileges to use hospital facilities within the scope of their licensure; 7.9 percent of bylaws provided medical staff voting privileges for clinical psychologists and 4.9 percent provided for their election to medical staff office.

   *Medical Staff Survey Report*, American Hospital Association Division of Medical Affairs, table 2, p. 2.
9. *Medical Staff Survey Report*, American Hospital Association Division of Medical Affairs, table 8, p. 8.

   For further information regarding credentialing of limited license practitioners see Zusman, pp. 79-90.
10. See note 6; also JCAHO, *AMH*, MS.2.15, p. 58.
11. JCAHO, *AMH*, 1992, MS.2.4.1.3, p. 56.
12. JCAHO, *AMH*, MS.2.4, p. 56; *Risk Management Handbook for Health Care Facilities*, Harpster, M. H., Veach, M. S., eds, p. 208.
13. JCAHO *AMH*, 1992, p. 68. "There is a mechanism to assure the same level of quality of patient care by all individuals with delineated clinical privileges, within medical staff departments, across departments/services, and between members and nonmembers of the medical staff who have delineated clinical privileges."
14. JCAHO, *AMH*, MS.2.4, p. 56; *Risk Management Handbook for Health Care Facilities*, Harpster, M. H., Veach, M. S., eds, p. 208.
15. JCAHO, *AMH*, MS.2.10, p. 57; Harpster, M. H., Veach, M. S., op. cit., pp. 208, 209; Weiss v. York Hospital 745 F 2d (3d Cir. 1984), cert. denied U.S. (1985); *Patrick v. Burgett* and other cases cited in *Medical*

*Staff Credentialing: Guidelines for Maryland Hospitals*, Maryland Hospital Education Institute, pp. I-1 to I-6, I- 10 to I-13, appendix III-5.

16. Jesse, W. F., Assessing and Monitoring Medical Practice in the Hospital, in *Hospital Privileges and Specialty Medicine*, Langsley, D. G., Signer, M. M., eds, Evanston, IL: American Board of Medical Specialties, 1986, p. 61.

17. Harpster, M. H., Veach, M. S., op. cit., p. 209; JCAHO, *AMH*, MS.2.12, p. 58.

18. Harpster, M. H., Veach, M. S., op. cit., p. 209.

19. JCAHO, *AMH*, MS.2.14, MS.2.15, p. 58; Maryland Hospital Education Institute, op. cit., appendix III-5.

20. JCAHO, *AMH*, MS.2.14, MS.2.15, p. 58.

21. Maryland Hospital Education Institute, op. cit., appendix III-5.

22. *Medicare: A Strategy for Quality Assurance*, vol. I, p. 21.

23. Roberts, J. S., Implications of Continuous Quality Improvement for Privilege Delineations, presented at Second Annual Medical Staff Credentialing Seminar, May 30, 1991, Katten Muchin and Zavis/Metropolitan Chicago Healthcare Council.

24. *The Minimum Standard*, American College of Surgeons' Hospital Standardization Program, 1918. Cited in Longo, D. R., Ciccone, K. R., Lord, J. T. *Integrated Quality Assessment*. Chicago: American Hospital Publishing, 1989, p. 3.

25. Longo, D. R., Ciccone, K. R., Lord, J. T. *Integrated Quality Assessment*. Chicago: American Hospital Publishing, 1989.

26. *The Role of Hospital Leadership in the Continuous Improvement of Patient Care Quality*. American Hospital Association Division of Quality Resources. January 1992.

27. *Clinical Practice Guidelines*. American Hospital Association Division of Quality Resources. March 1992, p. 1.

28. AMA Policy 93.017S; AMA Policy Compendium, A-90/I-90/A-91 Supplement, p. 73.

29. Ball, J. R., Credentialing, Privileging and Performance: View From the 90's, in *Hospital Privileges and Specialty Medicine*, 2nd ed., Langsley, D. G. and Stubblefield, B., eds., Evanston, IL: American Board of Medical Specialties, 1992.

30. *Clinical Practice Guidelines*. American Hospital Association Division of Quality Resources. March 1992.

31. Personal communication, AHA Division of Quality Resources.

32. JCAHO, *AMH*, MS.5.1, pp. 63-73.

33. Lang, D. A., *Medical Staff Peer Review: A Strategy for Motivation and Performance*. Chicago: American Hospital Publishing, Inc., 1991, pp. 67-78.

34. Statistical reports have been a useful complement to case review for some time. Hospitals are now developing sophisticated analytical techniques that can sometimes substitute for labor-intensive review of individual medical records. For example, the statistical review of antibiotic usage described triggered a detailed review of Dr. A's patient case-mix. With sufficient computer support, this review could be completed without turning to individual records. The peer review process is critical, however, in analyzing reports. Peers must make judgements based on data, but data cannot stand alone.

35. The Quality Indicator Project is a multi-institutional study sponsored by the Maryland Hospital Association. Member hospitals and health care systems share clinical outcome data on several indicators, creating a large database for reference and comparison.

36. Lord, J. T., The Medical Staff, in *Risk Management Handbook for Health Care Facilities*, op. cit., p. 67.

37. *Corrective action* is used by QM professionals to mean a remedial response to an identified problem or opportunity for improvement. The response could be a policy or procedure modification, education for an individual or group, increased supervision of an individual, purchase of new equipment, and so forth. A wide range of nonpunitive and punitive actions are available. See Lang, D. A., *Medical Staff Peer Review: A Strategy for Motivation and Performance*, op. cit., pp. 68-78.

    Attorneys use the term more narrowly to mean adverse actions taken against an individual practitioner (for example, denial, restriction, or removal of clinical privileges). This chapter uses the former definition. Adverse action will be used for the latter definition.

38. Summary suspension is not to be used lightly because it does not afford the practitioner a hearing prior to suspension. It can be appropriately used when patient safety is in imminent danger. Harpster, M. H., Veach, M. S., op. cit., p. 209.

39. Adams, M. A., Dabelstein, L., and others, *Medical Legal Survival: A Risk Management Guide for Physicians, University Hospital Consortium, 1991, p. 7.*

40. *See note 38, p. 7.*

41. *Harpster, L. M., Introduction to Risk Management Handbook for Health Care Facilities, op. cit., p. 3.*

42. Troyer, G., and Salman, S. L. *Handbook of Health Care Risk Management.* Rockville, MD: Aspen Publishers, 1986, p. 153, cited in Hagg, S. R., Elements of a Risk Management Program, in *Risk Management Handbook for Health Care Facilities*, op.cit., p. 28.

43. Cases cited in *Medical Staff Credentialing: Guidelines for Maryland Hospitals,* Maryland Hospital Education Institute, pp. I-1,2.
44. U.S. Department of Health and Human Services, Public Health Service, Health Resources and Services Administration, *National Practitioner Data Bank Guidebook,* pp. 3-4; *Risk Management Handbook for Health Care Facilities,* op. cit., p. 3.
45. See note 43, pp. 3-4
45. Mark Kadzielski's ten hot tips for dealing with the data bank, National Practitioner Data Bank reaches its terrible twos, *Hospital Risk Management,* December 1991, p. 157.
47. Several excellent textbooks listed in the bibliography present an overview of IC, including accounts of its history far beyond the scope of this chapter.
48. Management of postoperative patients is an example of a clinical process that may involve increased risk of nosocomial infection. Management often includes the use of ventilators, sometimes for prolonged periods, in patients who are in a weakened state. Some patients develop ventilator-associated nosocomial pneumonia. Examining the clinical pathway or process of managing postoperative patients may find opportunities to reduce the use of ventilators. This might then reduce the rates of ventilator-associated nosocomial pneumonia.
49. Longo, D. R., Ciccone, K. R., Lord, J. T., op. cit., pp. 78-79.
50. See note 48, pp. 80-81.
51. Generic screens are used by peer review organizations (PROs), hospital utilization management staff, and others to identify cases for review regarding possible patient care problems. Screens may include discharge with patient's temperature above a specified level, unplanned return to the operating room, and so forth.
52. Longo, D. R., Ciccone, K. R., Lord, J. T., op. cit., pp. 65-74.
53. In certain situations this can be done without physically moving the patient; the hospital and payer simply agree to a lower reimbursement based on less intense service. In other circumstances, the patient may be moved to a hospital-based skilled nursing facility (SNF).

## Bibliography

*AMH: Accreditation Manual for Hospitals.* Joint Commission on Accreditation of Healthcare Organizations, 1992.

*Delineation of Clinical Privileges.* National Association Medical Staff Services, 1991

Gassiot, C. O. and Starr, P. J. *Principles of Medical Staff Services Science.* Education Council of the National Association Medical Staff Services.

Harpster, L. M., and Veach, M. S., eds. *Risk Management Handbook.* American Hospital Publishing, Inc., 1990.

Lang, D. A. *Medical Staff Peer Review: A Strategy for Motivation and Performance.* Chicago: American Hospital Publishing, Inc., 1991.

Langsley, D. G., and Signer, M. M., eds. *Hospital Privileges and Speciality Medicine.* Evanston, IL: American Board of Medical Specialities, 1986.

*Legal Status of the Medical Staff.* Office of the General Counsel of the American Hospital Association, 1986.

Lohr, K. N., ed. *Medicare: A Strategy for Quality Assurance; Volume I.* Washington, DC: National Academy Press, 1990.

Longo, D. R., Ciccone, K. R., and Lord, J. T., *Integrated Quality Assessment: A Model for Concurrent Review.* Chicago: American Hospital Publishing, Inc., 1989.

*Medical Legal Survival: A Risk Management Guide for Physicians.* University Hospital Consortium, 1991.

*Medical Staff Credentialing: Guidelines for Maryland Hospitals.* Maryland Hospital Education Institute.

*Medical Staff Survey Report: Division of Medical Affairs.* American Hospital Association, 1991.

*National Practitioner Data Bank Guidebook.* U.S. Department of Health and Human Services, Public Health Service, Health Resources and Services Administration.

Second Annual Medical Staff Credentialing Seminar. Katten Muchin and Zavis and the Metropolitan Chicago Healthcare Council, 1991.

Zusman, J. *Credentialing and Privileging Systems.* American College of Physician Executives, 1990.

## Appendix

> ### Table 1. The Minimum Standard
>
> 1. That physicians and surgeons privileged to practice in the hospital be organized as a definite group or staff. Such organization has nothing to do with the question as to whether the hospital is "open" or "closed," nor need it affect the various existing types of staff organization. The word "staff" is here defined as the group of doctors who practice in the hospital inclusive of all groups such as the "regular staff," "the visiting staff," and the "associate staff."
>
> 2. That membership upon the staff be restricted to physicians and surgeons who are (a) full graduates of medicine in good standing and legally licensed to practice in their respective states or provinces, (b) competent in their respective fields, and (c) worthy in character and matters of professional ethics; that in this latter connection the practice of the division of fees, under any guise whatever, be prohibited.
>
> 3. That the staff initiate and, with the approval of the governing board of the hospital, adopt rules, regulations, and policies that specifically provide:
>
> (a) That staff meetings be held at least once each month. (In large hospitals the departments may choose to meet separately.)
> (b) That the staff review and analyze at regular intervals their clinical experience in the various departments of the hospital, such as medicine, surgery, obstetrics, and the other specialties; the clinical records of patients, free and pay, are the basis for such review and analyses.
>
> 4. That accurate and complete records be written for all patients and filed in an accessible manner in the hospital—a complete case record being one that includes identification data; complaint; personal and family history; history of present illness; physical examination; special examinations such as consultations, clinical laboratory, X-ray, and other examinations; provisional or working diagnosis; medical or surgical treatment; gross and microscopical pathological findings; progress notes; final diagnosis; condition on discharge; follow-up and, in case of death, autopsy findings.
>
> 5. That diagnostic and therapeutic facilities under competent supervision be available for the study, diagnosis, and treatment of patients, these to include, at least (a) a clinical laboratory providing chemical, bacteriological, serological, and pathological services; (b) an X-ray department providing radiographic and fluoroscopic services.

**Table 2**

Statement of the American Hospital Association
with Respect to the Profession of Chiropractic and Hospitals

In this statement, the American Hospital Association sets forth and reaffirms its policy regarding the practice of chiropractic in a hospital setting.

It is the policy of the American Hospital Association that individual hospitals themselves determine whether chiropractic services are to be provided in a hospital setting. This determination is made by the hospital's governing board taking into consideration, among other legitimate factors: state law, the needs of the patient constituency of the hospital, and appropriate procedural rules and regulations, having in mind protection of the legitimate interests of the patient and the hospital. Such considerations are no different with other licensed health care professionals. The American Hospital Association notes that, in line with such considerations, hospitals that are members of the American Hospital Association have incorporated chiropractic care into a hospital setting, where other licensed health care practitioners and doctors of chiropractic work in a common setting.

The American Hospital Assocation specifically disavows any unlawful effort by any private, competitive group to "contain," "eliminate," or undermine the public's confidence in the profession of chiropractic.

The Association has no objection to a hospital granting privileges to doctors of chiropractic, where consistent with law, for the purpose of: (1) administering chiropractic treatment to patients who wish to have such treatment, whether administered in conjunction with or separate from other health care treatment or services administered by medical doctors or other licensed professional health care providers; (2) furthering the clinical education and training of doctors of chiropractic; or (3) having new diagnostic X-rays, clinical laboratory tests, and reports thereon made available to them, by individual pathologists or radiologists employed by or associated with such hospital, upon the request or authorization of the patient involved.

Those hospitals that are interested in learning more about chiropractic and the practice of chiropractic in a hospital setting may contact either the International Chiropractors' Association, 1901 L Street, N.W., Washington, DC 20036, or the American Chiropractic Association, 1701 Clarendon Boulevard, Arlington, VA 22209. These groups can also provide, upon request and with the hospitals' consent, a list of some of the hospitals that currently provide chiropractic servies or that have granted privileges to doctors of chiropractic.

# The Use of Specialty and Sub-specialty Credentials for Hospital Privileges

Donald G. Langsley, MD

Those concerned with hospital medical staff privileges often depend on credentials. Each Credentials Committee would prefer to use a nationally accepted external standard rather than to make individual judgments and defend those judgments. National or state-wide standards do exist for accreditation of training programs, certification of individual specialists and licensure of individual physicians and may be useful to those making decisions about staff membership and privileges. Board certification by one of the 24 American Board of Medical Specialties (ABMS) and American Medical Association (AMA) recognized boards indicates that a physician has completed an accredited residency, has been examined by respected examiners in the specialty, and has met high national standards. A certificate of successful completion of an Accreditation Council for Graduate Medical Education (ACGME) accredited residency program means that the physician has completed training in which the program itself (but not the individual trainee) has been evaluated and judged to meet published national standards. A license to practice medicine (it usually reads "medicine and surgery") indicates that the physician has met certain standards designed to protect the safety of the public. Though licensure demands only a minimal level of competence in comparison with specialty certification, it does set standards for medical education and medical knowledge. Those licensed are given authorization to practice. Although licensure sets minimal standards, certification is evidence that the physician has met a higher standard. The requirements of advanced training, a period of prac-

**67**

tice as a specialist (in some fields), a thorough review and verification of credentials and passing an examination demonstrate the qualifications necessary for specialty certification. The examination will always include a written component, and for 15 of the 24 boards, include an oral examination.

The ABMS position on the use of certification for credentialing or delineation of clinical privileges has been that certification or subcertification should be considered as only *one* of several valid and important criteria. This position was officially adopted in 1983, but has been the posture of ABMS for many years. The original purpose of certification and the role of the specialty boards was the "improvement of medical care through the setting of professional standards" and the "surveillance of medical qualifications". These purposes are listed in the ABMS Bylaws. But there has always been opposition to requiring certification and subspecialty certification in order to participate in patient care. Certification is an important benchmark, but only *one* of other criteria to determine eligibility to practice. Like the Joint Commission on Accreditation of Healthcare Organizations (JCAHO) standard, the delineation of clinical privileges should be based on training, experience and demonstrated current competence. One way to judge current competence uses the judgments of peers who know the clinical work of the candidate under consideration. This is the task of each hospital's medical staff Credentials Committee. Unfortunately, such judgments may be tainted by local competitive conditions or the personalities of the individuals involved.

### How Specialty Boards are Recognized

Since 1933, the official recognition of specialty boards in medicine has been achieved by the collaborative efforts of the American Board of Medical Specialties (originally the Advisory Board for Medical Specialties) and the AMA Council on Medical Education. In 1934 those efforts were formalized through the establishment of the Liaison Committee for Specialty Boards (LCSB) and the publication of the *Essentials for Approval of Examining Boards in Medical Specialties*. By 1948, 14 new specialty boards had received approval, bringing the total number to 18. Between 1948 and 1969, no new boards were approved, but in the next decade (1969-79) the remaining five specialty boards were approved, bringing the total to 23 boards. In 1991 another Board (Medical Genetics) was approved, bringing the current total to 24 boards.

Subspecialization has been a characteristic of the past decade. During the 1940s seven subsidiary boards for subspecialty certification were formed under the aegis of existing specialty boards. By 1970, areas of recognition of subspecialties had doubled, by 1980 they had quadrupled and now have increased eight-fold. In 1973 the ABMS revised its Bylaws to provide policy guidelines and procedures for the approval of subspecialty certification called Certificates of "Special Competence" (later renamed "Special Qualifications"). Subspecialty areas could be administered through a committee of the appropriate primary board(s) when approved by the ABMS. Currently the 24 Boards of ABMS issue certificates in 32 different kinds of general certificates and 70 types of subspecialty certification. Some boards offer general certification in more than one area. For example, pathology offers a general certificate in Anatomic Pathology, another in Clinical Pathology and another in Anatomic and Clinical Pathology. Radiology offers general certification in Diagnostic Radiology, or in Radiation Oncology. Psychiatry and Neurology offers general certification in Psychiatry, Neurology and in Child Neurology.

The 24 boards also offer certification in 70 subspecialties, as noted above. Subspecialization has raised concerns because it is alleged that subspecialization fragments medical care by involving several subspecialists in the care of a single patient, rather than having the patient treated by a single "primary care" physician. Others suggest that subspecialization increases the cost of medical care, but the high quality of medical care we now enjoy is a consequence of the advancement of medical science. Those who become thoroughly expert in a special field of medicine find that they can master a limited area. They limit their practice (and their research) to a narrow field. The consequence of this is that groups with similar interests form national specialty societies and since they want to clone themselves (teach another generation), form training programs called "fellowships". Out of this limitation of practice comes the wish to be recognized for that special expertise. The subspecialist wants to be credentialed to achieve recognition of "special qualifications". No one expects the science of medicine to stand still and one can expert further requests for credentials as new subspecialties develop.

## Added Qualifications

Two issues have prompted the ABMS to develop a third route to certification called "Added Qualifications". Recognizing that new areas of medical practice based on scientific developments are constantly emerging, but that these new areas may not be so extensive as to justify subspecialty status, ABMS has authorized certificates of Added Qualifications. Such certification must, as with all other types of certification, be approved by the ABMS before a board is authorized to issue it. The recognition of added qualifications is a modification of the approved general certificate to reflect the fact that a candidate has satisfactorily completed full time formal training of at least one year in length and has satisfactorily completed an additional examination in that field. The training program must be one associated with an Accreditation Council on Graduate Medical Education (ACGME) or Canadian equivalent residency program. It must incorporate a specific and identifiable body of knowledge that may include certain procedural skills or practice modes, but is not meant for isolated technical skill areas. To be approved as a new field for Added Qualifications, there must be documentation of the existence of a body of scientific medical knowledge underlying the area which is generally distinct from or more detailed than that of other areas in which certification is offered. There must also be a group of physicians concentrating their practice in the proposed area, national societies interested in the proposed area, as well as acceptable educational programs in the field.

Added Qualifications is an integral part of the primary discipline involved, but it may be part of one or more specialties., Thus, the term Added Qualifications may represent a qualification in horizontal areas which cross existing specialties. It is meant to recognize the practitioner's identification with the primary discipline from which he comes, as well as the added preparation. An example is the recently approved certification of Added Qualifications in Geriatric Medicine which has been authorized for the two specialties of Internal Medicine and Family Practice. In each case, the notation of added qualifications is part of the general certificate so that the certificate would read "Certified in Family Practice with Added Qualifications in Geriatric Medicine" or "Certified in Internal Medicine with Added Qualifications in Geriatric Medicine". It is hoped that this mechanism will discourage additional administrative structures such as new divisions in hospitals or medical schools.


### Recertification

Another aspect of credentialing concerns recertification. From a point early in its history, the ABMS has recognized that provision should be made for updating the evidence that a specialist has kept abreast of current methods of diagnosis, treatment and prevention. Currently, 17 of the 24 Boards issue only time limited certification which has the effect of mandatory recertification.

## Determination of Certification or Recertification

How does a hospital determine whether or not a physician is actually certified, subcertified or recertified? The only authoritative way is to inquire of the board involved or the ABMS. The ABMS receives data on all certifications or recertification.

A convenient way to determine this information is to consult the ABMS Compendium of Certified Medical Specialists or one of the 25 ABMS individual specialty directories. There are 25 such because Psychiatry and Neurology are published separately. These directories are published every two years and are available from the ABMS. Included in each entry is the name, type of certification (and or subcertification and/or recertification), year and place of birth, medical school and year graduated, internship, residency and fellowships served, academic and hospital appointments, professional associations and office telephone. The entries for each specialty are listed alphabetically, and there is a geographic index as well as a master index for all diplomates in the COMPENDIUM. This basic reference is prepared from the data on certification submitted by Boards, but the biographic information about graduate medical education and practice is provided by the diplomate himself. ABMS makes every effort to publish an accurate directory and devotes considerable research to correct addresses since seven percent of all physicians change addresses each year. The ABMS no longer recognizes the publication called *Directory of Medical Specialists* as an official biographic directory (though we used to). The only authorized directories at this time are the ABMS published ones.

## Board Eligible Status

The concept of being "board eligible" has long been used to indicate that a physician has completed the residency necessary to be admitted to the certification process. Hospitals have also used the term. Agencies who employ physicians have used this status to award a difference in salary. Unhappily, it is an inexact term and "has been given such diverse meanings that it has lost its usefulness." Some physicians have used the term year after year while making no perceptible progress toward certification and it has sometimes been accepted improperly as a permanent alternative to certification. The requirements for admission to the certification process change from time to time making this term susceptible to changes in meaning. The ABMS has recommended that the use of the term "board eligible" be disavowed. Information about the certification status of any individuals may be sought from the respective specialty board. Information about whether a physician has satisfactorily completed an ACGME accredited residency should be sought from the program director of the residency program presumed to have been completed.

## Self-Designated Boards

As one reviews the usefulness of board certification, it is necessary to ask "which boards?" Applicants for hospital staff privileges may present credentials from a variety of types of organizations called "boards." There are no legal restrictions on any person or group establishing a board and at this time the ABMS is aware of the existence of at least 120 self-designated boards which are not recognized by the ABMS or the AMA. The recognized boards are the 24 which have met the requirements for ABMS membership. To become recognized a "board" must apply to the Liaison Committee for Specialty Boards (LCSB) and must meet the requirements of a set of criteria published as the *Essentials for the Approval of Examining Boards in Medical Specialties.* Unless the board is approved by the LCSB (the ABMS and the AMA), there is no way to evaluate the standards or the products of that board. There is great variation in the standards of these self-designated boards. A few do require established and accredited fellowship training and have a rigorous exam. Many have no training requirements or are willing to waive the requirement. Some waive the examination or give an examination that has no rigor or meaning. Recently one such self-designated board advertised its willingness to waive training and the exam. It would not waive the fee, of course. This particular organization was found to be engaging in deceptive advertising and was denied the use of the US mails. For these reasons and for the sake of using only the high standards of the ABMS boards, hospitals should recognize only the ABMS boards and realize the dangers of using credentials of any organization calling itself a board.

## Evaluation of Physician Performance

Physician credentialing has generally depended on satisfactory completion of accredited training and passing a written and oral examination. The written exams are in the form of multiple choice questions which can measure knowledge and some aspects of problem-solving and/or clinical judgment. Such tests are easy to administer and objectively score since optical scanners and computers simplify the mechanics of that scoring. As a general rule, a norm-referenced method of standard setting is used by boards which establish a cutting score based on a selected group of examinees such as first time takers of the exam who are graduates of Liaison Committee for Medical Education (LCME) accredited medical schools. However some Boards are shifting to criterion-based scoring. This type of test has the advantage of ease of administration and general acceptability in the profession as well as the courts. In using criterion-referenced approaches, scoring would probably be similar to the norm-referenced exam except for standard setting.

The problem with this type of examination is that it is a cognitive cross-sectional evaluation. The cross-sectional feature measures knowledge that exists at a given time. With the rapidly changing base of medical knowledge, one would have to repeat this cognitive test periodically to determine that the physician has kept up with the changing science. Thus, the rationale for time-limited certification and recertification will offer some answers, but there is significant resistance from practicing physicians when they are asked to take a cognitive test repeatedly. The objections are that the cognitive test is stressful and that it may cover a knowledge base not especially relevant to the present day practice of that physician. What specialist wants to have his recertification dependent on demonstrating knowledge in a basic science which is not part of his day-to-day practice?

The other objection to repeated cognitive tests is that they do not measure performance. Though knowledge is necessary for effective performance, it does not assure it. The tradition of assessing knowledge at nodal points in a physician's career is giving way to a call for demonstrated competence and performance assessment. As recertification moves toward an evaluation of practice, there is a call for competence evaluation that will also examine practice performance. This may use a battery of techniques such as chart-stimulated review, multistation tests with standardized patients, standardized oral examinations or peer ratings. The most satisfactory approach to performance measure in today's world is the judgment of competent peers. Such judgments are made by viewing the day-to-day work of a given physician which is easier to do during residency than during practice. During residency (or fellowship), the person being rated is constantly under supervision and is in a student role where ratings are expected as part of the learning process. During practice, the physician cannot as easily be observed in his work. The practitioner does not wish to feel that he is returned to a student status.

Another concern about performance rating is the lack of a standard system for rating performance. One recent development has been the ratings by residency programs in Internal Medicine. The American Board of Internal Medicine (ABIM) has worked out a system for making such ratings part of the certification process. A candidate for certification in Internal Medicine must receive satisfactory performance ratings in order to be admitted to the written (certifying) exam. The ratings are done on a standardized scale in which the definitions of various levels of performance are predetermined. Efforts to train the raters and check the use of the rating system are accomplished by periodic visits to each of the 430± IM programs by current or prior members of the Board. The ratings measure ten skills on a nine point scale and have achieved wide-spread acceptance. Other specialty boards require ratings by program directors as part of their certification procedures, but not all assemble performance ratings.

Since the accreditation standards of JCAHO call for medical staff privileges to be awarded on the basis of competence (see the chapter by Roberts), it is necessary to explore avenues to determine medical competence. Educators differentiate competence from performance, suggesting that competence represents *potential* for performance. A physician with demonstrated knowledge and skill *is able* to perform with those tools, but competence does not *guarantee* satisfactory performance. Those concerned with certification are aware that board examinations are cross sectional evaluations and that they do not guarantee a level of future performance, but only the potential for it. The issue of the predictive validity of certification exams is a topic under study, but there is insufficient firm evidence to be sure that certification will assure the public of the continued high level of performance needed to pass the certification exam at any given point in time. This is one of the reasons for the support of recertification by the ABMS.

The other effort to assure continued high quality medical care has depended on Continuing Medical Education. In another chapter, Bashook reviews the evidence that CME does change patterns of practice. If the goal of quality assurance is to be met, the Credentials Committee of the Medical Staff and the hospital governing board may choose to use one or more of the following approaches:

1) *The use of credentials* such as specialty or subspecialty certification. The problem with this approach is that it is a cross-sectional measure of performance. The ABMS policy points to the fact that though certification is an excellent benchmark, it should be only one of several measures used by the group considering the hospital medical privileges.

2) *Recertification* is another effort to assure ongoing competence and expresses the view that periodic recertification (using an approach

which is appropriate to the physician's actual practice) is a better predictor of performance over the long run. Time limited certification is being used more frequently and is now the practice in 17 boards. Recertification using performance measures rather than repeated cognitive testing may be more acceptable to practitioners.

3) *Required Continuing Medical Education* is a third approach to the ongoing assurance of quality and the concern for practitioners to keep abreast of changes in science and practice. The evidence that CME can alter performance is reviewed by Bashook in another chapter of this book.

4) *Performance Evaluation* is a fourth approach and the one most likely to yield useful data if the method is standard, feasible, and valid. As noted above, one of the few standardized approaches to performance evaluation is that done during the residency. The performance evaluation must be ongoing rather than cross sectional. The oral examination of the certification process may be a performance evaluation (as in the live patient examinations of the American Board of Psychiatry & Neurology), but it has not been validated as a predictor of future performance.

Performance during practice is the key issue in privileging. Credentials which represent assessment in the past may be useful to decisions about medical staff appointments, but privileging and the renewal of privileges, should focus on actual performance which awards the privileges. Credentials are not a substitute for an assessment of ongoing performance. The challenge to our field is to use measures of performance which are valid and reliable and which are easy and inexpensive to administer in the hospital. To date, no system of evaluation meets all of those requirements but some systems of evaluation are currently available and the next few years will see improvements. Some of the more sophisticated methods are more likely to be used by national evaluation organizations because they require computerized or elaborate methods. One of the more promising approaches, the use of simulated/standardized patients, is not likely to be used by community hospitals. However, there are simpler, yet useful systems of assessment which could be used by small hospitals. The advances in technology of information about health care treatments make it likely that community hospital will find it easier to do performance assessments. The computer technology which hospitals use in the Diagnosis Related Group (DRG) era will make it possible to use information about individual physicians which had not previously been available.

## Approaches to Physician Performance Assessment

To review the methods currently available for assessment of physician performance, one should consider:

1. Direct observation and ratings
2. Medical record review
3. Computer simulations
4. Simulated patients
5. Effect of continuing medical education
6. Utilization review
7. Patient satisfaction and patient behavior (compliance)
8. Cognitive tests
9. Decision analysis
10. Technical skill assessment
11. Interpersonal skill assessment
12. Malpractice claims or Risk Management
13. Outcomes of diagnosis and treatment

## Direct Observations and Rating

Ratings of performance by experienced clinicians is a classic method of evaluating physicians. It begins in the clinical years of medical school and is used extensively during the residency. Such ratings are part of the oral examination in the certification process. Though Psychiatry & Neurology are the only specialties which continue to use live patients in the oral exam, ratings of problem solving and judgments are made in other oral exams. Such ratings are most useful when they are standardized, i.e. when there is a clear definition of what is to be rated and when the raters are trained to the point of satisfactory inter-rater reliability.

Ratings of physicians practicing in hospitals and/or other settings are generally not so well standardized. It is part of the medical tradition to observe and make judgments, but not all judgments are put to paper. Practitioners are understandably reluctant to judge the performance of their colleagues and peers lest they themselves be judged. Neither are they possessed of careful definitions of that to be rated or trained to make the ratings reliable. It is "easier" to have ratings done outside the system and hospitals would prefer to have that luxury. Among other reasons are fears of lawsuits. However the responsibility for performance ratings by peers at the individual hospital could become more acceptable if external scales, definitions, and standardized instructions were available. This is the challenge to the specialty societies and boards—to make such ratings available. Systematic ratings of performance should be based on standardized methods developed by national groups and rater-training could be accomplished by regional resources such as medical schools.

## Medical Record Review

Chart audit (sometimes called "medical audit") is an evaluation of the process of medical care. This type of assessment reviews a physician's performance in terms of what is or not done—at least as revealed by records in patient charts. Some favor this approach because of the difficulty in using valid patient outcome measures and because there is no firm evidence about the association between process and outcome. This is not to denigrate the importance of outcome, but rather to point to the need for evaluation of process in its own right. One can examine certain processes in patient care by comparing data in the chart with an agreed upon set of criteria which define satisfactory quality. One study selected six processes: (1) taking patient history; (2) conducting physical examination; (3) ordering laboratory services; (4) ordering roentgenology services; (5) prescribing therapy; and (6) providing special management services. The criteria to be used must be agreed upon by a suitable population of experts as well as by the physicians who will be audited. Certain primary diagnoses are also selected to conduct such a review. In another study, eight were chosen. They were selected because they had a high incidence rate, the condition was self-limited, it responded to therapeutic intervention, was not unduly influenced by patient compliance, required some effective preventive care and exhibited a range of variation in physician performance indicators. A sample of case records for each diagnosis were selected and trained medical record abstractors compile the data using a detailed instruction manual so that the abstractor does not have to make value judgments. There should be a demonstration of inter-rater reliability among the abstractors. The rate of compliance with the agreed upon criteria may then be calculated and the data represent a measure of performance. The usual medical audit or medical record review can then be discussed with the physicians audited, some corrective measures can be taken, and there can be a repeat audit of the same subject and same physicians at a later date.

In *Chart Stimulated Recall*, the audit method is modified to use an examiner with a prepared list of criteria similar to the one which is given to the chart abstractor. The difference is that the examiner is an "expert" who uses the opportunity to explore the treatment and management of the cases reviewed following the check-list outline, but going beyond it.

For a chart-stimulated recall evaluation of performance, a number of cases of a given diagnosis are reviewed and the results are recorded in the same manner as the audit except that the evaluator has more opportunity to review the conditions in a clinical fashion.

## Computer Simulations

The technology of the computer has made it possible to simulate the clinical situation by evaluating complex problem-solving and decision-making skills. One of the most promising approaches at this time is the Computer Based Examination (CBX) developed by the National Board of Medical Examiners (NBME). It is an unstructured, uncued simulation of medical practice. Using an individual microcomputer plus interactive video, the physician is presented with a clinical problem and may carry out a diagnostic evaluation and manage the case in the same fashion as in clinical practice. The "patient" in the computerized problem will respond to the activities of the physician as he interacts with the computer. Complications, adverse reactions and new medical problems may be programmed to arise during the simulation. The physician has available the full range of diagnostic tests and therapeutic modalities which can be found in a modern hospital or office. The computer maintains a record of the actions taken by the physician and this data is available for evaluating effectiveness as well as cost. In a report made at the meeting of the National Board in April, 1985, it was noted that studies of practicing internists and family physicians demonstrated significant correlation between the CBX situations and performance in actual practice.

Testing centers could accommodate a number of candidates each day. With the CBX it is not necessary for the test to be given at a single time since each candidate interacts with the test in a different fashion. The security of the system has been carefully planned. The pilot studies have been so promising that the NBME hopes to use CBX as one method for Part III of the National Boards.

The CBX experience gives encouragement to those who are interested in the possibility of computer based evaluation of performance for recertification or for hospital privileging. The possibility of regional centers or of establishing some type of test center at a given hospital (with advancement in the technology) suggests that this may be a feasible approach to quality evaluation. Nevertheless, the studies which determine that performance on the CBX are representative of actual practice must be extended. The validity issue is always the most challenging part of developing any type of evaluation instrument.

## Simulated/Standardized Patients

The past decade has seen the development of evaluation using simulated/standardized patients. Simulated patients may be trained to respond to a history in a fashion characteristic of certain disorders or may be used for physical examination. Standardized patients may also be trained to make evaluations of the physician who is examining them, thus lending an additional type of evaluative data. Simulated patients have been used for both teaching and physician skill evaluation. One could use simulated patients as part of an Objective Structured Clinical Examination (OSCE) which uses a series of stations. Each station covers a defined task. At each station, the examinee performs a focused clinical activity. It may be to take a brief history from a simulated patient, perform a focused physical examination on a simulated patient, interpret laboratory findings, or to provide health maintenance education to a simulated patient. At each station, examinee performance is observed and graded on check-lists by examiners recruited and trained for this task. A typical 20 station exam could be done in two hours. The OSCE has been used in Scotland, Canada, and the USA. Canada has used a variant of the OSCE with Chart Stimulated Recall (CSR) for practitioners. To date, the OSCE has been used mostly for medical students and CSR for practitioners; a recent pilot study by the ECFMG with foreign medical graduates as well as recent LCME school graduates, showed evidence that a similar test of clinical skills could distinguish between the two groups. Standardized patients have also recently been used by Stillman and Swanson in a pilot study funded by the American Board of Internal Medicine. The Educational Commission for Foreign Medical Graduates (ECFMG) has recently completed a Test of Clinical Competence and the National Board of Medical Examiners (NBME) is working on one. Both use standardized (simulated) patients.

## Continuing Medical Education

On the assumption that Continuing Medical Education (CME) will update a physician's knowledge and keep him abreast of quality care, the past quarter century has seen the development of systems for accrediting CME and for recording it. Twenty-two states and some specialty societies have required CME for re-registration of licenses or maintenance of membership in the society. Of the ABMS member boards who are engaged in recertification, nine require CME as part of the process. It has been suggested that CME be required as part of the process of renewal of hospital credentials and privileges. Indeed CME is part of the tradition of medicine. Medical education is a life-long process which does not stop with the awarding of the MD degree or the specialty board certification. It is part of the value system of the medical profession and medical education attempts to instill the practice of life-long learning.

All of this effort to systematize CME would be received more comfortably if there were firm evidence that CME does influence practice and maintains high quality clinical activity. The evidence is not widespread, and is more convincing for cognitive knowledge than clinical skills. Nevertheless a group of studies suggesting that CME can influence practice is reviewed by Bashook in another chapter of this book. It is likely to be more convincing for procedural skills than in other areas, but nevertheless does show encouragement. Assuring that this trend continues, some form of assessment could be the process of satisfying CME requirements.

## Utilization Review

The present system of hospital reimbursement is moving toward prospective payment. This has already been accomplished for Medicare and Medicaid by adopting a system of Diagnosis Related Groups (DRG) for payment. Instead of reimbursement for actual cost of whatever is considered medically necessary, the hospital is reimbursed a standard amount for the given condition (the DRG). Hospitals which give treatment costing more than the allowed reimbursement under DRG must absorb the loss. This system has stimulated hospitals to develop sophisticated computerized accounting systems which keep records on each class and the costs associated with that case. The records are necessary for reimbursement, but are also being used to keep track of each DRG (there are 476 of them) and profile of each physician. Economic factors are beginning to be used in review of privileges and maintenance of medical staff membership. A hospital argues that it cannot have its economic existence jeopardized by permitting all members of the medical staff to order any procedure or keep the patient in the hospital beyond the allowable number of days.

This technology now permits the hospital to maintain records on utilization of hospital days and of tests or procedures. It can be done by physician and by DRG. Physicians can be compared to other physicians on the medical staff and the outlier physicians can be easily identified.

This approach to evaluation on the basis of utilization of the hospital and/or its services as a measure of quality is often challenged by physicians who were educated with the view that whatever the patient needs for good care should be provided. The medical staff will resist the use of such criteria for evaluation of medical competence, but there is no doubt that hospitals will press for the use of such data. Today's focus on cost/effectiveness begins to look more at cost than effectiveness in the view of some, but effectiveness will not be ignored.

## Patient Behavior

Another approach to the evaluation of the physician is a type of outcome study. Such an approach looks at patient satisfaction with medical care. Additionally, one can examine the patient's compliance behavior in following the advice of the doctor. As an approach towards evaluation, these methods make the assumption that if the doctor is successful (competent) it will show in the patient's behavior. One can raise certain philosophical objections to such an assumption because the combination of a highly competent physician and a troubled or difficult patient may not show the outcome of satisfaction or compliance. Is it fair to ascribe that to the physician or have it reflect on his competence?

Nevertheless, as one aspect of evaluation, it is useful to look at this type of outcome data. In using it however, it should be realized that the outcome as so measured is a response to the total system of health care, the hospital, the personality of the patient, and the family or other persons in the patient's environment. All of these factors influence the outcomes noted above.

## Cognitive Testing

Cognitive testing is commonly used in the evaluation of physician qualifications. From the earliest phase of his education, the physician is given tests of knowledge, mostly in the form of multiple choice questions (MCQ's). Such examinations are useful in measuring the base of knowledge and may be constructed to estimate clinical judgment. Variations of cognitive testing such as the Patient Management Problem (PMP) have been developed and used to be thought to approach the clinical process but have been abandoned by some testing agencies. MCQ's are used by licensing boards and certifying bodies. They are commonly used as part of the recertification process though other factors are also used.

Schmidt and Norman find that the experienced practitioner uses prototypical and actual patients, a different cognitive system than that used by medical students who rely on memory of lists of symptoms. The practitioner's cognitive processes uses "illness scripts" and "instance scripts" If tests can be constructed which use the cognitive processes of practitioners, this may be more useful than the type of factual recall on which MCQ's are based.

The difficulty in constructing valid MCQ's should not be underestimated. Organizations such as specialty boards and licensing boards use testing services which are very experienced in test construction and psychometric analysis. The National Board of Medical Examiners is probably the best known of such agencies in the medical world. It uses panels of nationally known experts for the development of test materials and has a very competent staff to develop, produce and administer tests, and to score and analyze the results. Security is no small concern in the use of such tests and requires sophisticated systems. It is not likely that any given hospital could duplicate the facilities of such testing services.

Whether difficult or not, cognitive tests have real limitations. They measure a base of knowledge. Though knowledge is necessary as a part of competence, it is not the totality of competence. Knowledge may not correlate with clinical skill. Though one cannot conceive of a skilled clinician who is not knowledgeable, it is also possible to master a knowledge base without mastering the clinical skills necessary to apply it. It is generally known that candidates for medical specialty boards may do well on the knowledge exams by virtue of hard study, but not be able to demonstrate good clinical judgment or the effective application of that knowledge.

The hospital which depends on cognitive tests for review of competence will also find considerable resistance on the part of the medical staff. Physicians, like many others, feel that tests represent a hurdle which must be mastered at a point in time. Passing a test means passing a required course. Passing another test may lead to certification or licensure. But few physicians would volunteer for repeated testing of knowledge, especially when they feel that the test is not necessarily related to their everyday practice. The resistance to recertification has often been based on objection to taking another exam which may have little to do with current practice.


### Decision Analysis

Decision analysis is an evaluation of the *process* of medical care. In a sense, it is very much like the medical record review. Although there is controversy about whether process or outcome data are most useful, the argument is specious. Both are needed, but outcome studies are not easy to do. They require follow-up (patients are not easy to follow) and measures which are not always simple. The proponents of process studies argue that the data should be available in the treatment setting. One study suggests that process studies may be more desirable when outcomes from poor care are infrequent, or when they are determined by factors outside of medical care, when patients have complex multi-system disease, or when numbers of cases are too small to draw conclusions. Process studies require criteria which are specific and can be measured. The criteria must provide for differences in patients with the same disorder. They should provide for the longitudinal aspects of disease—a special requirement for chronic disorders. The process assessment must reflect the medical decision-making process. For example, the criteria list should require that there be interpretation and follow-up of test results if a test is required. Another problem with process studies has to do with the inadequacy of medical records in doing evaluations. One of the problems with medical records for process studies is that physicians rarely record the complete data base and omit negative findings.

This approach to the evaluation of performance is described for completeness, but it will readily be apparent that sophisticated decision analysis or process studies are not feasible for every hospital. These are more likely to be used in research studies and in the evaluation of the outcome of educational programs than everyday practice in a community hospital.


**Technical Skill Assessment**

Technical skills or psychomotor skill assessment is another aspect of performance. It is more likely associated with certain specialties than others and the surgical specialists are the most obvious. Engineers in industry have developed skill assessment for certain types of positions. Since the motor skills required of a physician have been only one part of practice, less work of this type has been done in medicine than in industry. However, there are examples which are reasonably common. Some involve the use of models for teaching medical students and residents. The same models may be used for motor skill assessment. A common example is the rususcianne model which is used to teach cardio-pulmonary resuscitation. Since many hospitals require that cardio-pulmonary resuscitation (CPR) skills be maintained by taking a review course annually, there is an opportunity for evaluation of this particular performance skill. For the most part, psychomotor skill evaluation has been done informally by the observation of peers and department chairmen. Since systematic evaluation methods are not always easy or available, a challenge for the future may be to find skill assessment techniques more adaptable to the community hospital.

## Interpersonal Skill Assessment

Interpersonal skills are far more difficult to assess than psychomotor skills. The National Board of Medical Examiners (NBME) spent several years on a study which reviewed the methods available. Though there are techniques including the use of the Interaction Analysis System, they are research instruments. The check lists used by other evaluators require rater training to assure inter-rater reliability. Validity studies are even more challenging. One of the specialty boards (the American Board of Psychiatry & Neurology) still uses a live patient interview as part of the certifying exam and retains this logistically difficult feature because of the importance of evaluating inter-personal skills—especially in psychiatry. Though this skill assessment is described for the sake of completeness, it is not readily done in the community hospital.

## Malpractice Claims or Risk Management

Though a grim reminder of the professional liability problems which medicine faces today, a malpractice claim assessment is another approach to performance assessment. However, it is complex and must be evaluated carefully. Malpractice claims are not necessarily a reflection of actual malpractice. Only a very small proportion of the claims are determined to be the fault of the doctor and a judgment entered. Even when that happens, it does not always reflect poor practice. It is not unusual for a jury member to phone the physician against whom a judgment was entered and say "I didn't think you were wrong doctors, but the patient needed the money." Furthermore, when a malpractice claim does arise from poor performance, it may reflect the far side of a continuum of performance ranging from acceptable to unacceptable. There should be more sensitive measures of performance and the medical staff should not have to depend on dissatisfied patients or lawyers to measure medical competence.

Certain indicators of inadequate performance are often the first recognized signals of trouble. As Breaden suggests, "Every resource available to a board or hospital should be used to identify the possibly unqualified or unfit physicians". Complaints are red flags and should draw the attention of Credential Committees and Department Chairpersons. In today's world, reports of the peer review processes of hospitals and other health care entities must be submitted to the National Practitioner Data Bank when there are actions which restrict hospital privileges, altered membership in the Medical Staff, malpractice settlements or awards, negative licensure actions or a change in professional society membership. While such problems in performance are late indicators, it is hoped that performance assessment as described in this chapter may identify problems before they result in such reportable outcomes.

## Outcome of Treatment

It has been suggested that outcome measures, although complicated and difficult to do, are the ideal measure of physician competence. After all, the outcome is the end result of a process. Outcome may be reflected in changes in subjective measures such as biochemical tests, or in measurable patient function such as changes in muscle strength or heart rhythm on the Electrocardiogram (EKG) or in X-Ray changes. Outcome may be measured by patient satisfaction, although that is not always associated with changes in function. Outcomes may be measured by utilization of health care services after treatment.

If competence is to be assessed by outcome, the criteria must be carefully developed. The standard against which a particular physician is to be measured should be a realistic one, and the outcome of a group of highly qualified subspecialists should not be the standard against which a group of generalists primary care physicians should be measured. The cohort of patients whose results are to be measured should be those similar to those who constitute the group which was the basis for the standard. Standards should preferably be national ones, but there truly are regional variations in the standard of practice. How to find the correct standard, and how a given hospital can institute an assessment of outcome for its own medical staff are problems which have not yet been solved, but the field of evaluation will continue to look for valid, reliable and feasible outcome measures.

## Issues

Certain issues about specialization and subspecialization must be considered as we move into a new era of health care. We have all been concerned about proliferation of new subspecialties and fragmentation of health care, but that is not going to stop. It is a consequence of the advancement of medical science and no one wants to stop that. Progress in medical science means reduction of suffering and conquest of disease. The consequence of progress has generally been increasing specialization because it requires special skill and attention to master new knowledge and new technology. One of the reasons for limiting practice when new technologies develop is that the physician must perform a given procedure or treat certain disorders frequently in order to develop and maintain skill. However, we must not weaken the bedrock and foundations of identification with the general specialty. This is not a simple problem. If one asks a general internist who is also subspecialized in cardiovascular disease what he is, the response will be, "I am a cardiologist". A psychiatrist who subspecializes in the treatment of children will give the answer, "I am a child psychiatrist". Physicians are inclined to identify with their subspecialty as the true identity and the group name which most specifically identifies them. To be part of the larger groups of general internal medicine or general psychiatry is not deemed so valuable as the identity of the smaller, more exclusive group. Subspecialty identification may contribute to the fragmentation which we seek to avoid. In dealing with this fragmentation, the ABMS must be a leader. We cannot be viewed as an anchor holding up progress. It is the responsibility of ABMS to authorize new forms of certification, but in doing so the review of appropriateness must be cautious. The answers found to date must not be considered "final" nor can new types of certification be considered the only solution. Continuing review of existing as well as new forms of certification must be carried on.

Data about medical manpower is essential. No single data base provides the answers about actual practice. We lack readily retrievable data about students in fellowships training. Tracking of physicians through medical school, residency, certification, practice and continuing medical education could be accomplished by interdigitating certain existing data bases, but it is only beginning. This does not suggest that planning should control manpower or training positions. The US has had its Graduate Medical Education National Advisory Committee (GMENAC) report, but our experience with government is that it predicts wide swings with resultant inefficiency. During the early 1960s, the US government predicted major shortages and called for doubling the size of MD graduating classes and instituted immigration preference to attract foreign physicians. Twenty years later, we hear of a significant oversupply of physicians and propose cutbacks. The ABMS and other voluntary agencies should not assume responsibility for manpower controls (or support government controls), but should make available valid data on medical specialists. The ABMS has developed an automated data base for biographic data on certified specialists and subspecialists. Data bases should also seek valid information about actual practice in more detail than is now available. Data bases such as those established by the AAMC, NRMP, AMA, ABMS and AHA should seek adequate intercommunication to combine the power of tracking medical careers.

In the US, corporatization of medical care, a shift to competition instead of regulation, the move away from solo practice on a fee-for-service basis, the entry of non-medical practitioners into medical practice, and the "physician glut" have created revolutionary changes in less than five years. These changes have affected and will create change in specialty practice and therefore the education, certification and evaluation of all specialists.

Recertification is a consequence of the rapid rate of change in medical science and the interaction between privileging and certification will pressure all specialties to be more active in this area.

Jurisdictional concerns and "turf" disputes will continue and probably be intensified in this period of competition and concerns about a physician surplus. It is also a consequence of changes in practice and therefore, changes in education. Both call for appropriate credentials. The ABMS is presently concerned with credentials in horizontal skills—fields of practice common to more than one primary specialty. This motivated the addition of the credential called "Added Qualifications." Whether this will diminish the intensity of jurisdictional disputes remains to be seen. Other ways of dealing with "turf" must be found. Turf issues must be differentiated from quality issues.

The field of specialization and special competence, and its evaluation, are of deep concern to those who take the responsibility for determining hospital privileges. To know the issues and problems is the first step toward their solution.

## References


Barrows, HS. *Newer Approaches to the Assessment of Clinical Performance.* Springfield, Ill: Southern Illinois University Press, 1985.

Borgiel, AEM, Williams, JI, Anderson, GM et al. Assessing the quality of care in family physicians' practices. *Can Fam Phys.* 1985, 31:853-862.

Breaden, DG. Markers and indicators of physician performance and fitness: an overview. *Fed Bull.* 1988, 75:67-73.

Carline, JD, Wenrich, M, Ramsey, PG. Characteristics of ratings of physician competence by professional associates. *Eval Health Prof.* 1989, 12:409-423.

Clyman, SG, Orr, NA. Status report on the NBME's computer-based testing. *Acad Med.* 1990, 65:235-241.

Conn, HL, Cody, RP. Results of the second clinical skills assessment examination of the ECFMG. *Acad Med.* 1989, 64:448-453.

Harden, RM, Gleeson, FA. Assessment of clinical competence using an objective structured clinical examination (OSCE). *Med Educ* 1979, 113:41-54.

Meyer, TC. The role of remedial CME. *Fed Bull.* 1990, 77:182-187.

Norman, GR. Reliability and construct validity of some cognitive measures of clinical reasoning. *Teach Learn Med.* 1989, 1:194-199.

*Physician Review Program (PREP).* Hamilton, Ontario: College of Physicians and Surgeons of Ontario, 1988.

Schmidt, HG, Norman, GR, Boshuizen, HPA. A cognitive perspective on medical expertise: theory and implications. *Acad Med.* 1990, 65:611-621.

Stillman, PL, Regan, MB, Swanson, DB, et al. An assessment of the clinical skills of fourth-year students at four New England medical schools. *Acad Med.* 1990, 65:320-326.

# Continuing Medical Education and Hospital Privileges

Philip G. Bashook, Ed.D.

Continuing medical education (CME) is a complex, substantial and misunderstood enterprise. Understanding the linkages between CME and hospital privileges requires a clarification of what is know about CME and how physicians use CME to alter their patient care practices. Also, important to consider in linking CME and hospital privileges are distinctions between initial applications for privileges, renewal of privileges, and requests to expand privileges. This chapter will address these points beginning with a description of CME based upon the research literature, followed by a discussion of potential linkages between CME participation and initial privileges, CME participation and renewal of privileges, and ending with recent developments in linking CME and expanded hospital privileges.

Deeply ingrained in medical practice is the expectation that physicians will want to continue learning, stay current with new medical developments, and use that knowledge in the care of patients (Manning and DeBakey, 1987). But, physicians attend continuing medical education programs not only to keep current; they also attend programs to see and speak with their colleagues and compare the veracity of their current patient care practices against reasonable alternatives being discussed in the programs and informally.

A second historical thread connects continuing medical education with expectations of clinical expertise through the recognition of a physician's clinical and teaching activities. As far back as the turn of the century and the famous report on the evaluation of American and Canadian medical schools by Abraham Flexner, hospital privileges have been offered to the clinician who brings "clinical facilities" (patients) to the hospital. Admitting many patients commands respect and influence (Flexner, 1910, page 111). Physicians who attract patients to themselves and maintain a large hospital practice are assumed to have the appropriate clinical expertise. Combining these historical threads it is reasonable to postulate that CME participation can serve as one measure, combined with other evidence of clinical expertise, to determine hospital privileges. However, continuing medical education is a complex and misunderstood enterprise. Many organizations and institutions sponsor pre-planned CME programs. Among the CME sponsors are medical schools, hospitals, specialty societies, health care agencies, and entrepenuers. Most, if not all, of these CME programs comply with accepted educational standards for teaching practitioners. For the individual physician CME occurs not only when they attend CME programs or "sit-in" on hospital conferences.

CME also occurs for most physicians in the clinical setting (office, clinic and at the bedside) during their daily interaction with colleagues (physicians and other health professionals) and patients. Moreover, effective CME is directly tied to an individual physician's actions in the care of patients.

## Realities of Continuing Medical Education

In the practice of American medicine today continuing medical education (CME) has become an integral part of almost every physician's practice. Physician specialists with hospital privileges participate in continuing medical education (CME) conferences as an essential part of their weekly routine. CME conferences sponsored by large hospitals usually last one hour, resemble a grand rounds lecture series or a case review small discussion group, and offer the physician participants a chance to listen to invited and peer experts discuss interesting cases and topics.

In teaching hospitals the house staff and faculty frequently organize and lead these conferences. Outside the hospital there are numerous CME conferences, courses, and retreat-type workshops that physicians can select to attend. Sponsors for these CME programs include medical schools, teaching hospitals, specialty societies, medical equipment suppliers, pharmaceutical companies, and entrepreneurs.

According to the Accreditation Council for Continuing Medical Education (ACCME), in 1991 there were 489 separate national organizations accredited to sponsor national or regional CME programs in the United

States. Another 1,826 organizations are accredited by local medical societies as sponsors of CME programs targeted only to local physicians (personal communication, 1991). Accredited CME sponsors are required to use appropriate educational planning methods and certify the number of CME credit hours a physician participant may claim from participating in one of the sponsor's CME programs.

CME credit hours have become the currency for proof of CME attendance in many arenas. Documented physician participation has been used for a number of years as part of the credentials process for licensure and membership in medical societies. For example, in 1991 there are 22 states that required proof of CME attendance for license renewal. Ten state medical societies had a CME attendance requirement for continued membership (Wentz et al, 1991). In addition to other more direct assessments of clinical expertise, some hospitals use CME participation as part of the evidence gathered in deciding upon continued hospital privileges.

An expanded conception of CME beyond just courses and conferences would consider the realities of CME involving informal self-directed educational activities physicians undertake to gather medical information. Some physicians in searching for information before considering participating in CME programs begin by consulting their personal library or speaking with colleagues (a specialist in their informal communication network, a physician in their informal communication network, or their partner or a physician they share office space with). Many review recent medical journals or as the hospital and medical school librarian for assistance. In each situation CME is a personal self-directed activity undertaken by a physician with a definite purpose in mind: to gather new or relevant information that may be of benefit in a patient care situation.

Complicating an appreciation of the CME enterprise are the confusing data from studies on the impact of CME on physicians' continuing clinical expertise. Research on the impact of CME programs (only courses and conferences) suggest these formal pre-planned programs have mixed success in demonstrating changes in physicians' behavior (Lloyd and Abrahamson, 1979; Davis et al, 1984; Haynes et al, 1984). These research reviews consider only experiments in which pre-planned CME programs were the CME interventions. The mixed messages from the research on the effectiveness of CME in changing physician behavior are quite understandable when one realizes the studies do not include as the CME interventions the very important factors, known from research on physician behavior change, that can influence use of CME as a source for learning. Some of these factors are: readiness of physicians to change their practice when they participate in CME courses (Geertsma et al, 1982; Lockyer et al, 1985), the social interactions among physicians resulting in informal learning (Friedson, 1970; Stross and Harlan, 1979) and colleague to colleague communications (Coleman et al, 1966; Rogers and Shoemaker, 1971; Maxwell et al, 1984, Hiss et al, 1979). What is surprising about the findings from the research on CME impact has been the evidence demonstrating the effectiveness of educationally sound CME programs to influence physician behavior.

A more careful analysis of how physicians use CME suggests that physicians change behavior in small increments (Davis, 1986). Furthermore, CME is part of a social context in which physicians use the opportunity of attending CME programs to meet other physicians, learn about their way of practicing medicine and compare their current expertise to their colleagues. Physicians employ a variety of information sources when they consider making changes in their practices (Coleman et al, 1966; Bashook, 1986; Richards, 1986b; Maxwell et al, 1984) and CME programs represent only one of many sources (Manning and Denson, 1979, 1980; Richards, 1986a; Cevero, 1981).

Obviously, CME is more than formal courses and conferences. It is continuing learning by physicians as self-directed adult learners (Richards, 1986a; Knox, 1980) Courses and programs are some of the many information sources and opportunities physicians use to stay current. The American Medical Association (AMA) has acknowledged the importance of self-directed learning by revising the AMA's Physician's Recognition Award (PRA) categories to encourage "self-directed learning" (Wentz et al, 1991).

Physicians can subscribe to a variety of CME programs that provide them self-study activities. These CME self-study programs are available from many sources in a variety of formats. Commonly available formats are CME videotape programs, self-assessment examinations, computer based CME programs, and CME programs using journal subscriptions with short quizzes.

Another self-study strategy to assist physicians helps them plan assess their personal learning needs, develop an educational needs prescription and recommend specific and appropriate CME interventions (Sivertson et al, 1973; Manning et al, 1980; Guillon et al, 1983; Stein, 1973; Bowler, for College of Physicians of Philadelphia, 1976, 1977; The Royal College of Physicians and Surgeons of Canada, 1991). Most of these CME plans include an educational needs assessment process to help physicians define the scope, range and educational challenges in their practice. Frequently, the needs assessment process uses record audits, patient logs, or sampling the physician's office and hospital activities to generate a practice profile.

Building upon the practice profile the physician completes a self-assessment test of knowledge and/or skills to evaluate clinical knowledge and practice strengths and deficiencies. The identified educational needs from the self-assessment test lead to recommended educational prescriptions of CME activities that physicians may initiate. The educational interventions recommended in CME prescriptions have included informal small discussion groups, attending CME conferences and courses, participation as a extern with a subspecialist colleague, and self-study programs including a combination of reading and the other activities. One study on the effectiveness of these CME plans for self-directed learning was designed for internists and family physicians (Professional Competence Assurance Program, PROCAP, Gullion et al, 1983). In addition to designing the CME plans the investigators assessed the impact of a CME intervention involving small discussion groups in a conference call format. Gullion and colleagues assessed ambulatory practices of 48 private practitioners to assess the office care of 953 hypertensive patients. A comparison group of physicians was not used in the study, but practice and outcome variables were assessed against consensus criteria developed by experts. They found through office record audits by medical record technicians the CME intervention resulted in significant improvement as compared to defined criteria in patient workups, prescribing behavior and patient education. One year after the CME intervention they also found a significant improvement in the number of patients with diastolic blood pressure at 90 mm HG or less; one of the commonly accepted standards for assessing success of hypertensive treatment.

Another form of self-directed learning as CME is reading medical literature. Physicians read extensively. An aphorism by William Osler expresses succinctly the general sentiment concerning physicians learning from reading, "to study the phenomena of disease without books is to sail an uncharted sea, while to study books without patients is not to go to sea at all" (Osler, 1904, page 210). A number of studies on physician reading habits report most physicians read medical literature on average 5 hours per week (Richards, 1986a). Nearly every physician adds to their personal medical library by subscribing to medical journals, ordering books and receiving free literature, books and magazines from various sources or as part of their specialty society membership (Manning and DeBakey, 1987). The American Medical Association's Physician's Recognitions Award (PRA) assumes that physicians are expected to read medical literature at least two hours per week and do not need the PRA as an incentive (Wentz et al, 1991).

Medical practice and CME occur in a social context (Friedson, 1970). Physicians rely on their colleagues for suggestions when contemplating clinical decisions and obtain information informally through "hallway consultations." They also learn from consultants when they refer a patient. In every medical community in which physician communication has been studied at least one local physician (not always a specialist) is the preferred contact by other physicians to learn more about new medical developments being considered for adoption into their practice (Hiss et al, 1978; Maxwell et al, 1984). These "educational influential physicians" (Hiss et al, 1978) and the informal communication networks that physicians develop among their colleagues (Stross and Harlan, 1979, 1981; Maxwell et al, 1984) serve along with other information sources as part of the CME enterprise. Physicians use the information to learn new ideas, test their knowledge and thoughts against those of their colleagues, and assess changes in their practice or plans for managing specific patients. Stross and colleagues at the University of Michigan demonstrated the effectiveness of "educational influential physicians" as an CME intervention to change the behavior of primary care physicians (Hiss et al, 1978; Stross et al, 1983; Stross and Bole, 1979, 1985).

## Linkage Between CME and Hospital Privileges

A physician's reputation as a clinician plays an important role in obtaining hospital privileges. From the physician's point of view hospital privileges are essential to practice good medicine. Unfortunately, in some hospital settings local pressures may overshadow clinical expertise to obtain hospital privileges. "Staff appointments made for personal or political reasons may of course be revoked for reasons that are no better" (Flexner, 1910, page 112). And, "the uncertainty of any one [hospital] connection constitutes a good reason for getting hold of as many as possible" (Flexner, 1910, page 112). For these reasons many physicians retain admitting and treatment privileges at two or three hospitals.

For many physicians their involvement in a hospital is limited to admitting a few patients and they development minimal collegial relationships with the other doctors on the hospital staff (Maxwell et al, 1984). Keeping in mind the social role of hospital CME programs and the community sense of local medical staffs organized around most hospitals (Hiss et al, 1978), the limited participation of some physicians in a hospital's CME programs or other medical staff activities creates problems in recredentialing these physicians. Some hospitals may only see these itinerant physicians when they make rounds on the few patients they admit to the hospital, consequently it can be difficult to assess the physician's clinical expertise other than by rumor or when there has been a serious adverse circumstance.

In these situations the physician's participation in CME at other hospitals and from other CME sponsors and their reputation in caring for patients must be considered.

There are three distinct situations to consider for hospital privileges: initial privileges, continuing privileges, and expanded privileges in order to perform additional medical or surgical procedures.

## Initial Medical Staff Privileges

Physicians may apply for initial hospital staff privileges at various stages in their medical career. Physicians just starting a practice provide the expected credentials based upon training and other requirements such as: medical school degree, unrestricted license, certificate of completion of residency training, specialty expertise and specialty certification. Experience and general competence are assessed through reports of other physicians or other hospitals. Most committees are looking for the good clinician who will attract patients to the hospital, fit into the current structure of hospital practice, fill needed expertise in the scope of hospital patient care services and in term attract additional patients to the hospital. For medical specialties where expertise in performing procedures is not essential, CME participation usually does not contribute to decision for initial hospital privileges. For the surgical specialties or medical specialties in which performing procedures is essential (e.g. Cardiology, pulmonary medicine, gastroenterology, etc.) evidence of current clinical expertise through participation in CME programs may be significant.

Physicians who have been in practice for a number of years and completed residency training or fellowship training years ago frequently are asked when applying for initial hospital privileges to demonstrate their expertise in performing procedures before being offered initial hospital privileges that include the procedures. These physicians may be required to document participation in CME programs that are designed to train them in the procedures. Documented CME participation refers to evidence of attendance at courses and conferences in which physicians receive Category 1 CME credit. In addition, some hospital committees will require the physicians to be supervised for a short time or while treating a number of cases when they perform the procedure.

Another situation in which documented CME participation becomes important in judging the physician's clinical expertise is when the physician does not have any demonstrated CME participation. All physicians are expected to keep current and continuously learn through CME. When there is a conspicuous absence of CME participation on the part of a medical colleague, the members of the medical staff become concerned and may question other aspects of a physician's credentials.

At the other extreme experienced clinicians often serve as faculty members for CME programs. The "Oslerian physician" frequently comes to mind in discussions about these "good clinicians" and teachers. These doctors are expected to be dedicated healers of the sick, scholars, and teachers (Osler, 1904, pages 131-145). It is very common for excellent clinicians to be invited to teach their colleagues as faculty members in CME programs.

Teaching colleagues enhances the reputation of both the clinician and the hospital, and the clinician demonstrates to colleagues a fundamental knowledge of the topic being taught. Through discussions of real cases seen by the physician and the care provided the clinician demonstrates his/her depth of clinical acumen. In CME programs that entail demonstrations of clinical procedures, the faculty member displays not only clinical acumen about the topic and the value and pitfalls of the procedure, but expertise in actually performing the procedure. Physician members of the hospital credentials committees who have witnessed the candidate's teaching may consider the application in light of the candidate's role in CME teaching.

## Renewal of Staff Privileges

When the good clinician and teacher ("Oslerian physician") applies for renewal of staff privileges this physician has credentials in the form of demonstrated expertise through teaching other medical staff. CME participation for these expert physicians has a different meaning. They document their expertise by reporting their role as faculty members in CME programs.

For most other physicians CME plays a less prominent role for renewal of hospital privileges. Most hospitals expect physicians to demonstrate acceptable performance with hospitalized care of patients, some evidence of clinical expertise, and little or no evidence of any challenges to their clinical competence.

A medical staff credentials committee might consider the following evidence of clinical expertise. The sequence begins with the most direct evidence for assessment of performance and moves to more inferential evidence.

1. Demonstrated expertise as documented by medical colleagues in the same in hospital based upon peer review of candidates' actual patient care (Hospital Quality Assurance Program, medical

record audit, risk management programs, tissue committee reports, etc.).

2. Reports from respected colleagues who have seen the physician's performance in other settings (peer review at other hospitals).
3. Certificates of participation in CME programs documenting evaluation of candidates meeting the program objectives in performing specific procedures, patient diagnostic assessments or treatment planning.
4. Reports from respected physician colleagues who have interacted with the physician outside the hospital but without evidence of witnessing actual patient care performance.
5. Documented attendance at CME programs.
6. Candidate self-report of expertise.

In considering renewal of hospital privileges most hospital credentials committees do not use CME participation as a factor unless the physician has adverse reports about his/her patient care practices. A common scenario involves looking at evidence from hospital peer review data, reports from colleagues within and outside the hospital and any adverse reports about the physician. However, participation in CME programs may be helpful when considering indirect evidence of keeping current.

CME participation is voluntary with most physicians participating in a variety of courses and conferences that interest them. Physicians are free to select any topic or course format they wish. Sivertson and colleagues (1973) found most physicians selected courses and conferences that reinforced their strengths, and rarely filled in gaps or strengthened their weaker areas of expertise. Using only a transcript of attendance records may not provide the best data for determining a physician's current expertise. Also, CME transcripts are maintained primarily to support relicensure applications and medical society memberships. As a self-directed learner, long-term repeated participation in CME programs should be an indication of a physician's commitment to keep current and intellectually active, but it is not proof of clinical expertise.

## Expanded Medical Staff Privileges

The challenges to credentials committees when considering expanded privileges based upon CME participation include: determining what evidence from participation in CME programs suffices to establish a physician's competence in performing the requested procedures; what documentation is needed to support the request; how to establish the veracity of the documentation; how to weigh the factors involved in situations when evidence is sparse or documentation is difficult or impossible to obtain.

Typical evidence available from CME courses as proof of attendance and potential expertise are: certification of participation or completion of the CME program, attendance records and certificates, evidence of passing a knowledge test, and evidence of participation in the few courses with workshop sessions to learn specific procedures with hands-on experience. All Category 1 designated CME programs offer certifications of participation and will report, on request, a description of the program including workshops and special hands-on experiences offered. There is no data on which CME programs offer evidence of tests completed or evaluations of participants' performance in completing hands-on practice sessions to learn clinical procedures. However, such data would be valuable to hospital credentials committees in assessing the benefit of CME participation these programs for purposes of expanded privileges.

The American Medical Association and the American Hospital Association are developing a mechanism for obtaining documented CME participation to learn new procedures as evidence in support of expanded hospital privileges. In 1989 the AMA Council on Medical Education adopted a resolution urging accredited CME sponsors to issue to physicians participating in CME documentation that could be used in support of a physician's application for expanded hospital privileges (American Medical Association, 1989). The resolution has been followed by a number of meetings among the relevant organizations interested in hospital privileges and CME to develop procedures and documentation forms that could serve the intended purpose. Starting in August 1991 the AHA and AMA have circulated draft versions of the "CME Performance Evaluation Document (CPED)" (American Hospital Association, 1991; see attachment) The CPED provides CME sponsors and the physician applicant a uniform document to record information about the designated course or conference and the physician's performance relative to the course objectives. If adopted by the CME community the CPED should provide further documentation that would be helpful to hospital credentials committees when they must consider expanded privileges.


**Conclusions**

Due to the nature of the credentials process in most hospitals physicians are faced with demonstrating their clinical expertise to renew privileges nearly every year. As competition increases among hospitals and among doctors some physicians are expanding the number of hospitals they use.

In turn they are required to initiate applications and renewal privileges more frequently. Continuing medical education participation becomes another source of evidence used by hospital credentials committees to determine a physician's clinical expertise. Peer review of patient care provides the best evidence for assessing clinical expertise needed for decisions about hospital credentials. CME participation becomes more valuable when considering expanded privileges or special privileges to perform procedures.

It should be kept in mind that CME participation in the context of privileges generally means formal pre-planned programs, not the major segment of CME activity physicians usually undertake in the form of self-directed learning. Also, based upon research on CME and how CME involvement benefits physicians in changing behavior suggests that CME is more than just formal courses and conferences. Physicians as self-directed learners are adult life-long learners. In the broader context of changing behavior CME is one of many information sources and social activities physician's engage in when they consider changing their patient care practices.

Participation in CME programs provides some of the evidence of sustained interest and continued involvement in lifelong learning. CME participation does not provide evidence of continuing clinical expertise without other proof of demonstrated competence. In place of direct evidence of successful performance or peer review of actual practice, most CME programs offer, at best, indirect evidence of potential competence through reports of attendance and descriptions of course content.

If the CME course director has assessed a participant's performance, the candidate achieves the course standards, and the CME director so certifies, then documented participation in the CME program might serve as evidence of clinical expertise in performing the course's defined objectives. This evidence from CME participation may be helpful combined with other data in determining expanded hospital privileges. The American Hospital Association and the American Medical Association are developing a mechanism and appropriate forms to support this process.

### References

1. American Hospital Association: Report by Committee on Privileging for New Procedures. Chicago, Illinois: American Hospital Association, August 27, 1991, 1991. Includes forms and commentary.
2. American Medical Association: Statement of the AMA Council on Medical Education Regarding CME Intended for Expanded Hospital Privileges. Chicago, Illinois, 1989.

3. Bashook P: Future Directions in Continuing Education. *Diabetes Educator* 1986;12 (Special Issue):215-218.

4. Bertram D, Brooks-Bertram P: The evaluation of continuing education: a literature review. *Health Education Monographs* 1977;5:330-362.

5. Bowler FL, Brading PL, Burg FD, Finestone AJ: A practice-related educational program. *Journal of American Medical Association* 1977;237:1346-1349.

6. Bowler FL: Maintaining physician competence through practice related individualized continuing education. Fifth Biennial Conference on Continuing Medical Education for State Medical Associations and Specialty Societies. Chicago, Illinois: American Medical Association, October 5-7, 1976.

7. Cervero RR: Factor analysis study of physician's reasons for participating in continuing education. *Journal of Medical Education* 1981;56:29-34.

8. Coleman J, Katz E, Menzel H: *Medical Innovation: A Diffusion Study.* New York: Bobbs-Merrill, 1966.

9. Curry L (ed.): *Learning style in continuing medical education.* Papers from Dalhousie Conference on Learning Style in Continuing Medical Education. Ottawa, Ontario, Canada: Canadian Medical Association, 1983.

10. Curry L, Putnam WR: Continuing medical education in maritime Canada: The methods physicians use, would prefer and find most effective. *Canadian Medical Association Journal* 1981;124:563-566.

11. Davis D: Evaluating continuing medical education: common sense and science. *Canadian Medical Association Journal* 1986;134:485-486.

12. Davis DA, Haynes RB, Chambers L, Neufield V, McKibbon A, Tugwell P: The impact of CME: A methodological review of the continuing medical education literature. *Evaluation and the Health Professions* 1984;7:251-283.

13. Escovitz GH, Davis D: A Bi-national perspective on continuing medical education. *Academic Medicine* 1990;65:545-550.

14. Flexner A: *Medical Education in the United States and Canada,* Reprint Edition (1972); A report to the Carnegie Foundation for the Advancement of Teaching (Bulletin *4). New York: Arno Press, 1910.

15. Friedson E: *Professional Dominance: The Social Structure of Medical Care.* New York: Aldine Publishing Co., 1970.

16. Geertsma R, Parker R, Whitebourne S: How physicians view the process of change in their practice behavior. *Journal of Medical Education* 1982;57:752-768.

17. Guillon DS, Adamson E, Watts MS: The effect of an individualized

practice-based CME program on physician performance and patient outcomes. *Western Journal of Medicine* 1983;138:582-588.

18. Haynes R, Davis D, McKibbon A, Tugwell P: A critical appraisal of the efficacy of continuing medical education. *Journal of American Medical Association* 1984;251:61-64.

19. Hiss R, MacDonald R, Davis W: Identification of physician educational influentials (EI's) in small community hospitals, Proceedings of the Conference on Research in Medical Education of the Association of American Medical Colleges. Washington, DC, 1978.

20. Knox AB: "Teaching Adults Effectively," *New Directions for Continuing Education*, Volume 6. San Francisco: Jossey-Bass, 1980.

21. Lloyd JS, Abrahamson S: Effectiveness of continuing medical education. *Evaluation and the Health Professions* 1979;2:251-280.

22. Lockyer JM, Parboosingh JT, McDougall G, et al: How physicians integrate advances into clinical practice. *Mobius* 1985;5:5-12.

23. Manning PR, Denson TA: How internists learned about cimetidine. *Annals of Internal Medicine* 1980;92:690-692.

24. Manning PR, Lee PV, Denson TA, Gilman NJ: Determining educational needs in the physician's office. *Journal of American Medical Association* 1980;244:1112-1115.

25. Manning PR, Denson TA: How cardiologists learn about echocardiography: A reminder for medical educators and legislators. *Annals of Internal Medicine* 1979;91:469-471.

26. Manning P, DeBakey L: *Medicine: Preserving the Passion.* New York: Springer-Verlag, 1987.

27. Maxwell J, Bashook PG, Sandlow LJ: The role of communication networks in physicians' adoption of innovations, Proceedings of Conference on Research in Medical Education of the Association of American Medical Colleges. Washington, DC, October 27-November 1, 1984.

28. Osler W: Books and men, in *Aequanimitas.* Philadelphia: Blakiston, 1904, pp 207-215.

29. Osler W: Internal medicine as a vocation, in *Aequanimitas.* Philadelphia, Pennsylania: Blakiston, 1904, pp 131-145.

30. Osteen A: Continuing Medical Education. *Journal of American Medical Association* 1986;256:1601-1604.

31. Richards R: Physicians' self-directed learning: A new perspective for continuing medical education, I. Reading. *Mobius* 1986a;6(2):1-13.

32. Richards R: Physicians' self-directed learning: A new perspective for continuing medical education, II. Learning from colleagues. *Mobius* 1986b;6(3):1-7.

33. Rogers E, Shoemaker F: *Communications of Innovations.* New York: The Free Press, 1971.

34. Sivertson SE, Meyer TC, Hansen R, Schoenenberger A: Individual physician profile: Continuing education related to medical practice. *Journal of Medical Education* 1973;48:1006-1012.

35. Stein LS: *Your personal learning plan; A handbook for physicians.* Chicago, Illinois: Illinois State Medical Society, 1973, (Mimeographed).

36. Stross JK, Bole G: Continuing education in rheumatoid arthritis for the primary care physician. *Arthritis and Rheumatism* 1979;22:77-81.

37. Stross JK, Bole G: Evalution of an educational program for primary care practitioners on the management of osteoarthritis. *Arthritis and Rheumatism* 1985;28:108-111.

38. Stross JK, Hiss R, & Watts C: Continuing education in pulmonary disease for primary care physicians. *Annual Review of Respiratory Diseases* 1983;127:739-746.

39. Stross JK, Harlan WR: Dissemination of relevant information on hypertension. *Journal of American Medical Association* 1981;246:360-382.

40. Stross JK, Harlan WR: Dissemination of new medical information. *Journal of American Medical Association* 1979;246:2622-2644.

41. The Royal College of Physicians and Surgeons of Canada: *The maintenance of competence (MOCOMP) pilot program;* Parboosingh, John (Project Director). Calgary, Alberta Canada: The Royal College of Physicians and Surgeons of Canada, 1991.

42. Wentz DK, Osteen AM, Gannon MI: Continuing Medical Education: Refocusing Support and Direction. *Journal of American Medical Association* 1991;266:953-956.

**AHA/AMA**
## CME Learning Assessment Form (CLAF)

This page is to be filled out upon completion of this course.

**Physician Participant:**

Name   (Last)                         (First)                         (Middle)

Address   (Office or Home)

City                                              State            Zip Code

**Assessment of Learning Outcome:**

Did the physician participant demonstrate achievement of the course learning objectives listed under number 3 on this form?

**Passing Criteria for Achievement of Objectives Met**

Cognitive Assessment          ☐ Yes          ☐ No

Skills Assessment             ☐ Yes          ☐ No

**Explanatory Comments:**

_______________________________________________________________

_______________________________________________________________

_______________________________________________________________

_______________________________________________________________

**Course Director:**

Decisions regarding privileging are the responsibility of the hospital. Therefore, the information on this form attests only to the attendee's performance at this course.

Signature

Name   (please print)

Title

Date

I personally attended all sessions of this educational program and attest that the information in the certification of the
_________________________________________________________ course is accurate and complete.

Signature of physician attendee

Name   (please print)

Date

**AHA/AMA** CME Learning Assessment Form (CLAF)

The remainder of this form can be filled out by the sponsor and duplicated for all participants, unless the content and/or activities of the course change. If the course descriptive brochure contains identical information to the requirements defined in this form, the brochure may be referenced and submitted in lieu of completion of this form. If the information contained in the brochure is incomplete, it may be necessary for the form to be returned for completion.

**CME Sponsor:**

Name                           Telephone Number

Address                        FAX Number

City               State      Zip

Accredited by ACCME?           ☐ Yes    ☐ No

Accredited by a state medical society?    ☐ Yes    ☐ No      Which state? ___________

**Program:**
(Please attach program brochure listing time schedule and faculty.)

1. Course Title: _________________________________________________

    Dates of Course: ______________________________________________

    Location: _____________________________________________________

2. Educational requirements: (Required of participant to enroll in course.)

    _____________________________________________________________

    _____________________________________________________________

3. Learning Objectives: (Please be concise and precise.)

    A. Cognitive:

       1. _______________________________________________________

       2. _______________________________________________________

       3. _______________________________________________________

       4. _______________________________________________________

       5. _______________________________________________________

    B. Skills:

       1. _______________________________________________________

       2. _______________________________________________________

       3. _______________________________________________________

       4. _______________________________________________________

       5. _______________________________________________________

**Program, continued:**

4. Educational Methods.   (Please be precise.)

Time Involved (hours)

A. Lecture:          ☐ Live        ___________________

                     ☐ Video       ___________________

B. Observation
·  of technique:     ☐ Live        ___________________

                     ☐ Video       ___________________

C. Hands-on laboratory work with animals:   ☐ Yes     ☐ No

   Brief description: _________________________________________________

   ________________________________________________________________

Time Involved (hours)

D. Discussion groups:   ☐ Yes   ☐ No        ___________________

   Topics: _________________________________________________________

   ________________________________________________________________

E. Other:   (Please specify.)

   ________________________________________________________________

   ________________________________________________________________

5. Assessment Methodology: How were participants assessed relating to attainment of educational objectives? List according to the learning objectives specified in number 3 on this form.

   A. Cognitive:   (Define criteria for achievement of objectives.)

   Methods of Assessment: _____________________________________________

   ________________________________________________________________

   ________________________________________________________________

   ________________________________________________________________

   B. Skills:   (Define criteria for achievement of objectives.)

   Methods of Assessment: _____________________________________________

   ________________________________________________________________

   ________________________________________________________________

   ________________________________________________________________

6. Which procedure, if any, was the participant expected to learn?

   ________________________________________________________________

   ________________________________________________________________

# Legal Aspects of
# Clinical Privilege Delineation

Donna D. Fraiche, J.D.

## Foreword

When Dr. Langsley called to ask that a chapter that I had written "Legal Aspects of Clinical Privilege Delineation" be updated for a new edition of *Hospital Privileges and Specialty Medicine*, I knew there would be a plethora of necessary new discussion. That chapter completed in 1985 predated many revolutionary changes. For example, the Supreme Court decision in *Patrick v. Berget*, 487 U.S. 94, 108 S.Ct. 1658, 100 L.Ed. 2d 83 (1988), and the Health Care Quality Improvement Act, COBRA and OBRA (patient anti-dumping laws) and, of course, that chapter preceded the computer switch which was turned on for the National Practitioner Data Bank in September of 1990. Even the Joint Commission was then referred to as the JCAH rather than the Joint Commission on Accreditation of Healthcare Organizations (JCAHO) and Resource Based Relative Value Scale (RBRVS) was a glimmer in a crystal ball when that chapter was published. The phrase *economic credentialing* had not yet been dared. The entire healthcare industry has undergone a breadth of policy-driven changes that have created new organizational systems which challenge legal precedent.

Medical staffs traditionally existed within the hospital. The hospital was a single building with beds and an emergency room. Now, hospitals are not just single institutions, but part of an ongoing continuum of health care delivery and, as such, the legal concepts relative to clinical privilege

**107**

delineation must also be reflective of the new broader settings within which health care delivery takes place in the United States.

The basic topics that were recognized as important in 1985 continue to be important today but must be re-focused. Because board certified practitioners usually rely on the hospital to provide a practice setting, equipment and ancillary services, reviewing legal changes within the context of today's institution is necessary. Dr. Langsley promised this revision effort might not take too long. One cannot see winks over a telephone line. So I agreed to this challenge.

## The Hospital as an Institution

The hospital as an institution was once easily defined as a matter of state law. Licensing created the entity, and statutes which defined the hospital as an institution appeared in most state laws. Medicare laws also addressed the hospital as an institution. Conditions of participation in that program further delineated requirements relative to the organizational structure. If met, the hospital could receive Medicare payments for treatment of Medicare beneficiaries. Drastic changes affecting the definition of a hospital over the last decade create a legal sensitivity to sources of law governing the operation of the institution. It is therefore helpful to begin with an historical perceptive.

### Historical Perspective

The hospital was defined as the building housing beds, departments, services with administrative and nursing care, often with an emergency room and diagnostic centers. It was traditionally governed by one Board of Trustees and an Administrator or Executive Director who acted in the absence of the Board to make the day to day delegated decisions. The hospital had a voluntary medical staff comprised of licensed physicians who organized themselves autonomously and elected their own governance. This organization was described in a document called the Medical Staff Bylaws. The then JCAH would review bylaws to assure that certain aspects of governance were in place to achieve certain quality care results.

### Major Changes

For the most part, the hospital as an institution still exists as a single entity. But the trend during the last decade has been toward systems and related organizations, joint ventures, cooperative endeavors and the continuum of a health care delivery system that includes more than just the building with the beds. The hospital or institution is often part of a larger operation that takes into account delivery of health care at every level, including primary and ancillary care, clinics, nursing, home health, rehabilitation and other services. The medical staff may serve each or all of these parts.

We find systems of delivering alternative health care are also governed by clinical privilege delineation decisions. The institution is a place where multi-disciplined and differently licensed individuals proceed to deliver care within the legal scope of licensure which is often dictated by independent state boards of professional examiners. In a multi-institutional setting, more opportunity is presented for the utilization of appropriately credentialed and independently licensed individuals. For example, if the institution includes home health services, the single medical staff may include licensed occupational and physical therapists.

Indigenous to the institution is its reliance on good business efforts. Hospitals do not exist on the kindness of strangers. Hospitals are legal entities that must be run as proper businesses with the legal safeguards applicable to businesses in place. Thus, there are laws governing the operation of hospitals too numerous to mention in this chapter, but which greatly affect the operation of the hospital. Corporate, tax, bond and health benefits are just a few areas of the law which affect how the hospital operates and may affect its governance. Hospitals as business institutions have become serious players in the business community, often participating in local Chamber of Commerce activities and often comprising the largest employment in a given region.

Why does this backdrop have particular relevance in light of the traditional triangular relationship of medical staff, board and administration? Because the crystal ball suggests even more changes in hospital-physician relationships as affected by external health care policy and internal business and health care decisions. More physicians and other licensed professionals may become employed by contract than a decade ago.[1] Recruitment practices have taken on whole new requirements for legal scrutiny and compliance in light of the evolution of Medicare/Medicaid fraud and abuse, professional ethics, tax exempt status and shifts toward managed care.


## Sources of Legal Relationships

The institution is organized to achieve its mission often through volunteers. The local board is often comprised of volunteers in the community. The institution may also have an employed staff, a contractual and a dependent staff. The board channels its efforts through a mission, goals, a charter and resolution. Corporate officers and directors owe a fiduciary duty to the institution they serve. Employment relationships are often governed by contracts or by at will relationships. Individuals or groups of individuals work together to achieve the mission of care and treatment in the context of the legal documents that attempt to generally reflect how this care is delivered. Examples of such documents include the charter (articles of incorporation of the institution); the job description of the chief executive of the institution; the written and oral contracts of the employees and independent contractors; and the medical staff bylaws and rules and regulations for those licensed independent practitioners who provide clinical care pursuant to the privileges which are delineated to them by the medical staff and governing board of the institution.

Because the non-employed medical staff, at least for the time being, continues to be responsible for nearly 80% of the resource allocation in the institution, the selection and retention of licensed practitioners is more key than ever. Selection and retention is usually governed by state law and the medical staff and governing body bylaws. Now, the federal law and regulations expressed in the Health Care Quality Improvement Act may also be adopted in the institution's bylaws providing additional procedures for the selection and retention of the professional staff. The external forces bearing upon the inner relationships of the institution are greatly felt by the professional staff. Those forces have included increasingly complex governmental regulation, increased medical malpractice claims, new reporting requirements, economic institutional survival and societal demands for unlimited access to the state of the art technology. These forces may create additional tension upon the voluntary staff relationship and affect the contracts of the non-voluntary professional staff.


## Evolution of Legal Theories

The standard discussion on medical staff legal issues usually begins with an historical perspective on *Darling v. Charleston Memorial Hospital*.[2] This case is usually incorrectly cited for the position that the hospital board is responsible for the negligence of its medical staff. In fact, the case arose out of a nursing staff incident and the court held that the governing board is accountable to patients for the health care delivered in the hospital under the doctrine of corporate negligence.

Years later the courts expanded the corporate negligence theory to address the duty that hospitals owe to the public to appropriately credential professionals who provide patient care services at the facility. In *Johnson v. Mis-*

*ericordia Community Hospital*[3] a hospital was found liable for the negligent credentialing of a physician on the medical staff who allegedly committed medical malpractice. The hospital was found to have failed to make a reasonable investigation into the physician's background before delineating his privileges.

Hence, the "knew or should have known" standard began to have applicability in a credentialing setting. This theme will be played out in the subsequent discussion relevant to the National Practitioner Data Bank (NPDB). The hospital is deemed to know that which it is charged with the responsibility of learning during the credentialing process. The "reasonable investigation" duty then evolved into a duty to perform credentialing functions adequately.[4]

What these courts would not dare to hold, at least not at that point in time, was that the hospital is directly liable for the medical malpractice of its non-employed medical staff.[5]

There is a line of cases which holds that independently contracted departments, such as radiology, anesthesiology and pathology, and professionals employed within them, may subject the hospital to liability. These cases expand the traditional notion of *respondent superior* liability *i.e.*, the employer is responsible for the actions of the employee in the scope of his or her employment. To recognize an apparent agency notion that attaches to the situation, hospitals must look at the way they hold out ancillary services to their patients. Courts have imposed liability for the professional negligence of a physician or a hospital where the hospitals and the medical staffs operating within them choose ancillary services directly and under exclusive contract by the hospital. In these situations the patient does not choose the physician or service, but the institution chooses or contracts for the physician or that service. Institutional liability for the actions of the contractor would arise out of a similar legal theory called negligent contracting. That is, the institution had the responsibility to check the background performance of the contractor it selects. Does the patient choose the medical staff member? Is this patient's care and treatment tied to a certain service? This new legal inquiry must be reflected in light of expanded notions of malpractice liability.

As the traditional voluntary, non-controlled independent medical staff member status changes through employment or contract, medical malpractice liability may expand on the part of the institution providing that direct patient care.

Despite the hospital's need to contract for the provision of certain professional services, it is the organized medical staff that continues to have the responsibility to check credentialing thoroughly, verify information and data, investigate the completion of information, thoroughly contact medical and other societies about individuals with whom the applicant has worked, studied, or maintained a professional relationship. The amount of investigation and quality of that investigation may change as the industry credentialing standard becomes higher. The same standard must apply whether an individual is being credentialed as independent and voluntary or as the contractee or employee of the hospital or a department.

With incredible emphasis on quality of care considerations through peer review standards for Medicare payment requirements and the ongoing medical malpractice crisis, hospitals will take credentialing activities to new heights of emphasis. Institutions will use credentialing professionals and national information sources to check references and qualifications of applicants. The reappointment process will take on more than rubber stamp renewal activity with medical staff offices and officers having increasingly more responsibility to monitor and document peer care. An internal institutional data bank which kept only incident reports and malpractice claims may now begin to include incidents of outbursts, personality and other clashes with peer and other staff working within the institution. These provide just a few examples of documentation that may be collected and reviewed before appointment, reappointment or during or as part of a disciplinary or corrective procedure. Not included in this list are quality assurance efforts or total quality management data and statistics that may not necessarily single out an individual. However, if an individual's professional care falls outside of the norm, it is possible that the underlying study producing that finding may also be used as a basis for reappointment determinations or even corrective action.

Bylaws, which often had "canned language" bought from a consultant or were amended simply to comply with Joint Commission standards, should now be looked at as a true indication of how the staff self-governs its credentialing activities.


### Medical Staff Membership is More than a Privilege

Medical staff membership was historically characterized as a privilege given and taken away at will. Courts have begun to recognize that practice and licensure may be a protected right that may be restricted or limited only if reasonable. The earliest reported decisions in the area of medical staff membership and privileges held that hospitals cannot arbitrarily and capriciously deny privileges and that such denial must be legitimately based on patient care considerations. Those cases usually held that the hospital must follow its bylaws at all times.

## The Role of Medical Staff Bylaws

In states where medical staff bylaws constitute a contract, courts will usually review medical staff disputes.[6] If courts find that the relationship of the medical staff member is more than voluntary and the documents governing the relationship are more than bylaws — for example, a contract — courts will usually treat the relationship much like a wrongful termination case under employment law or as a breach of contract under contract law.[7]

Since medical staff and clinical privilege cases turn on specific facts, it would be advisable to review each case on its own merits before falling into a premise-like attitude toward judicial review in general. Where, for example, the courts have reviewed summary suspensions of privileges based on allegations of a threat to patient care, courts have been more likely to uphold the suspension action.[8] Summary suspension should be defined in the bylaws. Examples of situations that could trigger summary suspension should be discussed during the creation and/or amendment of the bylaws. Once summary suspension is defined, so should the procedures particularly applicable to it since time is of the essence and other time periods relative to review by the specific medical staff committees are usually shortened for this summary type of review. Procedures must address what happens to the patients of the suspended practitioner in terms of their ongoing treatment.

Bylaws must be followed whether considered by courts to constitute a contract or not. It has generally been held that bylaws establish a binding contract between the hospital and staff delineating the scope of procedural and substantive due process protections.[9]

Court involvement in clinical privilege decisions is referred to in the legal context as *judicial review.* Courts usually do not get involved in the internal affairs of a hospital unless a suit is filed characterizing the actions of the party or parties sued as one or more of the following:

1. arbitrary;
2. capricious;
3. out of compliance with bylaws;[10]
4. unfair; in bad faith; a subterfuge;
5. unfairly discriminatory;[11]
6. constituting a conspiracy or conspiratorial activity;[12]

7. bias on the part of a committee or individual members thereof;[13]

The "rule of limited judicial review" of a hospital medical staff decision has evolved in a minority of cases.[14] The minority rule is that courts *will review* a credentialing decision of a private hospital to determine whether the decision is supported by substantial credible evidence.[15] In other words, courts will hear the facts rather than simply adjudge the fairness of the hospital's afforded hearing procedures. Courts once made a distinction between private and public hospitals for purposes of judicial review and due process inquiry in credentialing determinations. If it were deemed to be private, courts were less likely to get involved in reviewing a hospital's determination. However, *private* hospitals have been found to be quasi-public if they are heavily supported by public funds or if the hospital is the sole provider of care in the community.[16] Majority rule is that courts *will always* get involved to review the credentialing decisions of a *public hospital* in order to determine whether the decision is supported by substantial and credible evidence.[17]

## Emphasis on Due Process

Courts may take a more expanded view of judicial review now that clinical privilege determinations have been declared by Congress to be a *right* owed to a licensed physician, rather than a *privilege.*[18] Despite this heightened awareness, courts will probably reluctantly intervene in the institutional review process. Courts generally do not substitute their own judgment for that of proper hearing committees convened under a proper set of bylaws. However, if the determination is challenged as having been based on individual, personality or economic considerations, courts may become more interested in specific review of that particular determination.

Due process procedures evolve from common and constitutional law.[19] Due process in laymen's terms simply means fairness on a substantive basis. Due process also defines what procedural rights will be required in the determination process. If and when a court becomes involved, the first inquiry will usually be the test of basic fundamental fairness. Was there a hearing or review? Was it conducted fairly? Did it follow the procedures set out in advance for its conduct? Was notice of the reasons for denial or reduction of privileges given? Was the affected practitioner given the chance to appear, be represented and give his or her version of the facts? And finally, was there an opportunity for an appeal to an unbiased group of individuals charged with the responsibility of ultimately making the determination affecting privileges?

If these very basic questions were answered affirmatively by a court or hospital, there is a great chance that the challenge to the process will fail. In those instances where the actions of certain members of the staff or of the institution are alleged to constitute a conspiracy to deprive an individual of practice, the courts may well become involved in the review.

## JCAHO Addressed Medical Staff Organization

As previously discussed, state laws and regulations contain specific requirements for licensure of independent and dependent practitioners as well as those who may be on a hospital medical staff. The JCAHO has no specific prohibition on the types of licensed practitioners who may practice in a hospital and acknowledges that its rules are superseded by the state laws of the institutions surveyed. JCAHO requires that there be a single organized medical staff that has overall responsibility for the quality of professional services provided by individuals with clinical privileges as well as for accounting therefor to the governing body.[20] Because the JCAHO standards also require that a mechanism be established to ensure that all individuals granted clinical privileges provide services within the scope of those privileges, that mechanism must be defined. It is usually defined by the medical staff bylaws and confirmed by the governing body bylaws. The governing body's bylaws indicate that it holds the medical staff responsible for the development, adoption and periodic review of medical staff bylaws, rules and regulations that are consistent with hospital policy and with any other applicable legal requirements.[21] The mechanisms for appointment of medical staff, including the receipt and review of applications for such appointments, and for the granting of clinical privileges, and the renewal or revision of those privileges, must be specific to the institution. Not all mechanisms or review processes need to be exactly the same but should follow general unbiased guidelines that meet the due process standards discussed herein.

There are basic minimum standards which must be met for membership on a medical staff, including current licensure, relevant training and/or experience, current competence and health status. In addition to the mandatory standards, there are permissive standards which have been legally upheld and used to establish a basis for membership and the granting of privileges. These standards are as follows:

(1) the ability of the hospital to provide adequate facilities and support services for the applicant and his/her patients;

(2) the patient care needs for additional staff members with the applicant's skill and training;

(3) applicant's current evidence of adequate professional liability insurance;

(4) geographic location of the practice in relationship to the facility.

Some subjective standards that often appear in bylaws[22] include the requirement that the individual be able to cooperate or get along with others. A number of decisions have linked cooperative behavior with patient care.

In addition to these grounds, courts have begun to review decisions based on business considerations. In a recent decision on this subject, *Bilek v. Tallahassee Memorial Regional Medical Center, Inc.,*[23] a Florida hospital was enjoined from revoking the medical staff privileges of an incumbent radiation-oncologist for reasons other than patient care. A radiation-oncologist from another state had been awarded an exclusive contract and the incumbent's privileges were terminated. The Court found that due process was violated, as the hospital's bylaws provided that privileges could be terminated only for cause.

## Clinical Privileging

During the appointment process clinical privileges are often determined by the use of standard forms creating levels of privileges that can be performed given an assignment to a certain department. For example, a check off list which is attached to the application is often used. That list reads like a code book of general procedures performed by different specialists that can be accommodated at the facility. Caution should be taken to prevent use of a form that is not reflective of the procedures at a specific facility. For example, an inpatient psychiatric facility would have little use for a check off form that includes open-heart surgery as a routine procedure.

Another type of clinical privilege form often used includes category levels by intensity of procedure. The categories are Types I through III and move from general to specific. Type I usually includes the most general non-invasive procedures, and Type III usually includes the highest level of tertiary or specialized procedures which may require additional experience, competence, equipment and training. Some institutions tie these categories to specialty certifications necessary in order to be granted the privilege to perform each particular procedure under that category. An example might be cardiovascular surgery falling into the Type III category. A legal consideration to use in reviewing privilege forms is whether they are fair and objective and whether they were created in a way such as to avoid exclusion of certain classes of physicians from certain procedures.

Departmental policies may require that only board certified cardiovascular surgeons be allowed to perform Type III invasive cardiologic procedures. This requirement goes beyond basic education, training and competence and adds a certification requirement. If challenged by a non-certified physician seeking privileges to do cardiovascular procedures, the institution would have to demonstrate that this additional requirement was reasonable; not discriminatorily applied; and relevant to the particular needs of the institution and the community. This type of requirement uses external criteria, for example, the examination process of the American Board of Medical Specialties. As such, it would be advisable for a record be maintained demonstrating that the institution, the respective departments and its medical executive committee reviewed the external criteria and applied them to the environment of the specific institution and the patient care needs of the community.

What happens if a practitioner does not check off a procedure for which he or she has demonstrated past competence and experience to perform, but simply does not wish to perform any longer? For example, an obstetrician-gynecologist no longer wishes to deliver babies. Is that self-reduction of privileges reportable? Probably not.

What happens if a practitioner feels uncomfortable about renewing a full gamut of privileges that he/she rarely uses and may feel a little rusty to perform? Is this self-determination and final reduction in privileges reportable? Probably not. However, caution should be used given the ambiguity surrounding this whole area of what constitutes disclosure and reportability of certain privilege delineation determinations. Forms for licensure application and renewal change from state to state just as medical staff appointment and clinical privilege delineation forms seek different responses that may well require full explanation of such self-reduction. It is the externally imposed reduction of privileges that may constitute the kind of event more likely to mandate reporting and disclosure.

Renewal of privileges usually occurs at the same time as reappointment to the medical staff, and according to JCAHO requirements, must take place at least once every two years; however, during two year intervals, there are situations which may occur that may require review of the list of clinical privileges originally granted. The types of procedures the physician performs may need to be expanded or reduced. There is some concern that reduction of the types of privileges may create an "adverse determination" such that due process procedures and the Health Care Quality Improvement Act would come into play.[24] It should be stressed, however, that current competence and current experience levels should be part of the indicia of demonstration of ability to perform the particular procedures sought to be expanded or reduced.

Because many specialized procedures directly impact the economics of a particular physician's practice, scrutiny must be given to the reasons for granting, limiting or denying the privileges. Whether they grant, limit or deny privileges, decisions should always reflect patient and quality care considerations. If decisions are tainted by a sense that individual practices are being economically protected, antitrust concerns may attach. There are very few cases which uphold limiting the number of specialists who may practice at a hospital within a geographic area as a legitimate criteria.

## Distinguish Medical Staff Membership from Delineation of Clinical Privileges

*Medical staff membership and delineation of clinical privileges* can be distinguished. The medical staff includes fully licensed physicians and may include other licensed practitioners permitted by law and by the hospital to provide services independently and in accordance with JCAHO standards. Clinical privileges include the specific treatment and procedures that the professional is trained, experienced and competent to perform as well as able to be accommodated by the facility. It is not necessary that every practitioner who can practice without supervision also be a member of the medical staff. Only members of the medical staff can *admit* patients to the institution, not all medical staff members must be granted full admitting and clinical privileges. It may be appropriate to require certain categories of non-physician practitioners to co-admit their patients with a physician. All independent practitioners should have the scope of their practice defined through delineation of clinical privileges. Privileges should be delineated in accordance with criteria outlined *in advance* in medical staff bylaws, rules, policies and regulations.

Often a problem is presented when an applicant seeks a new privilege for a procedure or procedures not yet performed at the institution. How does a medical staff with little exposure dealing with those procedures review the application? If the hospital can effectively and professionally staff and accommodate the procedures but the medical staff feels uncomfortable engaging in peer review and supervision or monitoring of an unfamiliar procedure, the committees charged with such review may and probably should request outside assistance in performing their responsibility. Is there a certifying board with literature on the subject that can be reviewed? Can an outside group of experts be called in to review the procedure, its quality and effectiveness? What is in the acceptable medical literature about the procedure or the procedures sought to be practiced? Can this type of practice be safely accommodated at the facility? What are the true patient care risks?

If the hospital denies the application because it is unfamiliar with the procedure, the reasons given for denial need to reflect that the application was denied not because of an adverse effect on patient care, but because the hospital will be compelled to report its denial to the National Practitioner Data Bank. The practitioner whose application was denied may thus be placed in a defensive posture as he/she will also be compelled to report the denial as an *adverse determination* on future applications for privileges and renewals or new applications for licensure. In these situations the medical staff and governing board may find themselves in the unfortunate position of making rules, policies and requirements that are specific to the individual applicant. Although every kind of situation can hardly be predicted prior to receiving an application for a new type of procedure, it is advisable for most types of procedures that can be accommodated within a given facility to be recognized and explored and for policies relating to those procedures to be developed in advance. Additionally, those policies should be reviewed on a periodic basis to determine their compliance and need for revision in light of applicable law.

Ultimately the hospital's governing body must decide, after considering the medical staff's recommendations, which individuals will be given access to the institution for the purposes of providing patient care. These decisions should always be made on the basis of criteria articulated in advance and not on the basis of the possible competitive effects on any individuals or group. A decision not to grant access to the hospital for certain practitioners may be challenged as discriminatory. If a lawsuit is filed, it may be based on application of State or Federal antitrust laws as generally discussed herein.


## Antitrust Concerns

Section 1 of the Sherman Act proscribes restraints upon commerce through illegal concerted actions, contracts, conspiracies and combinations. Section 2 prohibits unilateral action or conduct which constitutes a monopoly.[25] Legal action to enforce compliance with antitrust laws may be brought by a private plaintiff, the United States Department of Justice, a state attorney general, or any of them. Actions seek three times the amount of economic damage and may include criminal enforcement, attorney's fees and costs, if successful. Broader than these provisions is Section 5 of the Federal Trade Commission Act ("FTC Act")[26] which prohibits unfair methods of competition. Many states have unfair trade or business practice acts which often parallel the FTC Act.

In the health care arena, there have been numerous antitrust cases brought privately and there has been increased emphasis on government enforcement. In the medical staff setting, one of the first cases was *Robinson v. Magovern*.[27] The court held that a hospital may deny privileges if the reasons were related to the hospital's legitimate goals.

### Antitrust Tests

### 1. *Jurisdictional—Commerce*

The jurisdictional test relating to impact on interstate commerce for purposes of federal antitrust law was explored at length in the Robinson case. How does practicing within a hospital setting have anything to do with crossing state lines or impacting commerce? The *Robinson v. Magovern* test was finally expanded in 1991 by the United States Supreme Court in *Summit Health Ltd. v. Pinhas*.[28] The case involved an ophthalmologist who was denied privileges and alleged a conspiracy to deprive him of the ophthalmologic marketplace by a hospital requirement that an assistant surgeon be used despite the fact that Medicare had stopped coverage for an assistant. The Supreme Court's analysis focused on existing National Practitioner Data Bank requirements and found that the jurisdictional test of interstate commerce impact in a privilege challenge case is met for purposes of the antitrust laws. The merits were not yet reached in that case.

### 2. *Conspiracy Requires at Least Two Entities*

In the original article on this subject, much emphasis was given to the then recent case, *Weiss v. York Hospital*.[29] The court in *Weiss* discussed the requirement that there be two separate and distinct economic entities recognized before an antitrust conspiracy can be found. Before *Weiss*, Pennsylvania courts found that physicians were competitors in a medical staff setting, but were only a part of a system of decision makers. As such, there were not two separate entities upon which a conspiracy allegation could rest. Since the credentialing decisions were based on sound reasoning, no violation of antitrust law was found.[30] Although the analysis used in these cases is often more excruciating, the courts are continuing to find that scrutiny should focus on the reasons for the credentialing decision and that if they rest on a sound basis, they will be upheld despite their anti-competitive effect.[31]

In *Weiss v. York*, the evidence was sufficient to establish a restraint of trade violative of the antitrust statute. Each case must be reviewed on its specific facts, yet the facts in *Weiss* present examples of what may be proper or improper credentialing techniques and motives. The plaintiff Dr. Weiss was an osteopath who had been denied staff privileges at York Hospital. He brought the suit both individually and as a representative of the class of all osteopathic physicians in the York medical service area against York Hospital and its medical and dental staff, as well as against ten physicians who had served on the medical staff executive committee and its judicial review committee. Dr. Weiss alleged that although allopaths and osteopaths are equally trained and qualified to practice medicine, his application of staff privileges was turned down solely because of his status as an osteopath instead of as an allopath. The court admitted that the case raised a number of complicated legal questions. It examined the history of discrimination against osteopaths, the application procedure for staff privileges, the application itself and the procedural history of the challenge to Dr. Weiss. The court held that in cases where there is an antitrust challenge under Section I of the Sherman Act, it is essential that the existence of a combination or conspiracy to restrain trade first be proved. Dr. Weiss contended that the hospital and its medical staff were legally distinct entities and therefore capable of conspiring for purposes of the Sherman Act, Section I. In so asserting, he alleged that the doctors who joined together to form the medical staff were separate economic entities who competed against each other so that, "as a matter of law," the medical staff was a single "combination" of doctors within the meaning of this section of the law. He also argued that the doctors were acting for their own benefit in discriminating against osteopaths and therefore fell within an exception to the ordinary rule enunciated by the Supreme Court in *Copperweld Corp. v. Independence Tube Corp.*,[32] which is that officers and employees of the same firm cannot conspire with each other for purposes of a Section I conspiracy.

The defendants argued that York Hospital and its medical staff were one legal entity and therefore incapable of conspiring. The U.S. Court of Appeal found that the medical staff is a combination of individual doctors who have independent economic interests in competition with each other and that any action taken by the medical staff as individuals satisfies the "contract, combination, or conspiracy" requirements of the antitrust law. However, the court agreed that the hospital *could not* legally conspire with its medical staff.

Thus, a medical staff should be considered part of the "umbrella" structure of the hospital. The "three-legged stool" or triangle is often used to describe the relationship of the administration, the medical staff and the governing board. A separately incorporated medical staff is a separate entity outside of the stool. As such, the conspiracy test could be more easily met if its credentialing decisions with the hospital are challenged.

The *legal entity* cases caused chills down the spines of many antitrust attorneys who represent hospitals. In 1988 the United States Court of Appeal for the Eleventh Circuit took up where *Weiss* left off. In *Bolt v. Halifax Hospital Medical Center,*[33] a physician whose medical staff privileges were revoked at each of three different hospitals brought an antitrust suit against the hospitals, their medical staffs and the local medical society alleging a conspiracy to drive him out of the medical community.

The court painstakingly reviewed the bylaws applicable at each hospital and included references to the specific processes for decision making, credentials committee recommendations and executive committee investigation. The court reviewed each medical staff determination which could be appealed through judicial-type review comprised of all active staff members. The court recognized that medical staff members are competitors. After its analysis, the court recognized three particular conspiracies:

1. the three hospitals and their medical staff members;
2. the hospitals among themselves; and
3. the hospital medical staffs and the community.

The court rejected the previous holdings that hospitals are legally incapable of conspiring with members of their medical staffs, which were based on the rule that a corporation cannot conspire with its officers and directors.[34] The court found this analogy at fault and declined to embrace it.

The FTC has also found a medical staff capable of conspiring with a hospital in efforts to keep podiatrists off the staff.[35]

Finally, a case worth reviewing because the United States Court of Appeal for the Fourth Circuit went to great lengths in describing the relationship between the hospital and medical staff in *Oksanen v. Page Memorial Hospital.*[36] The Court looked to the "degree of control" the hospital exercises over the staff during the peer review process in order to ascertain whether two separate entities exist for purposes of a conspiracy. The Court found that the Governing Board, while heavily reliant on medical staff recommendations, could modify those recommendations at any time and that " . . . it retained ultimate responsibility for all of the hospital's credentialing decisions." This authority was found enunciated in the medical staff bylaws. The Court also looked to the realities of the marketplace and found that the hospital's interests would not be furthered by engaging in a conspiracy among doctors as hospitals have an incentive to maximize the number of physicians who are granted clinical privileges. In conclusion, the Court made a statement worth reproducing here:

> "The antitrust laws do not prevent physicians from taking legitimate disciplinary action against unprofessional or incompetent practitioners. Many professions have long placed considerable faith in self-regulation, and it would be a blow to public confidence in these professions if the utility of these measures were impaired by an unjustifiable expansive reading of the antitrust laws with their concomitant burden of discovery."

### 3. *Defenses to Antitrust: State Action*

In a United States Supreme Court decision clearly attracting national attention, a defense often applicable to peer review decision making was analyzed and found not applicable.[27] The Supreme Court extensively reviewed the facts of a Ninth Circuit decision overturning a jury's antitrust damages award of $2 million. Dr. Patrick, the plaintiff, an Astoria, Oregon surgeon who declined to join the Astoria Clinic Physician Multi-Specialty practice as a partner, set up his own competitive practice. The clinic physicians thereafter utilized "peer review" proceedings to terminate Dr. Patrick's privileges at Astoria's only hospital on the ground that his practices were below acceptable standards. The Court of Appeal reversed the jury's finding of antitrust liability holding that the Oregon Peer Review Statute constituted an "articulated state policy" which could be asserted as a defense to the antitrust action. The United States Supreme Court reversed in favor of Dr. Patrick despite numerous *amicus curiae* briefs from organized health care associations taking the position that peer review activities should be immune. The United States Supreme Court couched the "policy argument" as follows:

> "effective peer review is essential to the provision of quality medical care and that any threat of antitrust liability will prevent physicians from participating openly and actively in peer review proceedings . . . "

However, despite this strong affirmation of peer review policy, the Court imposed antitrust liability. Justice Marshal's opinion pointed out that one of the partners of the clinic was on the State Board of Medical Examiners which issued a letter of reprimand to Dr. Patrick. Despite its retraction of said letter, the Supreme Court noted the obvious presence of bias in the termination review procedures resulting from the fact that the same author of the letter also served on the hospital medical executive committee whose vote terminated Dr. Patrick from the staff. During his medical staff appeals at the hospital, Dr. Patrick voluntarily surrendered his privileges and filed suit for violation of the antitrust laws. Finally, the Supreme Court found that the Oregon statutory scheme requiring notification to the Board of Medical Examiners of a decision to terminate or restrict privileges[38] does not constitute a state program of active supervision over peer review decisions so that the state action doctrine did not apply as a defense to Dr. Patrick's antitrust action. The Supreme Court found that the State of Oregon does not actively supervise the termination of hospital privileges and that no state official has or exercises ultimate authority over private privilege determinations. Because the Oregon law does not give Oregon's health division such authority, it has no power to review private peer review decisions or overturn a decision that fails to accord with state policy. State action as a defense to antitrust in peer review cases will thus probably be ineffective in a medical staff antitrust case, depending on the particular state statute involved.

## Health Quality Improvement Act

During the rolling tide of *Patrick*, a certain congressman from Oregon reacting to the upheaval in his state introduced the Health Care Quality Improvement Act of 1986.[39] Chapter 117 of the United States Code Public Health and Welfare Title is called "Encouraging Good Faith Professional Review Activities." This law thrust Congress into its first true foray into medical staff selection and retention issues.

The Act generally provided immunity from antitrust suits brought by an affected practitioner against an institution or others acting for or on its behalf who conducted peer review and authorized the establishment of the National Practitioner Data Bank. The preamble to the Act reflects Congressional concerns expressed as follows:

1. The increasing occurrence of medical malpractice and the need to improve the quality of medical care have become nationwide problems that warrant greater efforts than those that can be undertaken by any individual state.
2. There is a national need to restrict the ability of incompetent physicians to move from state to state without disclosure or discovery of the physician's previous damaging or incompetent performance.

3. This nationwide problem can be remedied through effective professional peer review.
4. The threat of private money damage liability under federal laws, including treble damage liability under federal antitrust law, unreasonably discourages physicians from participating in effective professional peer review.
5. There is an overriding national need to provide incentive and protection for physicians engaging in effective professional peer review.

For immunity to obtain, the action taken must constitute "peer review" as defined in the statute and in subsequent regulations.[40] This law applies to hospitals, professional societies, health maintenance organizations, state licensure boards, certain group practices and individuals who participate in peer review. The peer review action, however, must take place in "reasonable belief that it is in furtherance of quality health care"; after a "reasonable" effort is made to obtain the facts; after notice and hearing procedures are afforded; and in "reasonable" belief that the action is warranted by the facts then known.[41]

Subchapter II of the Act includes the reporting requirements[42] and received even more attention through its requirement that a national data bank be established under contract and that it receive data as to the "adverse actions" taken against physicians by peer review entities as well as to payments made under a policy of insurance, self-insurance or otherwise in settlement of or judgment in a medical malpractice action or claim. The Act authorized the Department of Health and Human Services ("DHH") to set out regulations to implement the Act which regulations were finalized October 17, 1991.[43] Collection of data began on September 1, 1990 when the electronic equipment began to accept information. At the time of this writing, the data bank has had difficulty with backlogs and with accessing inquiries for information.

The reporting requirements also included an interim step regarding dissemination of the "adverse actions" to respective state licensing boards within fifteen (15) days of finality. State boards must in turn report such "adverse actions" to the National Practitioner Data Bank within an additional fifteen (15) days. Failure to report may cause loss of immunity under the Act as well as possible fines. The DHH has also issued a guidebook for users of the Data Bank setting out the procedures and time periods. Insurance carriers and others who pay medical malpractice judgments or settlements in any amounts are required to report such payments within thirty (30) days directly to the National Practitioner Data Bank.

If a hospital fails to request or query the Data Bank for information during credentialing of a physician, it is presumed to know in any medical malpractice action related to that physician the information contained in the Data Bank. The Johnson v. Misericordia finding discussed earlier herein also found that the hospital could be negligent under a theory of negligent credentialing if it "knew or should have known" certain matters that proper investigatory technique could have established.

The information within the Data Bank is afforded certain confidentiality except that it may be disclosed to a plaintiff's attorney in a medical malpractice case if a hospital is a defendant and if it is alleged that the hospital failed to properly credential and query the Data Bank as to the physician in question. There are numerous unresolved and unclarified issues relative to the Data Bank.

There are very few decisions to date that address the Health Care Quality Improvement Act. An early decision, *Austin v. McNamara*,[44] found that the Act immunized a hospital and individual physicians on the medical staff from federal antitrust liability for their conduct in connection with the suspension and subsequent conditional reinstatement of a neurosurgeon's staff privileges as the actions were in the interest of furthering quality health care and were taken after extensive evaluations and monitoring of the patient care.

### The Contracted Medical Staff

The concept of contractual arrangements with professionals to provide certain services is not altogether new. The effect of contracting for staff, whether professional or administrative, should be reviewed. If there is a departmental contract for an ancillary service, the contract should require that each professional independent sub-contractor or employer be subject to the medical staff bylaws. Does that mean each individual must be credentialed? A Florida court in *Hospital Corporation of Lake Worth and Hospital Corporation of America v. Raul Romaguera, M.D.*[45] reflected upon the contract rights of an individual in view of medical staff bylaws, in particular the amendments thereto. The court awarded damages to a physician who alleged that the bylaws were not followed when his contract status at the hospital was terminated and he was not allowed to practice at the hospital thereafter. The action alleged tortious interference with a business relationship. The court found that amendments to the bylaws provided that the termination of contracts with physicians would not terminate their staff privileges.

The traditional notions of medical staff privilege delineation will likely change as and if the practitioner's status within the institution moves toward a contractual relationship. In order to assure that certain services can be provided within the community, institutions are increasingly contracting to get those services. Seeing the same familiar medical staff members performing the same procedures on a routine basis may become a thing of the past as the need to provide certain services attracts transient, guest or occasional practitioners whose services are often provided by contract. Being sensitive to quick and thorough reference checks and having a system in place before the potential for these new contract services is presented is necessary for the efficient administration of the review process used to delineate the clinical privileges granted to contract practitioners. Contractual relationships should also take into account medical staff and governing body bylaws and the amendments thereto since consistency is necessary for legal compliance. Institutions need to be in a position to check contracts for compliance with medical staff credentialing requirements.

## Conclusion

As hospitals and systems take a new look at themselves they must review their medical staff relationships with a view toward effective collaboration. The bodies of law that apply to those relationships evolve often after the relationship is conceived. A proactive approach toward analyzing the legal authorities that govern the institution and medical staff can help to strengthen relationships. Education is critical to keep the medical staff informed of the regulatory legal changes affecting their selection, retention, and credentialing responsibilities. As the continuum of healthcare widens, the institution must reach out to embrace the needs of its primary and specialty care networks, its voluntary and contracted staff, its governing board, executive leadership and the community. Effective and good faith peer review can help smooth the bumps of this current transition.

## References


1. *Hospitals,* "Compensation, Social Trends Alter Hospital-MD Relations." Cover story (November 20, 1991). More M.D.s opt to become employees. 22.6% in 1987 as compared to 25.2% in 1990. Source: AMA Center for Health Policy Research, 1991.
2. 33 Ill. 2d 326, 211 N.E. 2d 253, 14 A.L.R. 3d 860 (1965) *cert. denied,* 383 U.S. 946 (1966).
3. 99 Wis. 2d 708, 301 NW 2d 156 (1981).
4. *Elam v. College Park Hospital,* Cal. App. 3d 332, 183 Cal. Rptr. 156 (Cal. App. 4 Dist. 1982).

5. Cf. *Thompson v. Nason Hospital,* 542 A. 2d 1371 (Pa. Super. 1988), *aff'd,* 591 A. 2d 703 (Pa. 1991). The Pennsylvania Supreme Court supported that a hospital may be liable for the negligence of a member of the medical staff.

6. *Gianetti v. Norwalk Hospital,* 211 Conn. 51, 557 A. 2d 1249 (Conn. 1989), reversing a thirty year precendent that established "non-review" of these decisions.

7. *See,* for example, *Fletcher v. Eagle River Memorial Hospital,* 441 N.W. 2d 297 (Wis. App. D. III 1989).

8. *Bouquett v. St. Elizabeth Corp.,* 430 Ohio St. 3d 50, 538 N.E. 2d 113 (Ohio 1989). Physician's summary suspension on grounds of conviction of conspiring to distribute controlled substances was upheld. The Ohio State Supreme Court held the bylaw phrase "best interest of patient care included not only a physician's technical skills and professional competence," but also his "perceived integrity." Physician had been afforded due process in the procedures. *See also Tasher v. St. Tammany Parish Hospital,* 1988 WL 10177 *aff'd* 862 F. 2d 873 (5th Cir. 1988), *cert. denied* 109 S.Ct. 3190 (1989).

9. *St. John Hospital Medical Staff v. St. John Regional Medical Center, Inc,* 90 S.D. 674, N.W. 2d 472 (S.D. 1976); *Lawler v. Eugene Wuestoff Memorial Hospital Assn.,* 497 So. 2d 1261 (Fla. App. 1986); *Berberian v. Lancaster Osteopathic Hospital Assn.,* 395 Pa. 257, 149 A. 2d 456 (Pa. 1958); *McElhinney v. William Booth Memorial Hospital,* 544 S.W. 2d 216 (Ky. 1976); *Miller v. Indiana Hospital,* 277 Pa. Super. 370, 419 A. 2d 1191 (Pa. 1980); *Anne Arundel Gen. Hosp., nc v. O'Brien,* 49 Md. App. 362, 432 A. 2d 483 (Md. App. 1981); *Stiller v. LaPorte Hosp. Inc,* 570 N.E. 2d 99 (Ind. App. 3 Dist. 1991).

10. *Jain v. Northwest Community Hospital,* 67 Ill. App. 3d 385 N.E. 2d 108 (Ill. App. 1st Dist. 1978); *Duby v. Jordan Hospital,* 369 Mass. 626, 341 N.E. 2d 876 (Mass. 1976); *Gates v. Holy Cross Hospital,* 529 N.E. 2d 1014 (Ill. App. 1st Dist. 1988). Court will reinstate privileges.

11. Courts will entertain Title VII Civil Rights Claims. *See Shah v. Memorial Hospital,* 1988 WL 161175, 1988 2 Trade Cases (CCH), Par. 68, 199 (W.D. Va. 1988); *Milo v. Cushing Municipal Hospital,* 861 F. 2d 1194, 56 U.S.L.W. 2622 (10th Cir. 1988). *Mitchell v. Frank R. Howard Memorial Hospital,* 853 F. 2d 762 (9th Cir. 1988); *See also "Exclusion of or Discrimination Against Physician or Surgeon by Hospital,"* 37 A.L.R. 3d 645. Recently a Pennsylvania court found that Title VII applies to staff privilege termination actions if based on national origin. *See Mallare v. St. Luke Hosp. of Bethlehem,* 699 F. Supp. 1127

(E.D. Pa. 1988); *Pardazi v. Cullman Medical Center,* 838 F. 2d 1155 (11th Cir. 1988).

12. Where there is a conspiracy to deprive or deny privileges, courts will review the action. *See Nashville Memorial Hospital, Inc v. Binkley,* 534 S.W. 2d 318 (Tenn. 1976); *Willis v. Santa Ana Community Hospital Assn.,* 58 Cal. 2d 806, 26 Cal. Rptr. 640, 376 P. 2d 568 (Cal. 1962).

13. For example, members of the credentials committee also serve on higher appeal committees, such as the medical executive committee and/or board of governors. *See Weiss v. York Hospital,* 745 F. 786 (3d Cir. 1984).

14. *Knapp v. Palos Community Hospital,* 531 N.E. 2d 989 (1st Cir. 1988).

15. *Barrows v. Northwestern Memorial Hospital,* 505 N.E. 2d 1182 (Ill. App. 1st Dist. 1987); See also, *Rosenblit v. Superior Court,* 231 Cal. App. 3d 1434, 282 Ca., Rptr. 819 (Cal. app. 4 Dist. 1991)[adequacy of fair hearing was questioned, court conducted the hearing]

16. *See,* for example, *Klinge v. Lutheran Charities Association of St. Louis,* 523 F. 2d 56 (8th Cir,. 1975). States following this theory: Alaska, Arizona, California, Colorado, Hawaii, New Jersey, New Hampshire, New Mexico, Ohio and Vermont.

17. *Truly v. Madison General Hospital,* 673 F. 2d 763 (5th Cir. 1982) *cert. denied,* 103 S.Ct. 214 (1982); *Dayan v. Wood River Township Hospital,* 18 Ill. App. 2d 263, 152 N.E. 2d 205 (Ill. App. 4 Dist. 1958). cf. The Michigan Supreme Court has ruled that private non-profit hospital medical staff decisions are not subject to review. *See Hottentot v. Mid-Maine Medical Center,* 549 A. 2d 365 (Maine S.Ct. 1988).

18. Health Care Quality Improvement Act, 42 U.S.C. §11101–11152, *et seq.* (1986)

19. " . . . nor be deprived of life, liberty, or property, without due process of law, . . . U.S.C.A. Const. Amend. V, §4; "Citizens of the United States; . . . or depriving any person of due process of law or equal protection of the laws." U.S.C.A. Const. Amend. XIX.

20. MS 1 of the JCAHO Accreditation Manual for Hospitals, 1992

21. AMH. GB1.1.9 (1991).

22. *See Everhart v. Jefferson Parish Hospital District No. 2,* 757 F.2d 1567 (5th Cir. 1985); *Miller v. Eisenhower Medical Centers,* 27 Cal.3d 614, 166 Cal. Rptr. 826, 614 P.2d 258 (Cal. 1980); *Mahmoodian v. United Hospital Center, Inc,* 404 S.E. 2d 750 (W.Va. 1991).

23. (Unreported) 2d Jud. D. Ct. (FA Apr. 29, 1991). This case is representative of a growing number of legal challenges to staff determinations made on the basis of so-called economic grounds.

24. *See* Health Care Quality Improvement Act discussion herein.
25. 15 U.S.C. §1; 15 U.S.C. §2.
26. 15 U.S.C. §5.
27. 521 F. Supp. 842 (W.D. Pa. 1981), *aff'd mem.*, 688 F. 2d 824 (3rd Cir. 1982), *cert. denied*, 459 U.S. 971, 103 S.Ct. 302 (1982).
28. 114 L. Ed. 2d 366, 111 S.Ct. 1842, 59 U.S. L.W. 4493 (1991).
29. 745 F. 2d 786 (3d Cir. 1984).
30. *Pontius v. Children's Hospital*, 552 F. Supp 1352 (W.D. Pa. 1982).
31. *Oksanen v. Page Memorial Hospital*, 945 F. 2d 696 (4 Cir. 1991), *in banc*
32. 467 U.S. 752, 104 S.Ct. 2731, 2741, 81 L.Ed.2d 628 (1984).
33. 851 F. 2d 1273 (11th Cir. 1988).
34. *Harvey v. Fearless Farris Wholesale, Inc*, 589 F. 2d 451, 455 n. 7 (9th Cir. 1979); *Weiss, supra*, 745 F. 2d at 815-17; *Buckner v. Lower Florida Keys Hosp. Dist.*, 403 So. 2d 1025, 1029 (Fla. App. 3rd Dist. 1981); *Copperweld Corp., supra*, 104 S. Ct. 2731, 2741 (1984).
35. *Healthcare Mgmt Corp.*, FTC File No. 841, 50 Fed. Reg. 41693 (Oct. 15, 1985).
36. *Oksanen, supra*, 945 F.2d 696 (4 Cir. 1991).
37. *Patrick v. Berget*, 487 U.S. 1243, 108 S.Ct. 2921, 101 L.Ed.2d 952 (1988).
38. Ore. Rev. Stat. §441.820(1) (1987).
39. Pub. L. 99-660, Title IV, §402, Nov. 14, 1986, 100 Stat. 3784, 42 U.S.C. §11101–11152 (1986).
40. 42 C.F.R., Part 60.
41. 42 U.S.C. §11112(a).
42. 42 U.S.C. §11131.
43. 42 C.F.R. Part 60.
44. 731 F. Supp. 934 (C.D. Ca. 1990).
45. 511 So.2d 559 (Fla. App. 4th Dist. 1987).

# The JCAHO Credentialing Process

James S. Roberts, MD

This chapter will address the elements of the current health care environment that by themselves and together have and will continue to force more effective evaluation of the quality of care and more accurate privilege delineation.

Table 1 lists the factors in the health care environment and within most health care organizations which enhance the importance of fair and accurate privilege delineation.

Taken together these factors provide powerful impetus to more effectively review the quality of clinical care, and, by so doing, to more accurately identify individual clinical performance and grant clinical privileges only in areas of current competence. It is in this context that I will discuss Joint Commission for Accreditation of Healthcare Organizations (JCAHO) standards for quality assurance and privilege delineation.

## The Evolution from Quality Assurance to Continuous Quality Improvement

Since 1979, the Joint Commission has been on a steady course of change in its quality assessment standards. The objective has been to stimulate health care organization to move from random, often unfocused and ineffective review to a facility-wide system of evaluation which is planned, systematic, meaningful, efficient and effective. The first phase of this evaluation was described by Roberts and Walczak and resulted in standards

**131**

which asked for a quality assurance system having the characteristics noted in Table 2.

---

**Table 1. Factors Heightening the Need for Effective Credentials Review and Privilege Delineation**

1. States allow a broad scope of practive by many professional groups.
2. Hospitals are expanding their services, often requiring types of practitioners that have not practiced previously in the hospital.
3. The state-of-the-art continues to evolve requiring careful attention to continuing competence.
4. Increasing sophistication of hospital services requires more precise matching of individual and hospital competency.
5. Despite the shrinking volume of inpatient care, medical staff membership and clinical privileges continue to be highly desired.
6. Antitrust and liability exposure requires that a hospital carefully define and follow and effective credential review and privilege delineation process.
7. The public continues to demand high quality, cost-efficient health care.

---

**Table 2. Characteristics of a Current Hospital Quality Assurance (QA) Program**

1. All major aspects of care are monitored and evaluated.
2. All clinical components of the institution are involved in the QA program.
3. Monitoring and evaluation consist of routine collection of important patient care information and periodic evaluation of that information.
4. Important problems are resolved and opportunities for improvement are taken.
5. Criteria based upon the literature and expert clinical judgment are used in monitoring and evaluation.
6. Findings of quality assurance are linked to delineation of clinical privileges.
7. The multiple QA mechanisms are coordinated across hospital departments and practitioner group.
8. The effectiveness of the program and each of its components are periodically evaluated, and, where necessary, strengthened.

Building on this base of systematic quality assurance, the 1992 *Accreditation Manual for Hospitals* represents the first step in the Joint Commission's evolution to standards that focus more directly on performance. They are designed to foster continuous improvement in the effectiveness and efficiency with which an organization performs those governance, management, clinical and support activities most important to patient outcomes. Over the next several years, this evolution will result in assessment and improvement activities having the characteristics listed in Table 3. The first and second characteristics listed in Table 3 deserve special attention. Some have misinterpreted the evolution to process-focused continuous quality improvement to justify inattention to the competence of individuals. In the interest of "moving the curve" some seem to believe that it is inappropriate to continue to address individual "outliers". Nothing could be further from the truth. Our professional obligation remains and we must deal decisively with incompetent or impaired colleagues. The shift to more concerted attention to process simply reflects the fact that process weaknesses are the root-causes of most quality problems. But individuals with important deficiencies in capability are still with us and must be prevented from harming patients.

As noted later in this paper, this balanced attentions to both the individual and the process/system will allow more sophisticated use of data and more accurate decisions about an individual's privileges.

## Credentials Review and Privilege Delineation

With this as background, let us review privilege delineation specifically. This chapter will try to identify four or five relevant and recent changes

---

**Table 3. Characteristics of Future Assessment and Improvement Mechanisms**

1. Focused more on processess/systems than on individuals.
2. Uses information in a less punitive manner.
3. Assesses important governance, management, clinical and support processes.
4. Involves ALL staff in assessment and improvement activities.
5. Fosters cross-departmental and cross-disciplinary review and improvement work.
6. Addresses both the technical and the patient perspectives of quality.
7. Uses both process and outcome information in assessment activities.
8. Tests improvements prior to their full implementation.
9. Has continuous improvement as the objective.

that the Commission has made in its medical staff standards. Then, I will pose ten questions which represent a summation of the key elements of our privilege delineation standards and which might be helpful as the reader analyzes the credentials review and privilege delineation process.

First, what has changed in this area of standards? In 1984, for the first time, the JCAHO added a standard to the governing body chapter of the *Accreditation Manual for Hospitals* asking the governing body to require the existence of processes designed to assure that "all individuals who provide patient care services are competent to provide such services". This is not limited to those who have traditionally been defined as medical staff members, but includes all the other individuals who provide care in hospitals. This can be accomplished through job evaluation or performance review enhanced to analyze the clinical activities of each of these practitioners.

In 1984, we also made a significant change in our medical staff chapter. This occurred after long and spirited debate resulting in a revised chapter focused on those individuals who are independent practitioners. There are those who are allowed by the state and the hospital to practice without direction or supervision. Those who initiate and carry out their clinical practice should be defined in terms of individual, facility-specific clinical privileges. These clinical privileges must be recommended through medical staff processes to the governing board in a manner described in the medical staff bylaws. At the option of the hospital, independent practitioners may or may not actually be members of the staff, but their competence is to be assessed and their privileges are recommended and approved through well defined medical staff and governing body processes.

While this was an important change, it was perceived to be more radical than it actually was. At the time we made the change, the widely held perception was that the standards limited medical staffs to physicians and dentists. As a matter of fact there are a large number of states, 20 or so, where a variety of other types of practitioners were (and are) allowed to be members of hospital medical staffs.

Because of the importance of accurate assessment of competence and relevant privilege delineation, we have also placed more emphasis on credentials review and privilege delineation in the survey process. About 40 percent of the hospitals we surveyed in 1984 received one or more contingencies concerning privilege delineation. The most frequent problem we found was that, as hospitals contract more and more of their services to outside groups, they were not assessing the competence and granting privileges for *each* of the individuals providing care under the contract. This is a particular problem in emergency medicine, radiology, anesthesiology and nuclear medicine departments. Another requirement resulting in a very high frequency of contingencies is that which asks hospitals to use quality assurance information as they consider the question of clinical competence for any individual practitioner. This natural bridge between performance review and privilege delineation, while logical, has proven difficult to build. Subsequent changes in the standards have centered on consolidation of similar requirements spread throughout the Medical Staff chapter. The 1992 *Accreditation Manual for Hospitals* (AMH) contains one standard for addressing all medical staff activities regarding credentials review and privilege delineation.

Those are the major changes in the survey processes and standards. What I would like to do now is to pose ten questions that you might want to consider as you look at your own process of privilege delineation. I am not going to talk about due process.

## Is the Process Defined?

Question 1 is fairly straightforward. Most hospitals have a well-defined privilege delineation process. It is described in the medical staff bylaws, and everybody has signed off on it. Hospitals often have problems, however, when the processes they have defined are not followed, when prescribed timetables are not met, when the steps of the process are not followed, or when obvious conflicts of interest are not avoided. On the other hand, rigorous adherence to the defined process has served hospitals well. The message—define a solid approach and follow it.

## Are All Independent Practitioners Included?

I mentioned the problem we are finding with contracted services. Other problems are with people who do not admit frequently or are consultants who infrequently provide care in the hospitals. Sometimes they tend to fall between the cracks. Also, there may be questions about whether certain practitioners are required to have privileges. These may be those practitioners who are new to the institution, and the hospital is not sure whether privilege delineation is the appropriate approach to delineating their practice. The key from the Joint Commission's perspective is whether or not the individual is an independent practitioner. If yes, then the privilege delineation process must be used. If not, often other approaches are acceptable.

## Are Responsibilities Defined, Understood and Fulfulled?

Question 3 is quite important. It is essential that all parties, department chairmen, medical staff or departmental committees, the medical staff executive committee, the governing body and support staff—have well defined privilege delineation responsibilities which they understand and fulfill. I want to focus on the department chairman since the primary responsibility for effective privilege delineation often falls here. While this is a multi-step process, the degree to which there is serious attention given to clinical competence often depends on the department chairman—his attitude and personal involvement. We find great variation in the department chairman's understanding of responsibilities and in the degree to which these responsibilities are fulfilled. As more and more attention focuses on the nature and quality of clinical practice in hospitals, the department chairman's capabilities will be an increasingly important ingredient affecting the quality of care. The department chairman's skills are critical to the success of a hospital with regard to the DRG's, professional liability, quality assurance and privilege delineation. It is a problem as we see it in hospitals and, contrary to popular belief, it is an issue for *all* types of hospitals, not just those whose chairmen are elected annually.

### Are Privileges Hospital Specific?

Question 4 highlights the need for privileges to be hospital specific. If a physician has endoscopy privileges in hospital A, should he automatically have them in hospital B? Not necessarily. It depends upon the capabilities of hospital B. As hospitals begins to aggregate more and more into systems there is a tendency for the privilege delineation process to cover multiple institutions even though the capabilities of those institutions to support given services may vary. Our response to this has been to insist that the privilege be hospital specific even though a hospital may operate in a larger organizational context. Ultimately, privilege delineation is a matching of an individual's specific clinical competence with the capacity and capability of the hospital characteristics which vary from one hospital to the next.

### Do You Verify Licensure?

This has been covered adequately in other sections of this book. I simply want to reinforce the importance of tickler files which help keep licensure and licensure verification up-to-date. An important innovation regarding this and the next issue is the use by several hospitals of a local or state-wide process of information-gathering. Often, using a single application form, the agency (often a state or county medical society or a hospital association) gather relevant documents and provide them to participating hospitals for their use in consideration of an applicant.

## Do You Know the Where and What of Training and Experience?

The sixth question affects both the person seeking privileges for the first time at a hospital and for current members of the staff who are asking for new privileges. Do you know not only where training occurred but what happened during that training. In those instances where someone goes away to gain additional training, what, in fact, was the content of the training? Did the person gain new competencies? Was hands-on experience obtained or was it book-learning? Remember, the new applicant or the individual seeking new privileges carries the burden to prove competence. Look into those situations where someone is applying for new privileges, and understand what happened at the two-week or one-month course away from the hospital. It's important!

## Have You Received and Considered Peer Recommendations?

Have you received and considered peer recommendations? It is tough to know the competence of somebody applying for membership for the first time. This is particularly true for types of practitioners not currently practicing at the hospital. Gather substantive information from knowledgeable peers about the individual's diagnostic and therapeutic competence and about that person's ability to work well with colleagues.

## What Do You Know About an Individual's Clinical Competence

Then there is the key question of clinical competence. How does one judge competence? To reach conclusions about competencies you need to know the nature and quality of the professional practice of the individual either before he got to the hospital or during the two years since you last considered him for privileges. If seeking privileges to do procedures, has the individual performed any of those procedures in the last two or three years? While a "no" to that question does not necessarily mean that you should deny privileges, it certainly ought to raise questions about the level of that person's continuing competence. If an individual has not cared for patients with particular important diagnoses, you should know this and raise questions concerning related privileges. In the major areas of practice for which the individual seeks privileges, what are the most important clinical skills—diagnostic and therapeutic, that the doctor ought to possess? Does the applicant have such skills? What information do you have about morbidity and mortality with regard to the individual under consideration? What are the findings from your Quality Asssurance program?

The capability to fully answer these questions implies a degree of sophistication and access to clinical information not possessed by many hospitals. Hospitals must continue to objectify their privilege delineation processes. Table I presents the reasons for doing so.

### Can the Hospital Support the Requested Privileges?

The ninth point is not a requirement of our standards but it is suggested. You ought to consider whether the hospital can support the type of practice that is being requested. Usually this is interpreted to mean the ability to handle a high technology kind of procedures, but it may also be as mundane as "do we have enough room in the operating schedule?"

The relevance of this issue is becoming apparent as hospitals evolve to the types of assessment mechanisms noted in Table 3. It is clear that patient outcomes and the efficiency with which they are achieved is influenced by both clinical and non-clinical processes. It may well be that a competent individual could not apply his/her skills fully if the support systems available in the hospital are not equally competent—a problem that could be created by insufficient or missing technology or personnel. This being the case, privilege delineation processes, over time, encompass sophisticated matching of individual and organizational knowledge and skills.

### Can You Demonstrate That the Process Works?

Finally, does it work? I end with this at the risk of reinforcing conceptions of the JCAHO as an organization obsessed with documentation. As a matter of good management you must know if this important process works. Privilege delineation is a key element of any hospital's effort to provide high quality care. You should assure yourself by periodic reassessment, that the process works well. As I meet with hospitals, I am surprised at how little evidence there is of good, solid review of clinical competence. I see a lot of judgments, and they may be accurate, but there is often no way to prove it.

# Previously Published Papers

# The Credentialing Process: Rational Decisions of Hospital Committees for Granting of Privileges in Gastrointestinal Endoscopic Procedures

James L. Achord, MD

Hospitals, through their Boards of Trustees, are held responsible for the actions of members of their staff, including physicians. Therefore institutions, as well as patients, are directly concerned with the competency of attending physicians. Nowhere is this more obvious than in performance of procedures. Physicians on hospital-credentialing committees perceive no problem in passing judgment on the adequacy of general training programs, but they may have trouble in subspecialty areas different from their own, or if that training has not been in a formally structured program leading to Board certification. For privileges in procedures, such committees generally have not placed enough emphasis on the importance of the cognitive training required for maximally safe and effective performance. If eligibility for certification has not been obtained, how are they to judge? Further, on what authority can they and the hospital (and its attorneys) rely to resist the very considerable pressure often brought on them to grant privileges in gastrointestinal (GI) procedures that they may suspect are not justified by the evidence of experience presented?

The problem, of course, is multfaceted. Successful completion of training programs in both general residency and subspecialty fields approved by the Accreditation Council for Graduate Medical Education (ACGME) implies, but does not explicitly define, competency in appropriate cognitive and certain procedural skills. Certification by the independent respective Boards defines a certain cognitive level but does not explicitly define competency in treating patients and does not address expertise in procedures. Approved programs do not train everyone to do every procedure available in gastroenterology. Specifically, many trainees from excellent programs have little or no essential hands-on experience in certain invasive procedures such as sphinctorotomy or placement of biliary stents. There is currently a strong move to require another year of special training for high-risk invasive endoscopic procedures. Therefore, clinical privileges, at least for procedures, should not be based solely on completion of some form of training program or on Board certification. Decisions must be based on demonstrated ability formally certified by the training program director. On strong recommendation of the GI Boards and under scrutiny of the program review activities of the ACGME, program directors now require GI trainees to log their experience wth procedures in much the same way as surgical trainees have done for years. Directors are required to certify these experiences and to document formal and periodic evaluation of the progress of their charges. Director's signatures are legally valid, and each is held responsible of the competency for their graduates.

Although those who are Board eligible in gastroenterology are not considered to be a problem for credentials committees, an indication of the procedures for which adequate experience has been gained by an applicant physician should be obtained and clinical privileges granted only in those for which the individual has been trained. Expertise in one procedure, such as upper endoscopy, does not define competency in another, such as colonscopy, despite the similar instrument technology.

It should be evident that not every physician who is trained to do so will want to perform procedures. Many excellent gastroenterologists prefer to concentrate their clinical efforts entirely in the cognitive aspects of our discipline. The GI Board expects candidates to be competent in upper and lower endoscopy, including biopsy and polypectomy, peroral small bowel and percutaneous liver biopsies, and esophageal dilation.

A major problem faced by credentials committees, however, is not the physician who has completed a formal training program in GI, but the one who wants to do gastrointestinal endoscopy and has not been through formalized training. It is clear that many have availed themselves of alternate pathways to competency, especially in the not so distant past, and it is not reasonable (or legal) to arbitrarily exclude them as a class. Indeed, many respected and widely published endoscopists fall into this category. What, then, are the minimal requirements that ensure a reasonably high probability of competency in GI procedures and justify the granting of hospital privileges? Some defensible *minimal* criteria must be available. The American Society for Gastrointestinal Endoscopy (ASGE) for some years has published guidelines approved by the American College of Gastroenterology (ACG) and the American Gastroenterologic Association (AGA), but these have had considerably less impact than they deserve. The American College of Physicians (ACP) has addressed this problem through its Clinical Privileges Project, the first two efforts of which are in gastroenterology and nephrology, and are now complete. The GI subcommittee included representatives of the ACG, the AGA, and the ASGE. The publication of the official statement of this project (GI) will appear in the *Annals of Internal Medicine*. It includes only four procedures: upper endoscopy, lower endoscopy, endoscopic retrograde cholangiopancreatography, and flexible sigmoidoscopy. It defines the currently accepted methods of training in GI endoscopy and points out that short courses with little or no "hands-on" experience are no longer considered an acceptable alternative path to competency, not only because such training it usually inadequate to allow for the immediate development of necessary manual skills, but also because it does not provide the necessary knowledge base with which to use them. It also addresses the problem of "old hands acquiring new skills."

It is important to note that, like all minimal criteria for competency, this statement requires thoughtful consideration in each case of application for hospital privileges. In recognition of the importance of the cognitive requirements necessary for safe and effective use of these instruments, the statement includes essentials of indications and contraindications for a very limited number of commonly used procedures. It is clearly intended neither to be comprehensive nor to be used as a standard of practice for any particular patient, especially in this rapidly changing field.

I recommend this statement to all credentials committees that have heretofore relied more on instinct, self-preservation, friendships, and allegiance to the profession to make their decisions—reasons that are sometimes difficult to defend.

James L. Achord, M.D., F.A.C.P., F.A.C.G.
*University of Mississippi Medical Center*
*Jackson, MS*

# Medical Staff Appointment and Delineation of Pediatric Privileges in Hospitals

American Academy of Pediatrics
Committee on Hospital Care

Medical staff credentialing, including the delineation of clinical privileges for each staff member, represents a cornerstone in the hospital quality assurance program. The process involves the evaluation and verification of a practitioner's professional competence and conduct based on his/her education and training, previous professional experience, personal background, and peer assessment. Once the practitioner's credentials have been confirmed and approved, clinical privileges are extended by the hospital, matching the practitioner's documented competence and skills with the standards and resources of the institution.

Because of the many significant differences between individual hospitals (ie, size, services provided, geographic location, population served, organization of the medical staff, fiscal and administrative characteristics), no one method for credentialing is universally applicable. The medical staff of each hospital is therefore responsible for establishing its own procedures for credentialing. There are certain elements, however, required in each hospital's credentialing process:

1. It must be thorough, fair, and timely and involve unbiased and good-faith peer review. Any possible malicious use of the peer review process is not acceptable.
2. The entire credentialing process must be clearly described in the medical staff bylaws. Included in this description should be mechanisms for



**145**

appeal and guaranteed due process for disputes concerning disciplinary actions and for changes in or revocation of privileges. The medical staff bylaws should also incorporate provisions of the federal Health Care Quality Improvement Act of 1986 as well as reference provisions of applicable state laws, to help achieve or describe available immunities and protection for the hospital and peer review committee members from various legal liabilities.

3. Criteria for specific clinical privileges must be well-defined, based on realistic national as well as local standards, updated at reasonable intervals to reflect advances in medicine, and used equitably for all applicants.

4. Confidentiality and protection against discoverability of information used in credentialing and peer review, subject to applicable law, must be incorporated in the process and adhered to rigidly.

5. The process should take into account the standards and characteristics recommended by the Joint Commission,[1] the Hospital Medical Staff Section of the American Medical Association, and state and/or federal regulatory agencies. Under state tort reform, for example, it is possible that a hospital may be required to report a termination or restriction of a medical practitioner's clinical privileges to the state medical licensing or disciplinary board.

6. The process must not allow conflicts of interest (economic or otherwise) to impair due process or duties the hospital may have under applicable law in managing the credentialing process.

When performed in an objective, systematic, thorough, and timely manner, the credentialing process is distinctly beneficial to the patient, the hospital, and the physician alike. The intent is to help protect the patient from receiving treatment by an incompetent or unqualified practitioner; to reasonably ensure that all members of the hospital's medical staff are clinically proficient, ethically sound, and capable of providing quality care that satisfies patients and reduces grounds for complaints or legal action; to provide the practitioner with a fair assessment of his/her clinical acumen, an assignment of hospital privileges that are consistent with his/her training and experience, and the right to an appeal and good-faith due process if disagreement arises.

## Credentialing Principles

The credentialing authority of the hospital to grant, change, or revoke clinical privileges is based on several principles.

1. The practice of medicine (pediatrics) within a hospital is not a right

of every physician, but rather a privilege extended by the hospital in accordance with applicable law.

2. The hospital (and its governing board) is legally and morally responsible for the safety of its patients and the quality of care provided by its staff.[2]

3. The hospital must ensure that all members of its health care team are competent and qualified to provide the services for which they have been granted privileges.

4. The organized medical staff of the hospital is entrusted by the governing board with the responsibility of recommending only competent practitioners to treat patients in the hospital. To meet this obligation in the credentialing of physicians, dentists and allied health professionals, the credentialing process should provide for *(a)* investigating and assessing the professional and personal backgrounds of every practitioner applying for privileges; *(b)* recommending to the governing board approval or denial of applicants, with assignments of specific levels of privileges appropriate for their training and experience; *(c)* monitoring of professional activities of each member of the medical staff through programs of quality assurance, utilization review, and risk management; and, *(d)* timely reappointment of each member of the medical staff based on ongoing assessment of performance measured by preapproved and published standards.

## Levels of Review Within the Hospital

To ensure that each applicant for medical staff membership is evaluated fairly and granted (or not granted) appropriate practice privileges, it is essential that multiple levels of review be included in the credentialing process. These different levels should specifically allow for professional peers with similar training and background to have meaningful input into the review. In small or rural hospitals, adequate peer review may require the involvement of physicians outside of the medical staff, but within the county or state medical societies. In large general hospitals, review by peers from medical disciplines other than that of the applicants may be needed to broaden the perspective of the credentialing process. Finally, when a candidate applies for practice privileges that extend beyond the purview of a single discipline, parallel credentialing by the separate departments involved may be required. In general, the credentialing process should include multilevel review by at least three of the following individuals or groups: department chairman, department credentials committee, hospital medical staff credentials committee, medical director, the medical staff executive committee, professional activities committee of the institution (often a subcommittee of the board of governors), and for final approval the governing board of the hospital.

The remainder of this statement examines in more depth the initial appointment process, the delineation of clinical privileges, and the reappointment process. Also, for ease of reference for the reader, a credentialing check-off list and a sample form for the delineation of clinical privileges are appended for use as a possible guideline should the hospital judge it appropriate.

### Initial Appointment

When applying to a hospital for the first time, a practitioner goes through two processes: the initial appointment and the granting of initial clinical privileges through a delineation of clinical privileges. The applicant's training, experience, and qualifications are closely examined, verified, and reviewed by peers. The applicant applies for one of several categories within the medical staff. In the process of applying, each practitioner who seeks staff membership must demonstrate the qualifications listed below, both at the time of appointment and continuously throughout his/her tenure on the medical staff.

### Licensure

A currently valid state license to practice medicine, dentistry, or the appropriate health care affiliation must be presented, unless this requirement is waived by the hospital board of governors in accordance with applicable law. Applicants should be required to report any loss of previ-

---

### Table 1. Initial Appointment Checklist

- ☐ Valid, verified state license.
- ☐ Drug Enforcement Administration number filed.
- ☐ Verification of Professional education and training.
- ☐ Board certification status.
- ☐ Felony convictions/loss or surrender of license to practice.
- ☐ Hospital suspensions/resignations.
- ☐ Letters of recommendation (number specified in bylaws).
- ☐ Alcohol/drug use/suspension: rehabilitation program verification.
- ☐ Health status listed and confirmed.
- ☐ Verification of medical liability insurance (if required).
- ☐ Release of liability form signed.

ous or current state licensure, including denials, probations, involuntary removal for disciplinary reasons, or the voluntary relinquishment of such licensure. Similarly, the practitioner's Drug Enforcement Administration certificate and number should be submitted along with information regarding any previous denials, revocations, changes, or voluntary relinquishment. The applicant should also be requested to provide details about any official sanctioning action.

## Professional Background and Performance

Professional education, training, and experience should be outlined by the applicants. The medical staff should request any additional information regarding clinical experience (eg, gaps in clinical experience, results of inpatient care) which will further assure the medical staff that the applicant is capable of providing quality patient care. Applicants must provide the following information: board certification/recertification; all professional experience including sabbaticals, leaves of absence, missionary work, military assignments, etc; medical society memberships, again including denials, revocations, terminations, or disciplinary actions; letters of recommendations from peers familiar with the applicant; concerns or unclear information should be further explored by telephone or written followup; filed, pending, or settled medical litigation involving the applicant, with confirming information provided by the practitioner's attorney or from court records; unfavorable peer reviews at previous or other currently used hospitals; felony convictions; voluntary/involuntary reduction of clinical privileges elsewhere; and voluntary/involuntary hospital staff resignations, suspensions, denials, or changes with explanation.

Verification of all submitted information by the hospital on behalf of the medical staff should be from primary sources, whenever feasible. In situations where the hospital contracts with a separate independent agency to collect information from the primary source(s) about the applicant, this arrangement is satisfactory as long as the hospital contracts with the agency and the agency gives the hospital all the information provided by the primary source. The hospital itself can then use this information to verify the information from the applicant.

In addition to information submitted by the applicant, hospitals are encouraged to seek additional information concerning the applicant from other sources, such as the American Medical Association's Physician Masterfile and the Federation of State Medical Boards Physician Disciplinary Data Bank (Fort Worth, Texas). With the institution of the Health Care Quality Improvement Act of 1986,[3] the development of a centralized data bank for physician quality assurance information is anticipated in 1989. These sources allow for further verification of information supplied by the applicant.

Causes for further investigation within the applicant review process should include high mobility of the applicant, graduation from a medical school of uncertain reputation, medical litigation, and professional disciplinary actions. In some instances there may be need for extensive written documentation and verification by telephone or other means. Throughout the credentialing process, the granting of appropriate privileges requires careful documentation to ensure that the applicant has the specific training and experience to perform the procedures and treat the diseases requested. Care should be taken in areas in which proficiency and safety are attained and maintained only by continuing experience. When delineation of privileges is based primarily on experience, adequate documentation of specific experience and successful results should be requested and verified.

## Attitude

All applicants should have demonstrated by their current attitude and performance their willingness and capability to work with and relate to other medical staff members, house staff and students (when applicable), members of other health care disciplines, hospital administration and employees, visitors, and the general community in a cooperative, professional manner essential to maintaining a hospital environment appropriate to quality patient care; participate equitably in the discharge of medical staff obligations appropriate to the assigned medical staff membership category; and adhere to recognized standards of professional ethics that prohibit, without limitation, illegal financial inducements and arrangements related to patient referral or treatment, delegation of responsibility for diagnosis or care of patients to a practitioner not qualified to undertake that responsibility, or failure to obtain informed patient consent to treatments when appropriate.

## Health Status

The applicant should be free of or have under adequate control any significant physical or behavioral impairment that could interfere with his/her qualification to provide optimal medical care. At the initial appointment, the medical staff should confirm satisfactory health status while respecting individual privacy. Any previous or current substance/alcohol abuse as well as enrollments in "impaired physician" or other treatment programs must be reported subject to state law at the initial application and on subsequent reappointment requests. When applicable, the applicant should submit documentation of successful completion of an impaired physician treatment program.

### Ability to Accommodate Hospital and Community Need

Hospital medical staff membership status and changes in clinical privileges are subject to the decision of the governing board. This decision is based, in part, on consideration of current and projected patient care, teaching, and research needs, as well as the hospital's ability to provide the facilities, staffed beds, and support services that will be required if the initial application is acted upon favorably. In addition, the effect, if any, that the addition of the applicant will have on the elective surgery schedule or on the availability of other hospital facilities must be taken into full consideration prior to final decision.

### Professional Liability Insurance

The hospital may require that each applicant be covered by a minimum limit of medical liability insurance from an acceptable insurer as a condition of membership on the medical staff. The applicant should be required to report any settled or pending medical litigation as well as the names of insurance carriers involved.

### Release of Liability

For the purpose of verifying information supplied in the application, the applicant should sign a statement releasing the hospital and references/sources from liability, assuming that the investigation of the applicant's background is done in good faith.

### Categories of Staff Membership

Although considered optional by the Joint Commission, most hospitals list various categories of membership, defined according to the role and hospital utilization of the practitioner. These categories have various names, such as Active, Courtesy, Associate, Senior, Consulting, Attending, Honorary, Adjunct, or Special. Resident or house staff designations may also be included. (In accordance with various state laws and the individual hospital, licensed independent practitioners may include psychologists, podiatrists, physician assistants, nurse practitioners, and others. Their role, breadth of practice, and supervision should be defined in the medical staff bylaws.)

For all categories, a defined initial period of provisional, probationary, or temporary status is important to allow for direct observation and validation of the practitioner's procedural skills, patient management style, and manner of care. When evaluating competency, direct observation of clinical skills is particularly useful in monitoring new members of the medical staff. Clinical data and patient care review (chart review) provide the basis for advancement decisions under peer review at the end of the provisional period. Specific written policies governing extensions of provisionary status, including the length of time and number of extensions allowed, should be included in the bylaws.

In most states where tort reform has been enacted, it is now required that the same standards applied to granting of provisionary or other categories of medical staff privileges also be applied to granting temporary privileges. Despite frequent pressures from medical staff members to conveniently provide temporary privileges (often in unreasonably short periods), temporary privileges should not be allowed until the requirements listed in the medical staff bylaws are satisfied completely.

## Use of Criteria

The methods for granting or restricting medical privileges should be reasonable, noncapricious, and avoid reliance on subjective impressions. Irrelevant, arbitrary, or inconsistent criteria should be avoided, and the criteria that are used should not be applied inconsistently to different individuals. Criteria must be avoided that are based on sex, race, creed, or national origin; membership in certain professional societies; or membership in a prepaid, closed-panel group practice. Courts have decided in favor of physicians who have sued hospitals when their appointments or clinical privileges were denied on the basis of such inappropriate criteria.

Privileges should not depend on any single criterion such as board certification or membership in a specialty society. Physicians from various specialties may rightfully be allowed to treat the same diseases and perform the same procedures if they meet appropriate criteria. Jurisdictional disputes should be discouraged in favor of rational granting of privileges. However, specialty board qualification and certification may serve as useful benchmarks in granting privileges.

Criteria should relate reasonably to standards of patient care and/or to the objectives and purposes of the institution. Several items beyond the scope of this statement have been reviewed elsewhere; exclusive arrangements between hospitals and physicians; exclusion of physicians on the basis of unavailable bed space or overabundance of certain specialists; moral, ethical and behavioral considerations; and the relationship of privileging to antitrust laws.

## Care of Children/Adolescents by Nonpediatrician Physicians

In hospitals where there is no organized pediatric department, the care of most children and adolescents will be managed by physicians other than pediatricians. Similarly, in many institutions where there are pediatric departments, children and adolescents may be cared for by specialists or generalists whose orientation may also include adult care.

At least two approaches to credentialing such physicians are in use: (1) each individual department credentials its own members, with approval by the Medical Staff Credentials Committee and/or Medical Staff Executive Committee, and (2) each department credentials its members with recommendations by the pediatric department as it applies to the care of children and adolescents. In either situation, each specialty could develop a listing of procedures and patient care situations (based on complexity of illness) involving children and adolescents, both specific to that specialty. For an example of such a listing, see Appendix II. Each department could then define what training and experience would be necessary to perform those procedures and/or provide a particular level of care.

Regardless of which approach is used, it is essential that the written guidelines within the hospital credentialing manual and/or medical staff bylaws be developed. It is essential that methods for granting or restricting medical privileges be reasonable and noncapricious and not be based on a single criterion such as board certification or membership in a specific medical specialty. Requirements for board certification, however, can serve as a good benchmark for use in determining such requirements.

When credentialing involves privileges considered within the purview of more than one department, the communication between departments and the role of the department chairman become critical.

## Due Pocess

Should a hospital organization decide to deny initial appointment or reappointment—or deny, curtail, or suspend privileges—it is imperative that due process and equal protection are provided in accordance with customary legal principles and, where appropriate, hospital bylaws. Two types of due process exist: substantive and procedural. Substantive due process is concerned with whether the rules and criteria stipulated in the bylaws are reasonable, fair, and not arbitrary, and whether the decisions made by a hospital medical staff or hearing panel are based on "substantial evidence," on the weight of relevant and reliable evidence, and only on that evidence which is presented to the medical staff or hearing panel. In various states, the courts may be unable to overturn a peer review decision that is supported by substantial evidence. Procedural due process is concerned with whether such rules are administered properly and applied equally to all staff members. A formal appeals process must be available to each candidate. In view of increasing litigation in this area, consultation with an attorney may help to guarantee due process before the final action is taken.

## Licensed Independent Practitioners

Interest on the part of licensed independent practitioners (exclusive of physicians and dentists) in obtaining hospital clinical privileges and medical staff membership, as opposed to affiliation only, is increasing. Many such professionals are being trained to provide services previously provided only by physicians. The evolving status of hospital privileges for these groups has been reviewed. The responsibility of the hospital organization to allow only competent individuals to engage in hospital health care also extends to this category of practitioner. Membership on the medical staff, subject to state law or regulation, is limited to physicians and dentists. However, all licensed independent practitioners should be credentialed through the regular physician staff mechanism, and final roles and functions should be recommended by the medical staff. The licensed independent practitioners must comply with the hospital bylaws, rules, and regulations.

Licensed independent practitioners should be assigned to appropriate clinical departments and should be subject to departmental policies. It may be appropriate for the staff bylaws to provide for staff affiliate status. Continuous monitoring of the nonphysician health professional's hospital activity should be implemented, as well as a mechanism for renewal of privileges. In the case of physician-sponsored practitioners, supervision should be defined consistent with authorization both by the law and by the hospital. It is recommended that any reappointment of licensed independent practitioners be done in conjunction with the sponsoring physician.

## Delineation of Clinical Privileges

The delineation of clinical privileges allows each medical staff applicant to request an individualized listing of hospital activities that the practitioner wishes to define as the nature of his or her hospital practice. In general, a request to the hospital governing board is made for a list of specific procedures and/or defined risk categories of care, allowing the practitioner to declare the breadth and depth of clinical services that he or she intends to provide in the hospital inpatient and outpatient setting. Guidelines for the delineation of clinical privileges are provided in the *Accreditation Manual for Hospitals*,[4] Standard MS.4 and Required Characteristics MS.4.1 through MS.4.6.

A precisely defined and specified structure and process for the delineation of clinical privileges is not provided by the Joint Commission. This process must be clearly defined in the medical staff bylaws for each individual hospital, using the guidelines established by the Joint Commission under MS.4.

Some of the essential elements to be considered in defining a hospital's delineation of clinical privileges include the following:

1. It must be assumed that each practitioner will practice within the scope of his or her skills and request consultation where appropriate.

2. Requests should be made based upon each applicant's individually documented training and practice experience.

3. Departmental recommendations must be based upon objective peer review of the application using criteria and guidelines clearly written into the medical staff bylaws or covered in the departmental rules and regulations.

4. Review and recommendations made by the department and criteria specified in the medical staff bylaws are consistently and uniformly applied to all applicants.

5. Qualifications of applicants requesting privileges must be verified by an individual familiar with the applicant's training and/or prior practice experience (eg, program director, practice colleague, or chief of staff from previous hospitals). As with other verifications at the initial appointment, all verification of requests must be from a primary source, whenever feasible.

6. Subject to applicable law, all requests must be discussed with strict confidentiality only within formal credentialing proceedings. The results of deliberations and recommendations by the department to the board of governors likewise should be handled in a confidential fashion.

7. Where potential departmental overlap might exist in the provision on any given clinical service or procedure, written guidelines within

the hospital credentialing manual or medical staff bylaws should be developed. These areas can be identified and resolved by the chairman of the respective departments.

8. Criteria upon which delineation of clinical privileges are based must be applied uniformly to all membership categories without bias toward, or prejudice against, any given group (that is, toward physicians, nonphysician providers, active or courtesy members). This guideline will ensure that the general public has access to a reasonable standard of hospital care based uniformly upon the qualification of the individual to provide that care.

## New Procedures/New Technology

Many new procedures, drugs, and clinical treatments become available each year due to rapidly advancing technology. The development of credentialing and implementation guidelines for new advances is essential to ensure uniform and quality application of the new technology. Besides developing specific criteria and qualifications for a new procedure or technology, the medical staff may recommend an on-site educational course or medical staff orientation to further familiarize the staff with the new application. The principles of objectivity and uniform application toward all practitioners on staff must be assured in credentialing a new technology.

## Different Approaches to Delineation

Because the Joint Commission does not specify precisely how delineation of clinical privileges must be accomplished practically, several different approaches have evolved.

### Category

Most often this delineation is based along specialty lines. Because no strict definition of the breadth of specialties exist and due to the variation between training programs concerning emphasis in certain areas of any given specialty, the bylaws should carefully define these limits when this method is employed.

### List

Although it is most adaptable to defining clinical privileges where procedures are involved, the "laundry list" approach is less adaptable where diagnoses or diseases are to be delineated mainly because of infinite number of possibilities to be anticipated.

## Severity/Complexity of Care

This approach is particularly adaptable to defining diseases to be treated, not by specific type but by the general severity of illness.

## Hybrid

Judging from methods most frequently used by hospitals today, a combination of the previously discussed methods is most often used in delineating the care provided to children.

An example of a delineation of clinical privileges is provided in Appendix I. The reader is encouraged to utilize this example in creating a format that is adaptable to the individual characteristics of his or her own medical staff.

## Monitoring Compliance

Compliance with defined privileges must be assured by all members of the medical staff in conjunction with the departmental chairman, medical director, or chief of staff. Privilege monitoring also occurs through the medical staff quality assurance program (eg, monitoring and evaluation of the quality and appropriateness of care) and may occur through the institution of an appropriate joint conference committee. Ready access to the credentialing files of medical staff members must be assured for the immediate use by the medical director, chief of staff, or designate should some question concerning privileges arise.

## Reappointment, Renewal, and Modification of Clinical Privileges

The reappointment process directs the routine reassessment of each medical staff member's hospital privileges. The process not only updates information submitted with the initial appointment request, but also adds the dimension of peer review of the individual practitioner's activities within the hospital since the last regular review period.

Many of the characteristics of the reappointment process resemble the initial appointment.

1. The Joint Commission delineated guidelines for the process of reappointment and reappraisal of privileges as found in Standard MS.5

and Required Characteristics MS.5.1 through MS.5.8 in the *Accreditation Manual for Hospitals.*[4]

2. The process of reappointment must be fully outlined and disclosed within the medical staff bylaws.

3. The medical staff, after review of the practitioner's record, makes a recommendation of acceptance, denial, or modification to the hospital board of governors, which in turn acts upon the recommendation. The governing board makes the final decision within the reappointment process.

The reappointment process also provides for the routine interaction between the hospital's medical staff quality assurance and credentialing programs. The process must occur at least every 2 years. The role of the department chairman or his/her designee in assuring that the reappointment system is fair, objective, and smoothly administered is crucial.

### Request for Appointment

The content of the reappointment request must be clearly defined in the medical staff bylaws. At a minimum, requests should require information from the practitioner in the following areas:

- Do you wish to be reappointed to the medical staff?
- Medical staff category requested (ie, active, courtesy, etc) as delineated in the medical staff bylaws.
- State licensure verification.
- Drug Enforcement Administration verification by submission of a copy of the current Drug Enforcement Administration certificate.
- Previously successful or currently pending challenges to licensure or Drug Enforcement Administration registration, including voluntary relinquishments of licensure or registration.
- Malpractice coverage verification if required for medical staff membership.
- Current status of medical liability suits filed, pending, and settled during the reappointment interval.
- Sanctions received (from medical disciplinary board, state licensing board, Professional Review Organization, etc).
- Any felony convictions since previous appointment.
- Change in medical staff membership and clinical privilege status at other hospitals where the practitioner is affiliated. Voluntary relinquishments or reductions of hospital privileges should be included in this request for change in status.
- Listing of all hospitals where privileges are currently or formerly maintained during the reappointment interval.

- Health status (ie, do health conditions exist that impair the practitioner's ability to practice?).
- Release of liability form signed, which should allow the hospital to verify that the practitioner supplied information as being correct.

This information should be supplied by the practitioner to the hospital in a timely fashion to allow for processing and peer review to occur before the end of the reappointment interval. In most hospitals, the information is reviewed in the same manner as during the initial appointment. It is reviewed first by the department, then by the credentialing committee, and finally by the medical staff executive committee prior to consideration and action by the governing board. Before any committee review, independent verification of accurate information is made by the hospital with the state licensure board, medical disciplinary board, and any other agency required by the medical staff bylaws.

## Individual Practitioner Clinical Activity Profile

Information regarding the practitioner's hospital activities within the reappointment interval is collected by the hospital's quality assurance program as well as other sources. When compiled, this information becomes the basis for the practitioner clinical activity profile. The AAP Committee on Hospital Care recommends that this be held confidential and nondiscoverable. The practitioner clinical profile and the request for reappointment

---

**Table 2. Reappointment Materials and Verification Checklist**

- ☐ Reappointment request completed and filed.
- ☐ Valid state licensure verification.
- ☐ Current Drug Enforcement Administration certificate and verification.
- ☐ Malpractice insurance verification (if required).
- ☐ Listing of medical liability suits: filed/pending/settled.
- ☐ Sanctions filed by medical disciplinary board, professional review organization, or state licensing board, if any.
- ☐ Felony convictions (if any).
- ☐ Change in delineated privileges (this hospital or any other) requested, listed, and verified.
- ☐ Listing of hospitals where privileges held.
- ☐ Health status listed/confirmed (if required).
- ☐ Release of liability signed.

form the basis for interaction between the hospital quality assurance system and the renewal of clinical privileges within the medical staff credentialing system.

The Committee on Hospital Care recommends that the following information be made available and reviewed: monthly medical staff monitoring and evaluation of the practitioner's clinical activities, surgical case review, drug usage evaluation, medical record review function, blood usage review, infection control information, utilization review, and mortality review. In addition, if specific areas of concern arise or information suggests an undesirable practice trend, the committee may request more specific information or ask to do a focused review of a larger sample of the practitioner's work.

### Individual Practitioner Clinical Activity Profile—Courtesy Staff

When a practitioner seldom uses a particular hospital facility, it is often difficult to generate a meaningful clinical profile at reappointment time. If the committee raises concerns about the granting of privileges to individuals who very seldom use the hospital, the committee may want to request a letter from the hospital principally used by the practitioner attesting to his active status in good standing in the areas of the clinical privileges requested. With the current trend of credentialing becoming more performance-based and outcome-driven, the practice of sharing hospital experiences, subject to applicable law, may become even more common place in the case of active staff membership.

### Medical Staff Review

Once the request for reappointment and the clinical activity profile are complete, the information is presented to the department or hospital credentials committee and opened to peer review. When requests for changes in clinical privileges arise, they can be reviewed and acted upon by the department and medical staff credentials committee.

Irregularities of the clinical activity profile may distinguish an individual's practice from the departmental norm. Once information is verified and the consensus of peer review suggest that irregularities do exist, additional information or explanation must be requested by the department chairman. The following guidelines should be followed to assure due process:

1. Always use hospital stationery and certified mail when corresponding with the practitioner.

2. Ensure that copies of any correspondence are not circulated outside the quality assurance system.
3. Do not include the patient name in any correspondence. Use other patient identifiers, such as social security or patient identification number.
4. State objectively the specific issues raised by the committee.
5. Always include a specific date for response.
6. Sign the letter after personal review for accuracy.
7. The practitioner's response should be received promptly by the committee.
8. After ratification and modification by the medical staff executive committee, the results of the review should be communicated in writing to the practitioner and also to the governing board, outlining the action plan and recommendations.

At any point in this process, the practitioner may appear before committees as designated in the due process portion of the medical staff bylaws. The committee should assist the practitioner in whatever way necessary and assure that all the issues raised and all information reviewed by the committee also be available to the practitioner.

The committee should be provided legal counsel by the hospital at all levels of the review process. The practitioner should be advised to consider obtaining his/her own legal representation.[3] (*Patrick v Burget*, 108 Sct 1658 (1988)).

Adverse action leading to a due process hearing procedure is an uncommon occurrence in most hospitals. The majority of concerns can be handled in such a way that consensus outcome and recommendation occur or voluntary solutions are designed and implemented.

The role of the chairman is crucial. Fairness, objectivity, assurance of peer review, and confidential dealings within the medical staff and the hospital are key considerations that must be protected and upheld at all times by the chairman and medical staff members.

COMMITTEE ON HOSPITAL CARE, 1989 TO 1990
David L. Dudgeon, MD, Chairman
Margaret C. Heagarty, MD
Michael A. Hogan, MD
Robert E. Myers, MD
James E. Shira, MD
Richard S. Wolf, MD

Liaison Representatives
Fred T. Brown, Jr, American Hospital Association
John B. Coombs, MD, American Academy of Family Physicians

Barbara-Jeanne Seabury, Association for the Care of Children's Health
Paul M. Schyve, MD, Joint Commission on Accreditation of Healthcare Organizations

AAP Section Liaison
Russell C. Raphaely, MD, Section on Critical Care Medicine
Theodore Striker, MD, Section on Anesthesiology
Consultant
Gerald Merenstein, MD

## Appendix I

### Pediatric Severity Categories: Delineation of Clinical Privileges

This delineation-of-privileges form is a sample for possible use in the independent judgment of a hospital. Application of this delineation form can be made to both the in-patient and out-patient settings in hospitals. This sample should be adapted to meet the individual needs of a specific hospital.

Departments other than the pediatrics department may adapt this format in delineating privileges applicable to the care of children within their specialty.

Select the category that best describes the severity of illness you expect to treat independently within the hospital and for which you are qualified to apply on the basis of your training or experience.

The assignment of actual disease categories should be created within each individual hospital, and it should be recognized that all staff physicians are granted privileges to perform emergency life-saving procedures. *Please check appropriate box.*

☐ Category I.  Treatment of illness, injuries, or conditions or the performance of procedures that carry low risk for the patient. *Criterion.* Training and experience with these conditions. Physician and nonphysician eligibility.

   ☐ <10  No. of children treated in this category.
   ☐ 10–50
   ☐ >50

☐ Category II.  Treatment of major or complicated illnesses, injuries or conditions in children with no significant risk to life. *Criterion.* Significant training in pediatrics. Experience in the care of these conditions. Board certification in pediatrics is not necessary.

      ☐ < 10  No. of children treated in this category.
      ☐ 10–50
      ☐ > 50

☐ Category III.  Treatment of major and/or complicated illnesses or performance of procedures that do carry a significant threat to life.

      *Criterion.* Extensive training and/or documentable experience in the care of these conditions. Board certification/eligibility with active (defined in the departmental rules and regulations) pursuit of certification in pediatrics a key benchmark.

      ☐ < 10  No. of children treated in this category.
      ☐ 10–50
      ☐ > 50

☐ Category IV.  Treatment of unusually complex or critical illnesses, injuries, or conditions or the provision of procedures for those that carry a serious threat to life.

      *Criterion.* Extensive post residency or subspecialty training or experience beyond board certification in pediatrics a key benchmark.

      ☐ < 10  No. of children treated in this category.
      ☐ 10–50
      ☐ > 50

**Newborn Severity Categories: Delineation of Clinical Privileges**

This delineation of privileges form is a sample for possible use in the independent judgment of a hospital. Application of this delineation form can be made to both the in-patient and out-patient settings in hospitals. This sample should be adapted to meet the individual needs of a specific hospital.

Departments other than the pediatrics department may adapt this format in delineating privileges applicable to the care of children within their specialty.

Select the category that best describes the severity of illness you expect to treat independently within the hospital and for which you are qualified to apply on the basis of training and experience. *Please check the appropriate box.*

☐ Category I.   Normal newborn care—uncomplicated.

      *Criterion.* As in Pediatric Severity Categories: Category I.

☐ >10  No. of children treated in this category.
☐ 0–50
☐ >50

☐ Category II.  Care of all newborns, including those with complicated but nonlife-threatening problems.
*Criterion.* As in Pediatric Severity Categories: Category II.
☐ <10  No. of children treated in this category.
☐ 10–50
☐ >50

☐ Category III.  Care of all newborns, including those with potentially life-threatening illnesses.
*Criterion.* As in Pediatric Severity Categories: Category III.
☐ <10  No. of children treated in this category.
☐ 10–50
☐ >50

☐ Category IV.  Care of all newborns, including those with any life-threatening condition.
*Criterion.* Subspecialty or significant postgraduate training beyond pediatric board certification (such as specialty qualified/certified neonatologist, pediatric cardiologist).
☐ >10  No. of children treated in this category.
☐ 10–50
☐ >50

## Appendix II

Hometown Medical Center: Delineation of Procedures/Privileges—
Department of Pediatrics

**Name** _______________________________________________

***Instructions:*** Place a check in Column 1 corresponding to the clinical privileges requested and provide the additional information requested in Column 2. Use a separate sheet if necessary.

| Procedure/Disease Classification | To Be Completed by Applicant | | Recommendations and Comment |
| --- | --- | --- | --- |
| | 1<br>Privileges Requested | 2<br>No. of Times Performed Within Past ☐ Months | |
| **Catheterization** | | | |
| Umbilical catheterization | ______ | ______ | ______ |
| Right heart (Swan-Ganz) | ______ | ______ | ______ |
| Cardiac | ______ | ______ | ______ |
| Insertion of Subclavian Catheter | ______ | ______ | ______ |
| Central line placement | ______ | ______ | ______ |
| Venous cutdown | ______ | ______ | ______ |
| Percutaneous arterial line placement | ______ | ______ | ______ |
| Peripheral arterial cutdown | ______ | ______ | ______ |
| ______ | ______ | ______ | ______ |
| ______ | ______ | ______ | ______ |
| ______ | ______ | ______ | ______ |
| **Other** | | | |
| Spinal tap | ______ | ______ | ______ |
| Hemo & peritoneal dialysis | ______ | ______ | ______ |
| Fluid/electrolyte management | ______ | ______ | ______ |
| EKG reading | ______ | ______ | ______ |
| EEG reading | ______ | ______ | ______ |
| EMG reading | ______ | ______ | ______ |
| Electrocardioversion other than during CPR | ______ | ______ | ______ |
| Temporary transvenous pacemaker placement | ______ | ______ | ______ |
| Order & monitoring of psychotropic drugs | ______ | ______ | ______ |
| Circumcision (neonatal) | ______ | ______ | ______ |
| Minor laceration repair | ______ | ______ | ______ |
| Incision & drainage of abscess | ______ | ______ | ______ |

## Appendix II—continued

Hometown Medical Center: Delineation of Procedures/Privileges—
Department of Pediatrics

**Name** ___________________________________________

*Instructions:* Place a check in Column 1 corresponding to the clinical privileges requested and provide the additional information requested in Column 2. Use a separate sheet if necessary.

| Procedure/Disease Classification | To Be Completed by Applicant | | Recommendations and Comment |
|---|---|---|---|
| | 1 Privileges Requested | 2 No. of Times Performed Within Past ☐ Months | |
| Chest tubes | _______ | _______ | _______ |
| Ventilator care | _______ | _______ | _______ |
| Vasoactive drug drip | _______ | _______ | _______ |
| Intubation | _______ | _______ | _______ |
| Exchange transfusion | _______ | _______ | _______ |
| _______ | _______ | _______ | _______ |
| _______ | _______ | _______ | _______ |
| _______ | _______ | _______ | _______ |
| _______ | _______ | _______ | _______ |
| _______ | _______ | _______ | _______ |

The above sample format constitutes only one of several alternate approaches. Others utilize patient diagnosis and severity of illness as a means of delineating clinical privileges. Regardless of the format selected, each hospital must define criteria sufficiently detailed to maximize the uniformity of their application and to minimize the exposure of the institution and the medical staff to potential liability.

## References

1. Eisele CW, Fifer, WR, Wilson TC. Medical staff credentialing. In: Eisele CW, ed. *The Medical Staff and the Modern Hospital.* Englewood, NJ: Estes Park Institute; 1985: 193–216
2. American Medical Association. *Delineation of Clinical Privileges, A Guide for Hospital Medical Staffs.* Chicago: AMA; 1985
3. Health Care Quality Improvement Act of 1986. 42 USC §11101
4. Joint Commission on Accreditation of Hospitals. *Accreditation Manual for Hospitals.* 1989 ed. Chicago: Joint Commission on the Accreditation of Healthcare Organizations; 1988

# Impartiality in Medical Staff Privileges Cases

Henry R. Arkin, JD

A basic element of due process is impartiality. In a medical staff privileges case, a failure to provide impartial decision makers for a physician whose privileges are being threatened would be a denial of due process as well as a violation of the principle of professional self-regulation. Challenges to the fairness of decision makers in privileges cases frequently take the form of antitrust actions, but impartiality as an element of due process encompasses a greater range of situations than the economic self-interest at issue in an antitrust suit. While the financial stakes and chilling effects are greater in antitrust litigation, due process suits challenging impartiality do occur, and an understanding of the due process requirement of impartiality is necessary for all physicians involved in peer review and privileges proceedings.

Impartiality, or bias, may be divided into general, but distinct, categories of 1) personal prejudice or animosity, 2) financial conflict of interest such that the decision maker stands to gain or lose by his decision, and 3) prior knowledge or prior participation leading to prejudgment. A fourth category recognized by some courts is where the decision maker has been enmeshed in other matters involving the person whose rights he is judging. Individuals falling within one or more of these categories should be disqualified from acting as decision makers, and a failure to remove such persons can result in a denial of due process.

Reprinted by permission of CONNECTICUT MEDICINE, Volume 51, page 225, 1987. Copyright Connecticut State Medical Society.

**167**

Impartiality decisions in privileges cases have been concerned mainly with prior knowledge and participation; with the latter, prior participation, comprising categories of prior participation by the decision maker as an earlier decision maker, as a member of an investigating committee, as a witness, or as a complainant or adversary. Simple knowledge is frequently a concern in a privileges case because it is not likely that physicians in a hospital will be unaware of alleged problems and deficiencies of a colleague. The smaller the hospital, the greater the likelihood of prior knowledge. Prior participation can be a problem because of a lack of experience or knowledge of procedural matters or, again in smaller hospitals, because of a small pool of physicians to perform all the necessary functions. As discussed below, prior knowledge or participation *per se* does not necessarily preclude impartiality. Rather, it is the degree and nature of the prior knowledge or participation that can disqualify a decision maker.

In privileges cases, as in other kinds of proceedings, courts recognize a presumption of impartiality for the decision makers involved.[1] A burden, therefore, is placed on the physician claiming bias or lack of impartiality. A simple allegation will not suffice: the challenging physician must present actual evidence of possible bias to overcome the presumption of impartiality. However, the physician must be given the opportunity to establish such evidence. In a recent California case, the court stated that the physician must be allowed to question designated decision makers in the manner of jury decision, or *voir dire*:

> . . . while the hospital's bylaws did not specifically provide for *voir dire* of the hearing panel, basic notions of fairness dictate that an individual, whose right to practice his livelihood at a particular hospital is being revoked, has a right to examine the members of the tribunal for possible bias against him. Fairness, according to the court, requires a practical method of testing impartiality, and *voir dire* is one such practical method.[2]

As stated, in the reported due process decisions, prior knowledge and participation have been the primary concern of the courts. Personal animosity has had little discussion in the reported cases. Financial conflict of interest has been at issue in the due process cases, but, again, this problem is much more frequently addressed from the more costly perspective of antitrust law. From the due process perspective, the courts, most implicitly, appear to follow the presumption of impartiality regarding competing physicians serving as decision makers. (However, with the enactment of P.L. 99-660 on November 14, 1986, changes may develop in this regard. This federal act creates the opportunity for immunity protection for physician decision makers in "professional review." One requirement for this protection is that individuals acting as decision makers may not be in "direct economic competition with the physician involved."[3] What this means precisely, and what, if any, changes in current practices this may require, is not clear at this time. One conclusion can be drawn: legal developments regarding financial conflicts of interest will likely emanate from legislation and antitrust law, not from judicial views of due process.)

Regarding the law of due process and prior knowledge and participation, ideally, as for judges and jurors, physicians serving as decision makers in privileges proceedings would have little or no prior exposure to the matter to be decided. However, given the nature of the hospital setting, near or complete unfamiliarity or lack of involvement is not required. Regarding simple prior knowledge, the attitude of the courts is that due process does not require that a physician be provided a hearing panel "made up of outsiders or of doctors who have never heard of the case and who (know) nothing about the facts of it or what they (suppose) the facts to be."[4] Similarly, in a 1979 case, the Oregon supreme court ruled that even though members of decision making committees were aware that things in the physician's department "had not been all sweetness and light," because the physician failed to carry the burden of showing prejudgment bias or basic unfairness, such general knowledge was not objectionable.[5]

Prior participation is more complex. Prior participation *per se* is not a violation of due process, but the particular nature and extent of a decision maker's prior participation could well be. In analyzing a prior participation problem, the first consideration must be the specific role in which the decision maker earlier functioned. Whereas prior participation as an adversary would automatically preclude impartiality, prior participation in another role may not. But, regarding such other, nonadversarial, roles, as a practical matter, the most prudent policy for a medical staff to follow would be that stated in 1971 Joint Commission on Accreditation of Hospitals guidelines for medical staff bylaws:

> No staff member who has actively participated in the consideration of the adverse recommendation shall be appointed a member of this hearing committee unless it is otherwise impossible to select a representative group due to the size of the medical staff.[6]

As stated above, prior participation of a decision maker can be divided into categories of prior participation as an earlier decision maker, as an investigator or as part of an investigating committee, as a witness, or as an adversary or prosecutor, or in some combination of these roles. Regarding prior participation as a decision maker—where a current decision maker would be sitting on a committee reviewing an earlier decision in which he participated—without question, it is preferable and advisable to avoid such overlapping membership on decision making bodies.[7] Even where an individual physician would be able to maintain objectivity in the matter, there could be an appearance of bias when the decision maker reviews judgments in which he had a part. In the handful of cases on this subject, the courts, after a careful review of the record, have taken a somewhat tolerant approach,[8] but overlapping membership should be avoided or, where necessary, minimized.

More troublesome than a combination of decision making at one level with decision making at a lower level is the combination of decision making with another function at a lower level—or for that matter the same level. These combination of functions problems can arise in a variety of ways, often unforseen. As a general proposition, a combination of decision making with an investigative or a witness function may be upheld by a court depending on the circumstances, but a combination of decision making with an adversarial or prosecutorial role is always improper. From a practical perspective, however, to reiterate, it would be prudent to try to exclude from a decision making role any medical staff member who has served even in an investigative role or as a witness if there was "active participation" in these functions.

Regarding the combination of a decision making, or adjudicatory, role with an investigative role, the most important consideration for privileges disputes is the 1975 U.S. Supreme Court decision in *Withrow v. Larkin*, a medical licensing case.[9] Here, members of the Wisconsin Medical Licensing Board held an initial "investigative hearing" to determine if there was probable cause to proceed to a charge and a revocation hearing. The actual investigation was performed by the staff of the board. At the investigative hearing, which was closed to the public, board members heard witnesses, and counsel for the physician was allowed to be present although not to cross-examine. The challenging physician claimed the board's involvement at the investigative stage destroyed its impartiality.

The Supreme Court disagreed. A combination of judging and investigating functions is not improper *per se*, the Court stated, and the simple assertion of bias in this regard would not overcome the presumption of impartiality. The Court went on, however:

That is not to say that there is nothing to the argument that those who have investigated should not then adjudicate. The issue is substantial, it is not new, and legislators and others concerned with the operations of administrative agencies have given much attention to whether and to what extent distinctive administrative functions should be permitted by the same persons. No single answer has been reached. Indeed, the growth, variety, and complexity of the administrative processes have made any one solution highly unlikely.[10]

Despite this caution, *Withrow* stands for the proposition that a combination of adjudicatory and investigative roles is not automatically unfair, and such combinations can be upheld depending on the particular facts of a case.

In a privileges case, a combination of adjudicatory and investigative or witness functions can take any number of forms. Two cases are illustrative. In *Ladenheim v. Union County Hospital District*,[11] the first of four procedural levels was a hearing before the executive committee of the medical staff sitting as the credentials committee. One of the three members of this committee had assisted the hospital attorney in preparing the written charges against the physician by interpreting a memorandum sent to him by the director of nurses. This degree of participation in the investigative stage, and familiarity with the evidence, was not found objectionable by the court, which distinguished between information acquired through participation in the case and that which derives from an "extrajudicial source," the latter being of a nature to disqualify a decision maker. In *Leonard v. Board of Directors*,[12] a combination of adjudicatory and witness functions of a non-physician member of the board of directors was at issue. Charges against the physician here included insubordination directed at the board, and for this reason a board member with the best first-hand knowledge of the facts testified before a hearing committee of physicians. The board member then participated first in the board's consideration of the hearing committee's recommendation of revocation and then on a joint conference committee. The court found this combination of functions permissible considering the board member to have acted only as a "witness developing facts rather than as an advocate or counsel" when he testified at the evidentiary hearing. Citing *Withrow*, the court suggested that even if the board member had assumed a role of an investigator, this may also have been acceptable. It must be pointed out, however, that the court apparently gave weight to the finding that the facts about which the director testified "were not conclusory facts and were, for the most part, undisputed by the plaintiff."

No firm or universal guidelines can be stated on the degree of prior participation in an investigative, or witness, role that a particular court will tolerate, and, as can be seen from the two preceding cases, these roles can take many forms. Certainly the Supreme Court's decision in the *Withrow* case should not be ignored, but Withrow does point to the threat to impartiality by a combination of functions.

Different from the *Withrow* situation of a combination of decision making and investigative functions is the combination of decision making and adversarial or prosecutorial functions. Due process and fairness require that this later combination of functions must always be avoided.[13] This rule is based on the simple proposition that "no man shall be a judge in his own cause."[14] Once an individual assumes an adversarial role, with its commitment, and obligation, to "win," impartiality is no longer considered possible. In a privileges case, this rule of "separation of functions" most obviously applies to a medical staff member who presents charges against the physician to a hearing panel. The rule would apply also to a hospital attorney and, obviously, to a medical staff or board member who may have initiated a complaint. It would apply in addition to physicians who because of close professional or personal relationships with those in an adversarial role may because of such relationships occupy an adversarial role themselves without intending or realizing it, for instance, physicians who are partners with or who receive substantial referrals from a physician in an adversarial role.[15]

A number of privileges cases have dealt with such separation of functions problems. A simple example is the recent case of *In Re Zaman*.[16] In this case, three physicians "with admitted bias" began the proceeding by submitting complaints to a hospital committee. The case proceeded to the executive committee of the medical staff and then to a joint conference committee consisting of four trustees and four physicians. Of the four physicians on this final panel, three were the original complainants. This the supreme court of South Carolina found to be improper: "Having three of respondent's original accusers sit also as his jury is a direct violation of respondent's right to a fair and meaningful hearing under the due process clause." Improper combination of functions was found also in *Hoberman v. Lock Haven Hospital*.[17] The medical staff member who initiated the charges here presented evidence to the medical staff executive committee and then participated in the committee's discussions and the decision. This combination of the functions of complainant, prosecutor, and judge in one person was found to be a violation of due process. The same view was expressed in *Storrs v. Lutheran Hospitals and Homes Society*,[18] where the chief of the medical staff summarily suspended the physician, presented the case against him, was a witness against him, and then was a voting member of a joint review committee ruling on the matter.

The principle of separation of functions would also apply to hospital attorneys. Just as it is improper for a physician who acts as an adversary or prosecutor to act also as a decision maker, it is improper for an attorney who presents a case, or who advises the physician who presents a case, to act also as counsel to the decision making body. For instance, in *Christhilf v. Annapolis Emergency Hospital Association*,[19] a federal court of appeals pointed out that a heavy burden had been placed on the hospital's counsel "who has been cast in the triple role of representing the hospital in court, advising the board about the discovery it should allow and the procedure it should follow in the administrative hearing, and presenting the charges against the doctor." The court suggested a change of hospital procedures or the appointment of a hearing officer.

In summary, impartiality is a concern in all privileges cases. With a small medical staff, it is all the more a potential problem. The courts express a somewhat tolerant attitude, not requiring the decision making process to be as "antiseptic" as a criminal prosecution,[20] but possibilities of bias—whether from personal animosities, financial conflicts of interest, or improper combinations of functions—must be guarded against at all times and avoided or minimized wherever possible.

## References


1. Kiracofe v Reid Memorial Hospital, 461 NE2d 1134, 1140-41 (Ill App 1984); Ritter v Board of Commissioners, 637 P2d 940, 946 (Wash 1981).
2. Lasko v Valley Presbyterian Hospital, 225 Cal Rptr 603 (Cal App 1986). See also Duffield v Charleston Area Medical Center, 503 F2d 512, 515-16 (4th Cir 1974).
3. "Health Care Quality Improvement Act of 1986," Pub L No 99-660, §412(b)(3)(A)(ii) and (iii).
4. Klinge v Lutheran Charities Association, 523 F2d 56,63 (8th Cir 1975).
5. Straube v Emanuel Lutheran Charity Board, 600 P2d 381, 385 (Or 1979).
6. Joint Commission on Accreditation of Hospitals, Guidelines for the Formulation of Medical Staff Bylaws, Rules and Regulations, art viii, §4(a) at 23 (1971). See also California Medical Association, Guiding Principles for Physician-Hospital Relationship (1974), in which is contained CMA-CHA Uniform Code of Hearing and Appeal Procedures, §2(e) at 10.
7. Id.
8. See Maimon v Sisters of Third Order of St. Francis, 458 NE2d 1317, 1320-21 (Ill App 1983); Miller v National Medical Hospital, 177 Cal Rptr 119, 125 (Cal App 1981); Ladenheim v Union County Hospital District 394 NE2d 770, 774 (Ill App 1979). See also, Duffield v Charleston

Area Medical Center, 503 F2d 512, 515-518 (4th Cir 1974) (where the court in tolerating overlapping membership stated that a key consideration is whether or not the prior knowledge came only from earlier participation in proceedings of the case, as opposed to "extra judicial" or outside sources); Woodbury v McKinnon, 447 F2d 839, 845 (5th Cir 1971) ("The consideration on a previous occasion of the plaintiff's qualifications would not demonstrate such bias as to constitute a denial of due process".) But see Applebaum v Board of Directors 163 Cal Rptr 831, 838 (Cal App 1980).

9. 95 SCt 1456 (1975).

10. Id at 1466-67.

11. 394 NE2d 770 (Ill App 1979).

12. 673 P2d 1019 (Colo App 1983).

13. A few courts, and implicitly JCAH guidelines (footnote 6), recognize that there may be situations where if enough decision-makers are excluded for reasons of bias, it may be impossible to proceed with a case. This would be a problem in hospitals with very small medical staffs where, presumably, substitution or use of outside physicians would not be possible or practical. A court in such circumstances may follow a "rule of necessity" and tolerate some degree of an otherwise impermissible combination of functions, feeling that disqualification because of bias should not be allowed to destroy the only body with the power to act. Leonard v Board of Directors, 673 P2d 1019, 1022-1023 (Colo App 1983); Duffield v Charleston Area Medical Center, 503 F2d 512, 519 (4th Cir 1974).

14. KC Davis, Administrative Law Treatise 18:2 at 340 (2d ed 1979). See eg, Poe v Charlotte Memorial Hospital, 374 F Supp 1302, 1310 (WDNC 1974).

15. Applebaum v Board of Directors, 163 Cal Rptr 831 (Cal App 1980).

16. 329 SE 2d 436 (SC 1985).

17. 377 F Supp 1178, 1186 (MDPa 1974).

18. 609 P2d 24, 28 n 12 (Alaska 1980).

19. 496 F2d 174, 181 (4th Cir 1974). But see Ladenheim v Union County Hospital District, 394 NE2d 770, 774-775 (Ill App 1979).

20. Suckle v Madison General Hospital, 362 FSupp 1196, 1210 (WD Wis 1973).

# Quality Assurance: Shaping Up Your Board

Barry S. Bader

Today's hospital board is on the hot seat regarding quality of patient care. Physicians may argue that quality of care is compromised by board frugality. "They won't hire enough nurses! The board's only interested in new business ventures and marketing, not quality," is a common physician complaint.

Externally, the requirements of accreditation bodies and state laws put the ultimate responsibility for quality of care and physician appointment squarely on the hospital's governing board. Increasingly, patients suing their physicians for malpractice also allege that the hospital board was negligent in granting credentials. The courts agree.

"The hospital stands as a buffer between the incompetent physician and the patient who has hardly any basis whatsoever for knowing the competence of any individual physician," said the presiding judge in *Johnson v. Misericordia*. A New York court even found that if a physician were part owner of the hospital and a member of the board himself, those circumstances did not relieve the other directors of their quality assurance responsibilities (*Raschel v. Rish*).

Finally, government and major institutional purchasers demand evidence of hospital quality. Self-insured employers, preferred provider programs, and HMOs engaging in selective contracting now routinely ask for more

Reprinted by permission of HEALTHCARE EXECUTIVE Volume 2, page 26, 1987, copyright American College of Healthcare Executives.

than a price list: They want information about the hospital's quality assurance, physician credentialing, and utilization review activities.

## Inescapable Responsibility

The governing board's accountability of the quality of patient care is inescapable. But under increasing external pressure, are directors up to the task? If they aren't, the hospital executive faces an uphill battle with the medical staff, accreditation bodies, external regulators, and the courts.

Unfortunately, governing boards are ill-equipped to get the job done. Many do not understand their responsibilities for assuring the quality of care. Lacking clinical training, hospital boards are uncomfortable second guessing the medical staff. "We've just got to trust the doctors," say many trustees.

Trusting the doctors is exactly what the board must do with regard to quality in general and physician credentialing in particular. But trust cannot be based on blind faith or ignorance. It must be based on valid information presented in terms the board can understand.

The role of the executive in this process can be difficult. On the one hand, the executive bears primary responsibility for educating the board about its responsibilities and for providing directors with the information they need. On the other hand, if the medical staff perceives that the executive is ganging up with the board to "get the doctors," the physicians may "sit down on the job." Medical staff boycotts of peer review responsibilities are symptomatic of this phenomenon.

There are no easy answers, but in my experience as a consultant and hospital trustee, there are several practical steps which executives can take to strengthen their board's role in quality assurance and physician credentialing.

## Action Steps

1. *Abandon the myth that "quality isn't measurable."* Hospital quality is in fact being measured every day; by government, third-party payors, and others. Everyone is measuring quality—except perhaps hospitals themselves. As JCAH President Dennis O'Leary recently wrote: "The health professions have been subjected to criticism for failure to develop the sophisticated statistical quality control methods that have long been a central feature of American business . . . . Recently, new performance evaluation methods have been developed and effectively applied to microsystems of care. Several sophisticated prepackaged quality assurance systems, with attendant software, are now on the market to meet a major need in hospitals; more will follow."

The real question for hospitals is not *whether* to measure quality but *how*: Which type of QA monitoring program should we use? What kinds of information on quality will be generated? What kinds of information should go to the board to ensure accountability for quality of care physician credentialing?

**2. *Educate the board on its quality assurance responsibilities.*** Boards should be familiar with the requirements placed on them by JCAH, state laws, court decisions, and the hospital's own corporate and medical staff bylaws. Executives should incorporate this information into new trustee orientation and reinforce it through periodic education.

Board members may be concerned about being sued for libel, slander, or antitrust as a result of their credentialing decisions. Generally, a board that pursues its responsibilities diligently and in good faith should not fear losing such suits. However, directors should be made aware of the protections they have. Does the hospital purchase Directors and Officers Liability Insurance? What are the policy coverages and limits? Do the hospital bylaws indemnify trustees? If so, does the hospital have the assets to cover a potential judgment? Does state law grant immunity to good-faith board actions? These protections vary, and in some states are frightfully weak, but directors have a right to know the extent to which they are protected— or vulnerable.

**3. *Work through the medical staff structure to provide the information which the board needs.*** This requires the medical staff leadership to recognize the board's quality of care responsibilities.

It may be useful to remind physicians about the benefits of having the board do an effective "end-stage" job of credentialing. When the medical staff recommends rejection of an applicant or termination of privileges, the aggrieved practitioner may claim the medical staff was not acting on grounds of quality, but trying to reduce competition to their practices.

The board lessens the antitrust liability of physicians by thoroughly reviewing the facts instead of rubber stamping the medical staff's recommendation. Similarly, by insisting on adherence to hospital policy and procedures, the board supports those physicians who, through the medical staff organization, are working to build a high-quality hospital.

A few physicians usually are key to effective quality assurance and credentialing. Typically, they are the medical director or chief of staff, the chairman of the medical staff quality assurance committee, and the chairmen of the major clinical departments. Whether these individuals are elected or salaried, they have the primary responsibility for seeing that QA and credentialing work. The executive should solicit their support and involvement in developing appropriate information for submission to the board. In many cases, these individuals should be the ones to present QA reports and credentials recommendations.

**4. *Consider forming a board committee on quality care.*** Most hospital boards have a finance committee, a strategic or long-range planning committee, and several other committees where the real work of the board is done. Hospital management provides reports and fields tough questions. The committees study viable options and make recommendations to the board—backed up by a concise presentation of facts and alternatives.

Contrast this to the way most boards are informed about new physician applicants or reappointments. Typically, they are read a list of names and specialties and told "these individuals have been approved by the medical staff." If serious questions are to be raised about a physician, a full board meeting is generally the wrong forum at the wrong time, so questions are almost never raised. Board approval is perfunctory.

One answer is to create a board quality care committee. In smaller hospitals, the joint conference committee or the board's executive committee may be suitable to perform the function.

A quality care committee is generally composed of several board members, including both physicians and nonphysicians. Exofficio, nonvoting members should include the medical director, chief of staff, and chairman of the quality assurance committee, as well as a representative of the medical staff body—usually the medical executive committee or credentials committee—which makes credentialing recommendations to the board.

It's useful to educate the board quality care committee on how the hospital's physician credentialing process works. Periodically, the committee on quality care and the medical staff's leaders should discuss the process for reviewing new appointments and reappointments: Exactly how does the medical staff verify education and training, proficiency in the privileges requested, and satisfactory performance at other facilities? What does the medical staff do if negative or questionable information is uncovered? A dialogue around questions such as these is mutually constructive and helps hold the medical staff accountable for a rigorous credentialing process.

The committee thoroughly reviews new appointments and reappointments prior to submission to the board. Each name should be accompanied by a brief description of the applicant (e.g., specialty, location of practice, years of experience, special qualifications) and a checklist showing that all the required background checks (e.g., education, training, license liability insurance, references) have been satisfactorily completed. When anything out of the ordinary has been uncovered regarding an applicant or reappointment, the committee should be briefed fully and have the opportunity to ask questions.

In addition to credentialing, the board committee on quality care should receive periodic information on the quality assurance and risk management programs. Information may include reports on problems identified and resolved as well as the status of potential and pending liability claims.

The confidentiality of these discussions should be strictly observed. When controversial issues arise, such as a problem physician, the board committee should never question clinical judgments. If the committee is uncomfortable, it should question the process by which judgments are made and send back recommendations for further consideration.

It might say, "We are not questioning your judgment that Surgeon X is negligent and his privileges should be revoked, but we want to know this: Have you followed your own bylaws? Have you sought expert outside reviews? Have you subjected other surgeons to the same review as Dr. X so that he cannot accuse us of unfair treatment?"

**5. *Develop physician performance profiles which can be used by the medical staff and which, in less detailed form, can be shared with the board committee on quality care.*** The physician performance profile goes to the heart of what the medical staff and the board need to know in order to make informed reappointment decisions. A good medical staff peer review program—which results in an objective, valid performance profile—is the hospital's best defense against allegations of antitrust, personality factors, and other non-quality motivations for adverse credentialing actions.

The physician performance profile is a summary of pertinent clinical activity and any peer review findings—positive and negative—with regard to a given practitioner. The profile is designed to assist the chief of the department and, secondarily, the credentials or medical executive committee during the periodic reappraisal for reappointment and renewal of privileges. The data on the profile should not be used in isolation. If the profile includes any negative information, the chief should be able to refer to the peer review findings or to the medical records, or seek additional consultation before making a recommendation.

What information on physician performance should the board committee on quality care see? The answer will vary widely. Some medical staffs provide the board with a statistical summary of clinical activity (e.g., number and types of admissions, operative invasive procedures, consults, etc.) and a summary of any negative findings from peer review of adverse occurrences, surgical case review, utilization review, mortality review, infection control, and other quality assurance medical staff monitoring programs.

From these summaries, the board committee can identify physicians whose performance patterns vary from the norm. A board should not draw conclusions from statistics alone, but these data provide a basis to hold the medical staff accountable for demonstrating the current clinical competence of practitioners recommended for appointment.

At the very least, the board committee should be briefed about practitioners in areas where performance problems have emerged. The chairman of the medical executive committee or credentials committee should explain the nature of the problem, the investigation which the medical staff conducted, and the rationale behind the recommendation being made—which may be reappointment with full or restricted privileges, required proctoring, or termination of privileges.

### Benefits Worth Risk

Most executives view the area of credentialing as a high-risk endeavor. If they push too hard, they may antagonize the medical staff and force a confrontation in which the doctors stay and the CEO packs his bags. However, an increasing number of executives recognize the importance of a fair but rigorous quality assurance and credentialing program that has top-level board support.

For one thing, the executive knows that building a high-quality hospital requires a high-quality staff of physicians. That's what QA and credentialing are supposed to achieve. The development of a board quality care committee and of physician performance profiles may be controversial, but they provide the executive with an essential board mechanism and vital information.

By strengthening the board's quality of care responsibilities, the executive also shifts some of the heat from his chair to the board's—where it belongs.

We trustees are not well paid. My salary, like most volunteer trustees', is $0 per year. But, we've accepted a seat on the board, and along with the prestige comes the responsibility to make tough decisions. Increasingly, hospital directors will make the right decisions, if they are provided with the appropriate information. And, in turn, a conscientious board will motivate physicians to take their peer review responsibilities more seriously. Concerned members of the medical staff will assume leadership and thus assure that the medical staff thoroughly pursues its quality assurance and credentialing tasks.

# Taking Care of the Doctors: The Hospital's Duty To Evaluate, Monitor, and Discipline Its Medical Staff

Constance H. Baker, JD

*Scenario 1:* In evaluating a new applicant for staff privileges, a hospital receives a neutral letter of reference from the chief at another hospital. The letter lacks any statement attesting to the physician's clinical competence. *Scenario 2:* Although numerous and repeated problems have been apparent to the hospital's risk manager and director of quality assurance throughout the initial appointment term of a physician, the department chairman fails to review these data. The physician's reappointment sails through and the board grants privileges. *Scenario 3:* A prominent obstetrician arrives in the delivery room, obviously inebriated. Discreetly, the resident handles the delivery and averts a crisis, but the obstetrician remains on the staff.

All three scenarios highlight the hospital's duties in the credentialing process. Scenario 1 concerns the hospital's duty to evaluate new applicants, Scenario 2 the duty to evaluate and monitor existing staff members for reappointment, and Scenario 3 the duty to monitor and discipline. It is these duties to evaluate, to monitor, and to discipline that are the heart of a hospital's credentialing responsibilities.

The courts clearly have established the duty of a hospital to evaluate its physicians and other health care providers.[1] Lawyers representing plaintiffs in medical malpractice suits are becoming more knowledgeable



**181**

about this independent duty of the hospital to evaluate and supervise. Indeed, hospital defense counsel have noted an increasing number of lawsuits that not only allege negligence of physicians or hospital personnel in the provision of direct patient care but also negligence of the hospital in its duty to evaluate and monitor.

The explosive growth of malpractice claims is one factor motivating hospitals and other health care institutions to evaluate and improve their credentialing and disciplinary procedures. In addition, the *Accreditation Manual for Hospitals* of the Joint Commission on Accreditation of Hospitals has specific requirements that pertain to medical staff privileges.[2] And as an increasing number of state legislatures enact comprehensive tort reform packages, they are simultaneously tightening hospital requirements for credentialing and risk management systems.

A hospital is not held to a standard of perfection in its credentialing and monitoring responsibilities, but rather to the standard of a reasonably prudent hospital.[3] The actual discharge of this duty is complicated by medical staff turf battles, tensions between the medical staff and administration, fears of antitrust liability arising from the exclusion of competitors, and the natural tendencies of individuals to shy away from awkward and sensitive situations.

This article is intended to assist hospitals and their medical staffs in fashioning reasonably prudent credentialing systems. The first section discusses a few key elements of an effective credentialing system, including the important role of the medical staff coordinator, the use of a physician proctor to evaluate new applicants, the investigation of applicants for initial appointment and reappointment, and the education and training of department chairmen. The second section offers some observations and practical suggestions for grappling with a few inevitable problems, including physicians who have trouble getting along with others and allegations of incompetence and impairment.


## Some Features of Effective Credentialing Systems

*The skills of the medical staff coordinator.* Often underrated in importance by hospital management, the medical staff coordinator should display several important qualities. The coordinator should be organized and able to process a vast amount of paperwork and should develop basic computer skills. Irreverence toward the status quo is another important quality: last year's application form certainly can and should be improved; the existing evaluation form undoubtedly can be redesigned to yield more useful and specific information; the reappointment form can be revised; and the reappointment process can always be more timely.

Naturally, the coordinator must cooperate with hospital management and key medical staff leaders, including department chairmen, the president of the medical staff, and the chairman of the credentials committee, and should continually communicate with them. This ongoing communication will aid the entire credentialing process; the absence of communication would inevitably hurt the hospital.

Finally, the coordinator should be persistent and attentive to detail, particularly in ensuring that the hospital has complete credentialing information for all applicants for initial appointment and reappointment. Applicants for initial appointment should not have any chronological gaps in their records. Did they answer every pertinent question on every form? Did all the hospitals listed on a new applicant's form confirm the physician's good standing? Was the training chief contacted? In *Johnson v Misericordia*, a hospital was held negligent in failing to properly evaluate a physician who had failed to answer all questions on his application form.[4] The court reasoned that if the hospital had checked thoroughly, it would have discovered his problems at other hospitals. Other hospitals and medical staff coordinators can learn a valuable lesson from *Johnson*. If the question is unimportant, it should not be on the form. If the question is on the form, it should be answered.

*The use of a proctor as evaluator of new applicants.* Physicians who apply for initial appointment may be virtual strangers to the hospital, and yet the hospital has a duty to evaluate them. How can it best discharge this duty? An emerging trend in the evaluation of new applicants in general, and in determining the appropriate delineation of privileges in particular, is the appointment of a physician/proctor to evaluate and observe new applicants. For surgical specialists, the proctor may actually observe the surgical procedures. For internists and pediatricians, prior discussion of treatment plans may occur. Chairmen of departments may serve in this role, or they may delegate this duty to a senior member of the department.

The use of proctors can be a real help to hospitals in evaluating new applicants. Nevertheless, the use of proctors raises the question of whether the proctor owes a duty of care to the patients of the physician being evaluated. Recently, a California court was confronted with a lawsuit against a proctor, a board-certified orthopedic surgeon, who was sued by a patient whose attending physician the proctor was observing.[5] According to the plaintiff, the proctor, having observed the attending physician's negligent conduct, owed the plaintiff the duty of actually taking over the surgery to prevent the malpractice.

The court disagreed and found that no duty of care was owed from the proctoring surgeon to the patient; hence, it found no breach of duty. This particular proctor, who had not even scrubbed to participate in the surgery, was only observing and reporting on the management of several cases. Because he did not participate in any direct patient care and because he received no fee for his evaluative services, the court reasoned that imposition of liability would be inappropriate.

As hospitals experiment with the use of proctors, they should carefully define the proctor's role. If proctors are to be held responsible for the management of patients they have never met, there is little likelihood of anyone serving in that role. A carefully defined and limited description of the proctor's role is prudent. Proctors should determine whether their malpractice insurance covers their proctoring responsibilities. In some situations, hospitals may need to assist proctors to arrange for coverage.

*The investigation of the new applicant.* How thoroughly should a reasonably prudent hospital and medical staff investigate a new applicant? Although the exact nature of the inquiry will vary depending on the facts and circumstances, hospitals generally should cover the following bases:

- verification of license;
- verification of all other hospital and institutional staff privileges listed on the application, including letters or completed evaluation forms from the appropriate department chairmen at other hospitals verifying good standing and competent practice patterns;
- verification from the state disciplinary or licensing authority that there have been no adverse findings and that there are no cases pending;
- a status report on any pending or past malpractice cases, including supplemental letters and statements from attorneys engaged as defense counsel;
- verification of competency during postgraduate training, preferably from the training chief or director of the training program;
- proof of malpractice insurance coverage in the amount and form required by the governing board; and
- other letters of reference or evaluation forms from persons who have closely observed or supervised the applicant's work.

If any of the information received is adverse or suspicious, the hospital has been put on notice and should follow up with additional letters or requests for clarification. For instance, if a chief at another hospital provides a letter of reference that states no opinion as to clinical competence, the hospital, credentials committee, and pertinent chairmen should recognize this as a red flag and should persist until they receive some information.

Notwithstanding this advice, the hospital's medical staff bylaws should clearly state that it is the applicant's burden to resolve any doubts that arise. If the investigation raises doubts that are not resolved, the hospital should deny privileges.

*The investigation of the applicant for reappointment.* A common mistake made by hospitals and medical staffs in the reappointment process is the failure to systematically utilize the in-house data that have already been generated. Unlike the new applicant, the physician requesting reappointment is no longer a stranger to the institution. Before a physician is reappointed, the reasonably prudent hospital should review its own data from all relevant sources, including quality assurance and risk management records, incident reports, and disposition of malpractice cases. Department chairmen should routinely review and analyze these data prior to making any recommendation for reappointment and should pay particular attention to delineation of privileges. Data for the past two years may indicate a problem with a certain procedure and may suggest the need for remedial training or supervision. The department chairman should not "look the other way" at reappointment time but, instead, should make a recommendation based on all of the data reasonably available.

*The education and training of department chairmen.* Department chairmen have a critical role in medical staff credentialing and discipline, yet they may receive no organized training or education. Chairmen should be educated to the extent possible before a crisis occurs; their orientation should focus on the importance of quality patient care as the major goal in running their departments. Participants in orientation sessions might include other medical staff leaders, key board members, the hospital risk manager, and legal counsel. Department chairmen should understand the legal obligations of the hospital in evaluating and monitoring its physicians, the importance of the decisions made in delineating specific privileges, the need to review data for reappointment, and the importance of peer review records and of maintaining their confidentiality. As hospital agents, they should learn that they jeopardize the institution by ignoring problems when they arise. Rumors should be followed up and clarified. Suspicion of erratic behavior should be investigated. If hospitals invest some time and resources in helping department chairmen learn how to do their jobs, the effort should pay off.

If chairmen need a little extra encouragement and motivation, their orientation might stress their role in minimizing or reducing the numbers of malpractice suits against physicians in their departments and, hence, the attendant trauma usually associated with malpractice litigation. Regardless of frequent protestations to the contrary, physicians who are sued (as is the case with nearly all defendants in litigation) do take it personally. The arrival of the sheriff or private process server at the door is hardly what one would order as an ideal career development.

The stress and trauma associated with litigation is vastly underestimated. A recent study assessed the impact of litigation on the personal and professional lives of physicians who were sued; the physicians reported symptomatic reactions to litigation usually associated with depressive and stress-induced illnesses.[6] It is hardly surprising that sued physicians reported significantly worse symptoms than physicians who were not sued. Symptoms reported include depression, irritability, insomnia, fatigue, loss of interest, difficulty concentrating, excessive alcohol use, suicidal ideation, drug misuse, and exacerbation of physical illness.

The likelihood of being named as defendant may be less if a department chairperson carefully limits the delineation of privileges, evaluates all reasonably available data, and acts promptly when problems arise.


## Grappling with the Inevitable Problems

Certain situations recur in hospitals and present challenges to all concerned. How should the reasonably prudent hospital react to an allegation that a certain physician simply cannot get along with anyone else? What should a hospital do when one member of a professional association alleges that a member of a competing group is incompetent? And how should the hospital respond to a physician's erratic behavior and rising error rate?

*Inability to get along with others.* Certain physicians simply have trouble working in harmony with other members of the team. Hospitals are social institutions, and no one takes care of patients in a vacuum. The courts have acknowledged that inability to interact well with others can have an adverse impact on patient care, and most courts have held that the inability to work with others is a sufficient basis to deny or terminate privileges, *provided* the evidence suggests that there is at least a potential threat to patient care.

Certain types of behaviors will not sustain a denial or termination, such as physicians' criticisms of staff conduct and hospital procedures, particularly when the court views the criticisms as warranted. In *Rosner v Eden Township Hospital District*, the court struck down the denial of privileges of a thoracic surgeon, who had criticized staff and hospital practices.[7] The surgeon had complained about an incompetent nurse, opposed the election of certain medical staff officers, and insisted on treating a gunshot victim when the proprietor of the hospital was adamant that nothing could be done (the patient survived). Moreover, the physician testified for plaintiffs in malpractice actions. The court was unimpressed with the surgeon's supposed "temperamental unsuitability" and found nothing in the surgeon's behavior that adversely affected patient care.

In *McElhinney v William Booth Memorial Hospital*, a Kentucky court struck down a hospital's termination of privileges of a surgeon who criticized the chief of pathology for giving too much responsibility to assistants who were not pathologists.[8] The surgeon also had criticized the performance of the x-ray department.

Departure from the majority rule occurred in *Miller v Eisenhower Medical Center,* in which the Supreme Court of California stated that evidence to sustain a denial of privileges would have to show that the physician's inability to work with others presented a "real and substantial danger" that patient care might be jeopardized.[9] The court maintained that the physician's inability to work with others must constitute "a realistic and specific threat" and the evidence must be concrete and specific.

In some cases, the physician's alleged inability to get along with others is only one of several problems. In *Theissen v Watonga Municipal Hospital Board,* the physician had a documented drug problem.[10] The physician in *Pick v Santa Ana-Tustin Community Hospital,* refused to supply information about relevant professional activities for a three-year period of time.[11] And in *Ladenheim v Union County Hospital District* the physician failed to take proper care of a surgical patient.[12] In all three cases, medical staff privileges were denied. Although all three courts placed some emphasis on the physicians' inability to work with others, it is unclear whether the courts would have decided differently in the absence of other problems, which were apparent.

How does a prudent hospital deal with complaints about uncooperative physicians? Because the ability to interact well with others is a subjective assessment, the hospital should avoid undue reliance on these complaints if at all possible. Other problems are often apparent, such as impairment. If other problems are not apparent, the hospital should develop documentation that demonstrates that the decision not to appoint or reappoint is not the result of bias or malice and that the physician's alleged inability to work with others is not a subterfuge to avoid appointment of an abrasive but otherwise qualified physician.

If the applicant's disruptive behavior consists of criticizing hospital procedures or the professional competence or medical practices of other staff, evidence of the possible adverse effect of such behavior on medical care must be sufficiently strong to preclude the conclusion that the applicant's inability to cooperate with others is being used as a subterfuge. The objective is to develop a record demonstrating by clear and persuasive evidence that the applicant presents a realistic and specific threat to the quality of medical care provided by the hospital. The following guidelines may prove useful:

• Document the physician's inability to work as part of the medical team;

- Document, where possible, that this inability has adversely affected patient care;
- Develop documentation confirming analysis that criticisms of other physicians, staff, or hospital procedures were abrasive and unwarranted;
- Demonstrate that outbursts of anger were unwarranted, by considering the physician's reasons;
- Document the physician's failure to abide by hospital procedures and policies; and
- Document other reasons for denying privileges such as questions related to professional competence or ethical issues or denial of privileges at other hospitals.

The importance of adequate documentation of a consistent pattern was a key factor in the recent case of *Cipriotti v Board of Directors of North-ridge Hospital Foundation Medical Center.*[13] The California Court of Appeals upheld the termination of the privileges of a difficult physician, whose disruptive patterns were well documented and whose individual incidents had been consistently called to his attention.

*Incompetence.* When one physician questions another physician's competence in the hospital setting, there often follows an allegation of personal bias or animus. For serious concerns about possible incompetency, it is prudent to consider the use of an outside independent expert to deflect the charges of personal bias and to assist the hospital in getting a fresh look at the situation. State and national specialty societies can assist in arranging reviews.

The outside expert should not have any stake in the outcome and should be totally independent, perhaps practicing outside the primary service area of the hospital or out of state altogether. The hospital should fairly compensate the expert at a negotiated hourly rate. It is not wise to skimp on professional fees. The expert should be willing to testify, if necessary, in an in-house hearing under oath and should be courageous enough to testify about a fellow physician's incompetence (if his or her opinion so indicates) under the rigors of cross-examination and the naturally intimidating atmosphere of a hearing.

The use of an outside independent expert may be beneficial in promoting an amicable settlement of a peer review dispute. Once the accused physician's attorney receives an adverse written report from an independent expert, amicable negotiations often follow. The use of an outside expert may well eliminate bias as an issue and may prevent false concerns from clouding a real problem of incompetence. On the other hand, the medical staff may resent an outside consultant who may be "forced" on it. To the extent possible, the medical staff should play a role in the determination to bring in the outside consultant.

*Impaired physicians.* The term "impaired physician" generally refers to a physician who abuses drugs or alcohol or both. When a hospital is informed that a certain physician is behaving erratically, when there is a troubling change in behavior, or when a theft of drugs is noted, the possibility of impairment should be suspected. Understandably, these situations are awkward and tense. Nevertheless, the following guidelines may be of help.

Some states require notification of the medical licensing board and have programs for impaired physicians. Hospitals should comply with such laws.

Many state medical societies have a committee dedicated to the rehabilitation of physicians. If there is such a committee and no governmental program is mandated, the hospital should promptly contact a committee member for advice as to evaluation and treatment. If no such committee exists, hospitals should consider enlisting the aid of the appropriate department chairman together with a psychiatrist who has experience in confronting suspected abusers. An impaired physician should be strongly encouraged to participate in an inpatient treatment program, perhaps one specializing in treatment of physicians such as the program run by the Medical Society of Georgia; health professionals who specialize in treating impaired physicians, depending on their evaluation, usually recommend participation in inpatient programs.[14]

The impaired physician should not be permitted to exercise any staff privileges during the period of treatment, whether by suspension or voluntary leave of absence. Hospitals have a duty to assure that the impaired physician will not provide patient care until the physician demonstrates fitness to do so.

After completion of the inpatient treatment program, the physician often enters into an "aftercare contract" providing for further treatment. Whether the physician is competent to practice during the aftercare period depends on a number of circumstances and should never be presumed without adequate proof. The phenomenon of impaired physicians often sets up a tension between the humanitarian instincts of fellow physicians, who will tend to favor treatment and full restoration of privileges, and the hospital's duty to provide high-quality care and to protect its patients. The hospital does not have a duty to rehabilitate a physician, to accord the physician the privileges necessary to aid him in his recovery, to conduct drug tests, or to provide therapy and psychiatric help. In contrast, the hospital does have a duty to its patients to provide high-quality patient care.

At the very least, any hospital that chooses to allow an impaired physician to remain on the staff should consult with the treating psychiatrist, have a mechanism to monitor the physician's attendance at group meetings, and receive reports of the results of frequent drug testing, both random and scheduled. Unfortunately, the rate of recidivism among impaired physicians is high.[15] Any physician who has a drug problem should be carefully monitored by the hospital, or its delegated physicians. A "business as usual" approach is inappropriate, can result in needless harm to patients, and could provide the basis for punitive as well as compensatory damages.

If a hospital assumes the duty to monitor these physicians, it must discharge it reasonably well. If a hospital requires periodic psychiatric reporting, it must ensure that these reports are received and that the reports confirm competence. If a hospital requires routine drug monitoring, the tests must be done promptly. Unless the hospital and medical staff intend to live up to the letter and spirit of these assumed obligations, it is better not to assume them at all.

Even though a hospital may carefully monitor a physician with a drug problem, it runs the risk of an unsympathetic jury that will not think the hospital acted appropriately in retaining the impaired physician. This unfortunate fact of life in today's litigious society should be considered, together with other criteria, in the hospital's response to an impaired physician.


## Conclusion

The previous discussion focuses on several features of effective credentialing and disciplinary systems that should assist hospitals in promoting quality patient care and in withstanding judicial scrutiny. It also discusses some common pitfalls in frequently recurring situations involving incompetent, impaired, and disruptive physicians.

If a disgruntled physician whose privileges have been denied or terminated challenges the action, will the record reflect that the hospital's actions were reasonably prudent? Were appropriate criteria applied? Will the evidence confirm that the hospital acted with the best interests of patients in mind? Will the hospital appear steady and evenhanded and not discriminatory? Did the hospital follow its bylaws? If the answers to the above questions are "yes," a court probably would conclude that the hospital has acted in a reasonably prudent manner in discharging its duty to evaluate, to monitor, and to discipline.


## References

1. Darling v Charleston Community Memorial Hospital, 33 Ill. 2d 326, 211 NE 2d 253 (1966), *cert. denied*, 383 U.S. 946 (1966).

2. Joint Commission on Accreditation of Hospitals: *Accreditation Manual for Hospitals*, 1987 ed. Chicago; Joint Commission, 1986, pp 109-127.

3. Johnson v Misericordia Community Hospital, 99 Wis.2d 708, 301 NW 2d 156, 171 (1981); Holton v Resurrection Hospital, 410 NE 2d 969 (Ill. 1980).

4. Johnson v Misericordia Community Hospital, 99 Wis.2d 708, 301 NW 2d 156 (1981).

5. Clarke v Hoek, 174 Cal. App.3d 208, 219 Cal. Rptr. 845 (1985).

6. Charles SC, at al: Sued and non-sued physicians' self-reported reactions to malpractice litigation. *Am J Psychiatry* 142; 437, April 1985.

7. 58 Cal.2d 592, 25 Cal. Rptr. 552, 375 P.2d 431 (1962).

8. 544 SW2d 216 (Ky. 1976).

9. 27 Cal.3d 614, 166 Cal. Rptr. 826, 614 P.2d 258 (1980).

10. 550 P.2d 938 (Okla. 1976).

11. 130 Cal. App.3d 970, 182 Cal. Rptr. 85 (1982).

12. 76 Ill. App.3d 90, 394 NE2d 770 (1979).

13. 147 Cal. App.3d 144, 196 Cal. Rptr. 367 (1983).

14. Talbott GD, et al: The Medical Association of Georgia's disabled doctors program—A five-year review. *J Med Assoc Ga* 70:545, August 1984.

15. Shore JH: The Impaired Physician, four years after probation. JAMA 248:3127, Dec 17, 1982; Green RC Jr, Carroll GJ, Buxton WD: Drug addiction among physicians: the Virginia experience. *JAMA* 236:1372, Sep 20, 1976.

# Quality Criteria for Medical Staff Admission: A Beginning


Bruce M. Bartels, FACHE
John W. O'Donnell



**Summary**

Pressures influencing the size and composition of medical staffs are increasing as hospitals and physicians respond to competition, market priorities, increasing numbers of physicians, and quality-of-care concerns. This article examines whether the quality of care provided by an applicant may be the primary criterion for admission to a hospital's medical staff. Methodological, legal, and organizational concerns that arise from this approach are reviewed. A quality criteria approach can assist in responding to increasing numbers of physicians, the transition to managed care, and the marketing interests of a hospital.


Much has been written concerning the reasonableness and legality of restricting medical staff membership based on facility limitations (White 1987). This article examines whether quality of care provided by the applicant may be the primary or sole criterion for admission to a hospital's medical staff.

The current health care environment poses many questions without obvious or conclusive answers—for example, the effect of a growing number of physicians. A traditional free market view would indicate that an oversupply of service providers will correct itself over time, and such tradi-



**193**

tional theories seem less applicable to the physician supply (Paris 1986). Pending the development of some balance, however, hospitals must deal with the current supply of physicians as a major consideration in the delivery of patient services.

The missions of many hospitals combine elements of patient care, education, and research. Patient care, however, remains central to all of these interests. The fulfillment of mission becomes increasingly complicated with the introduction and implementation of such changes as prospective payment and managed care systems. As a hospital attempts to assure quality patient services, the constraints and demands of the current health care environment may, in fact, be exacerbated by a medical staff open to all minimally qualified physicians. A hospital with medical staff membership determined by rigorous standards or by invitation only may be better able to serve the hospital and patient interests of quality care and competitive costs. Evaluation of the policies and procedures for determining medical staff composition is required in considering this issue.

## Open Medical Staffs

Until recently, most hospitals have maintained open medical staffs (Trustee 1985). In typical open-staff situations, the hospital medical staff recommends and the hospital board actually grants membership based on several basic criteria. These criteria, at the least, include graduation from an accredited medical school, a minimum period of time spent in graduate medical education, and current licensure in the relevant jurisdiction. In many instances, the hospital medical staff performs a quality assurance role by requiring higher qualifications for hospital practice than the state has required for the practice of medicine in general. Over time, greater specificity has been required of medical staff applicants, especially as concerns for quality assurance, risk management, and accreditation have increased. In general, however, the basic approach of these hospitals is to allow free access to the medical staff for any qualified applicant.

## Restricted Membership

A second approach involves restricting the membership of a medical staff. Such restriction may be based on an organizational relationship between the hospital and another entity, which is common among academic medical centers that are owned by universities or serve as the primary teaching sites for medical schools. In these situations, medical staff membership often is open only to those physicians serving on the medical school faculty or affiliated with a faculty practice group. Hospitals owned by physician practice groups, such as clinics or health maintenance organizations (HMOs), have similarly restricted medical staff membership. In these instances, medical staff membership is limited to those physicians who are members of the affiliated organization.

A hospital's capacity to deliver care to the number of patients generated by its medical staff remains a separate reason for strict restriction of medical staff membership (Joint Commission on Accreditation of Healthcare Organizations (JCAHO) 1988). In situations where their physical capacity and resources have been strained by the number of patients, hospitals have either closed the medical staff entirely or instituted moratoria on the admission of certain categories of practitioners who are directly involved in the area of limited resources. Such restrictions based on facility constraints have generally been upheld by courts reviewing challenges to the practice.

## "Quality" Criteria

A third option for determining medical staff membership, although not yet tested, is the restriction of membership based on predetermined "quality" criteria for admission and successful reapplication. The objectives of such a system would be to balance the considerations of the quality of the medical staff with the economic benefits of a large number of providers in a competitive setting. In effect, such a system approaches what might be found in a managed care system. The major emphasis, however, is on the quality of the physicians and their activities rather than on the simple number of physicians on the medical staff.

As mentioned above, quality-of-care information has been used in the medical staff admission process in increasing detail and quantity for many years. Each year medical staffs seek additional information from applicants as well as seeking verification of their credentials from multiple sources. A common practice had been to ask an applicant for places and dates of education and experience, and at one time this information was taken virtually at face value. Today that information must be confirmed through independent verification (JCAHO 1988). Additionally, data on continuing education experiences, statements from persons in positions to comment objectively on current competence, malpractice claims history, personal interviews, special practice interests, relationships with fellow physicians and other health care personnel, board status, frequency of relocation, health status, and much more are commonly sought from all applicants. Overall, assessment of an applicant's credentials is much more thorough than in the past. Generally, however, if the information is acceptable to the reviewing body, no other limitation on the number of qualified physicians is expressed as a criterion.

The issue of what a qualified physician may do once gaining admission to the medical staff has changed as well. Once an applicant meets the admission criteria that exist, the privileges a physician might expect were once bound only loosely by a common understanding of the medical specialty in which an individual practiced. That practice, too, has given way in the face of growing complexity. Currently "laundry lists" of privileges or some version of them exist in many hospitals. Demonstrated and continuing competence has become an expectation for retention of medical staff membership and specific privileges (JCAHO 1988).

The use of "quality" criteria for determining medical staff membership may be viewed as an extension of this current practice of increased scrutiny of credentials and patient care information. The difficulty of this approach is to continue the advancement and refinement of the processes of evaluating credentials while at the same time identifying and implementing other valid, currently less quantifiable or verifiable measures of "quality." If done properly, such an approach should result in a medical staff whose membership is based on concerns for both the care for the patient and the efficiency and organizational integrity of the institution.

Measuring "quality" is central to the question of using it as the primary basis for determining composition of a medical staff. Techniques that are currently available may not be sufficient to determine quality and achieve the balance of appropriate care at a reasonable cost. A basic assumption for such a process is that the quality of care rendered by members of a medical staff is sufficiently measurable to allow discriminating decisions about who remains a part of or joins that staff. These decisions, while relating directly to quality, will indirectly respond to the impact of increasing numbers of physicians and the competitiveness of hospital/medical staff services.

## Determining Medical Staff Membership

Several issues must be identified and resolved in any such system. The major concerns fall into three areas—methodological, legal, and organizational. The most difficult area—methodological—identifies the processes and standards by which decisions on medical staff membership would be made. The legal component addresses the constraints imposed by courts on medical staff membership decisions. Organizational issues concern the implementation of such a system and the manner in which these decisions conform or conflict with institutional goals and objectives. Though obviously interrelated, each area raises special concerns.

## Methodology

An accepted methodology for determining the quality of practice has not yet been developed. The few measures currently available can be factors in the medical staff credentialing process, but they are not sufficient for anything other than gross evaluations. Consequently, a blend and balance of a variety of information from other existing sources is necessary to begin the integration of quality measures and medical staff privilege determinations.

Most hospital medical staffs have developed and used utilization data to meet externally imposed requirements. Many have initiated outcome data collection as well. Still unclear is the relationship between varying degrees of utilization and different outcomes. In separate efforts, several professional societies have identified volume ranges of activity for certain technical procedures that should translate to sufficient proficiency to continue performance (American Society for Laser Medicine and Surgery, Inc. 1984; *Medical World News for Obstetricians, Gynecologists, Urologists* 1986). This quantification as a quality measure, however, can blur in application. Are senior orthopedists with 20 years of experience in performing total joint replacements less qualified to perform such a procedure if they reduce the number to 10 below the suggested minimum in an effort to balance workload? Are aggressive, newly trained cardiologists who substantially exceed these types of targets merely successful at acquiring patients or are they performing marginally justified catheterizations?

It is clear that data collection on utilization and outcome is a starting point in measuring quality. Guidelines for procedural proficiency are another. Presently, each evaluation might involve individualized qualitative judgments combining these simple measures for determining competence. As with many new approaches, experimentation will have to occur to develop a justifiable system. Criteria such as mortality, infection rate, or procedural frequency, while useful, are only preliminary efforts.

Several approaches to quality measurement beyond those previously mentioned are now gaining acceptance. These methods are based on the analysis of care rendered by large numbers of physicians for a particular population. Analysis of such data will inevitably be extended and linked to individual experience and thus is relevant to developing a quality base for extending privileges.

Broadly speaking, these analytical techniques fall into three categories: case review, statistical profiling, and process and structural review. Each approach has its merits, and ultimately a widely accepted approach is likely to include elements of each.

## Case Review

The traditional case-based review undertaken by peer review organizations (PROs) and other utilization review organizations is unlikely to diminish. Case-based review is less likely to reveal patterns of practice than other forms of review because of the absence of continuous data relative to a practice and the absence of a comparative component. Nevertheless, a physician's experience with case-based reviews should comprise an element of evaluation for privileges since such measures are so commonly employed by a number of payers.

## Statistical Profiling

The JCAHO has initiated a movement away from its traditional process and structure review, which consisted of assessing an organization's capacity to render quality care but not determining its actual quality of care. The Joint Commission embarked on a several-year-long process of identifying clinical indicators that can be used to evaluate the quality of care rendered by members of an organization. While these indicators will be used to gauge institutional performance, they will also be, by extension, guideposts for initiating review of individual performance. The addition of indicator-based statistical profiles of an organization will generate major revisions in the concept of a survey.

Small area variance analysis is another statistical profiling technique even more accepted as a way to identify differences in patterns of practice from one locale to another. Developed and popularized by Dr. John Wennberg of Dartmouth College, this approach can also be used to compare individual performance, although, as with most such analyses, caution must be exercised to qualify differences based on severity of illness or on a small sample size.

A review of quality measurement efforts would be incomplete without reference to the Health Care Financing Administration's efforts. The mortality tables that have been issued for the last two years are admittedly inexact expressions of quality. However, they represent a serious attempt to develop and promulgate health care quality data to support consumer decision making, as well as only the initial portion of a broader release of such data. Another phase of this review is the recently announced intention to provide Medicare billing data to research organizations and possibly to release similar data for individual physicians.

Each health care organization should also be developing its own indicators as well as relying on data from pooled sources such as that described or as that being developed by national alliances. This will permit a process of evaluation sensitive to local concerns. Examples of baseline indicators that may be useful are: frequency of performing a particular procedure, length-of-stay trends, severity trends, morbidity and mortality data, nosocomial (hospital-acquired) infection rates, medical record completion compliance, patient survey data, meeting participation rates, unplanned readmission rates, and rates of ancillary service utilization. These indicators fall generally into the category of organizationwide or specialtywide reviews. Additionally, indicators can be developed on a procedure-specific basis, which provide the most pointed reviews. Examples of such indicators would include complication rates from heart valve replacement procedures and cesarean section rates.

Even though much of the methodology is still developing, sufficient baseline measures of quality exist to at least initiate the process of incorporating these measures into the granting of medical staff membership. Such good faith determinations could be made on the basis of the currently available indicators that address the degree of physician activity necessary for maintaining the highest quality hospital practice. Some of the criteria will need to be reevaluated as the environment and technology change. Five years from now today's ratio of angioplasty cases will not mean the same. Still, with care, these indicators can be used now.


## Process and Structural Review

Many issues accompany the implementation of quality measures in medical staff credentialing decisions. One involves the treatment of current staff members and the reappointment process. Practically speaking, equity would indicate some degree of "grandfathering" for physicians who joined the medical staff prior to this new process. That decision, however, should not be one of total insulation or exclusion (Horty 1984). Instead, the same criteria-based review should be undertaken and mechanisms developed that will assist in developing conformity with new guidelines. Attainment of standards acceptable to the medical staff and contemporary practice should occur within a reasonable period of time. Failure to achieve these standards would cause some additional action, such as a reduction in privileges or termination from the medical staff.

Another practical problem is the application of any accepted quality standards to individuals new to a hospital. Data may not be available to physicians making application to a different hospital after some years in practice elsewhere. Physicians just completing their training likewise may not have either the data or the experiences required to comply with the information needs of a quality evaluation mechanism. These instances may best be addressed for now by a structured review of each applicant during the provisional time on the staff.

A final point regarding methodology is the maintenance of quality. The review of quality once initiated will not be static. Measuring quality is still in its infancy, and growing pains will certainly accompany its application. This evolutionary nature will cause much introspection as different approaches are tried. Delaying or deferring this initiative, however, may well be counterproductive; not only will others perform this analysis of care, but a key opportunity for early implementation of important quality assurance efforts may be lost.

## Legal Issues

Any limitation on medical staff membership almost certainly means that some applicants will be denied membership. Denials of admission to medical staffs have generated a large number of legal cases challenging the validity of those actions. Changes in hospital use and occupancy rates and the concomitant effects on medical staffs will result in further litigation regarding the process of selecting and maintaining a medical staff. In general, however, reviewing courts have allowed private hospitals considerable discretion in determining medical staff membership as long as the process used was not applied in an arbitrary, unreasonable, or discriminatory manner (*Sussman v. Overlook Hospital Association* 1967).

It is beyond the scope of this discussion to examine all the federal and state causes of action used as the basis for challenging medical staff membership decisions. Federal and state antitrust, substantive and procedural due process, equal protection, and a number of other constitutional, statutory, and common law arguments have been used in litigation concerning the issue. Even with this array of challenges, federal- and state-level courts have upheld limitations on medical staff membership when those limitations are shown to be reasonably related to efforts to maintain or enhance the operation of the facility. For example, the hospital may require that all medical staff serve on a rotating basis in the emergency room (*Yeargin v. Hamilton Memorial Hospital* 1972) or that medical records be completed within a certain time period (*Peterson v. Tucson General Hospital* 1976). Less clear is the willingness of courts to recognize restrictions on medical staff membership that attempt in some way to link medical staff admission and retention with quality indicators. Specialty board certification or eligibility, as one indicator, has been upheld as a criterion for medical staff membership (*Khan v. Suburban Community Hospital* 1976), but quality criteria, with the exception of dismissal for incompetence, have not yet been the subject of definitive court decisions.

Concerns about quality of care have arisen in several antitrust cases. In *National Society of Professional Engineers v. United States* (1978) the U.S. Supreme Court was reluctant to recognize concerns about competence as valid justification for the anticompetitive effects of restrictions on a professional practice. Recently, the Supreme Court also touched on the issue in *FTC v. Indiana Federation of Dentists* (1986), questioning whether the Indiana Federation of Dentists' quality-of-care concerns were legally cognizable as a defense for a concerted refusal to deal with an insurer. As with the development of a methodology for quality criteria, the lack of commonly accepted, objective indicia of quality will probably hinder courts reviewing decisions as much as the institutions that are responsible for making the decisions in the first place.

While the case law in this area provides no definitive guidance, courts do seem willing to continue the policy of deference to the decisions of the hospitals regarding medical staff membership when those decisions are reasonably related to the mission of the hospital. As quality becomes an increasingly prominent concern for these institutions, particularly for those with a research and education mission in addition to that of patient care, quality criteria will certainly be scrutinized when said criteria form the basis for a denial of an application. The legal challenge for the hospital will be to develop and implement quality criteria reasonably related to the mission of the institution that will survive the allegations of being arbitrary, discriminatory, or unreasonable.

## Organizational Implications

Third, organizational implications of using more sophisticated quality criteria in determining medical staff composition are considered in determining medical staff membership. The close involvement, complete understanding, and ultimate decision making of the board of trustees are important and necessary not only as part of a defence to any legal challenge, but also to assure consistency and objectivity among clinical departments as criteria for medical staff membership are developed.

## Board Interests

The board's interest is in having a medical staff associated with the hospital that supports the highest reasonable quality criteria and is sufficiently responsive to the medical care requirements of a given area. A quality criteria approach to medical staff composition may conflict with the latter. The board needs to assure itself that the criteria developed consist of elements that are aimed at the quality of service rather than the limitation of practice or economic opportunities of the current medical staff. Obviously, the board also needs to be involved in the application of these standards, including the final decision on admission.

## Medical Staff Concerns

While the board's involvement and ultimate decision making are essential, so too is the agreement of the medical staff regarding the worth of the effort. Most physicians would agree that quality measurement is important and would therefore support the concept. The major issues regarding acceptance are the imprecision by which quality is currently measured and the potential for misapplication or misunderstanding of the available data.

It is difficult to convince medical staff members to subject themselves to scrutiny by reviews that are not yet of demonstrated or accepted validity. A most persuasive argument concerns the defensive value of self-imposed quality review processes in a hospital setting. If a medical staff chooses not to develop and refine its quality approach, there are growing numbers of external forces that will attempt to accomplish the same end without the staff's involvement. Virtually all large volume purchasers of health care, whether governmental or private, have begun efforts of this type. Consumers also will be even better informed users of health care services. As more data moves into the public domain, it is only prudent to begin using such reviews in anticipation of its use by others. Medical staffs would prefer to enter into a discussion of quality with information based on their own experiences and developed by them rather than relying on information based on someone else's experiences. As the focus of review of health care broadens to include quality as well as price, the best prepared medical staff will be the one that has moved assertively to demonstrate its quality.

A final, critical appeal for the medical staff must also be to serve the best interest of the patient. As understanding health care quality moves from a case-based, individually focused process to one of better-defined expectations expressed in the form of indicators or standards, the patient will benefit.

## Market Initiatives

The last element of organizational concern is that of medical staff composition conforming with market initiatives. The use of quality criteria could slow entry into a particular market if generalized standards are so high that only a minority of potential medical staff applicants can achieve them. This choice will need to be made on an institution-by-institution basis depending on what it defines desired quality to be. Over time, the emphasis on quality should serve market initiatives well as the prominence of the notion of value increases and is recognized by the medical care consumer.

The many pressures facing hospitals and their medical staffs can be addressed by more vigorous pursuit of quality standards. Many hospitals not facing capacity concerns still wish to influence the specialty representation and number of physicians on their staffs. An effective option in medical staff development that can be employed is the elaboration and raising of quality criteria for membership. This mechanism can assist in managing the increasing numbers of physicians, the transition to managed care, and the marketing interests of a hospital. Most important, the basic missions of the hospital can be served as well.

## References

American Society for Laser Medicine and Surgery, Inc. "Standards of Practice for the Use of Lasers in Medicine and Surgery." Wausau, WI: The Society, 1984.

*FTC v. Indiana Federation of Dentists,* 476 U.S. 447 (1986).

Horty, John. *Action Kit for Hospital Trustees.* (May-June 1984): 1,3-4.

Joint Commission on Accreditation of Healthcare Organizations. *Accreditation Manual for Hospitals.* Chicago: The Commission, 1987.

*Khan v. Suburban Community Hospital,* 45 Ohio St. 2d 39, 340 N.E. 2d 398 (1976).

*Medical World News for Obstetricians, Gynecologists, Urologists.* "Procedures: Who Will Do Them?" (14 August 1986): 6-7.

*National Society of Professional Engineers v. United States,* 435 U.S. 679 (1978).

Paris, Ellen. "Hippocrates Meets Adam Smith." Forbes. 10 February 1986.

*Peterson v. Tucson General Hospital,* 114 Ariz. 66, 559 P. 2d 186 (1976).

*Sussman v. Overlook Hospital Association,* 95 N.J. Super. 418, 231 A.2d. 389 (1967); see also *Griesman v. Newcomb Hospital,* 40 N.J. 389, 192 A.2d. 817 (1963).

*Trustee.* "Closed Medical Staffs." 38 (September 1985): 58.

White, Daniel. "Exclusion of or Discrimination Against Physicians/Surgeons by Hospital." *American Law Reporter Third* 37, 645 (1987).

*Yeargin v. Hamilton Memorial Hospital,* 229 Ga. 870, 195 S.E. 2d 8 (1972).

# Effective Physician Credentialing
## Properly Monitoring Medical Staffs
## Can Protect Hospitals from Liability


Stephen M. Blaes, JD
Gary E. Knight, JD



**Summary**

Healthcare facilities today are finding themselves increasingly liable in malpractice suits if they have hired incompetent physicians or allowed them to remain on the medical staff. Thus appropriate processes for physician credentialing are important.

The hospital medical staff has the authority to evaluate medical staff membership status and clinical privileges and to take disciplinary and corrective action. If the medical staff fails to do its job, however, the hospital governing board is responsible for making sure the credentialing process is carried out properly. The same rules apply to the reapplication process.

The hospital must associate its credentialing process with its prevailing concern for high-quality patient care and document that ideal. Preservation of market share and elimination of competition must never enter into the credentialing process.

Well-framed hospital bylaws will help provide protection from liability, if they are followed correctly. If a hospital deviates from its bylaws when processing an application or granting clinical privileges, it risks a lawsuit. Congress has passed the Health Care Quality Improvement Act of 1986-an act that not only protects patients from incompetent practi-



Reprinted by permission of HEALTH PROGRESS, November, 1990, page 60, Copyright Catholic Health Association.


**205**

tioners but also can help limit the facility's risk of liability by requiring facilities and third-party payers to report any adverse actions taken against physicians. The National Practitioner Data Bank is an information clearinghouse opened in September 1990 that hospitals must use to report and obtain professional information about physicians

Today, a hospital may be held liable for its failure to properly monitor and control its medical staff's professional activities. A patient can hold a hospital accountable if it knows or should have known a physician was unqualified to be granted clinical privileges or was incompetent to practice medicine in accordance with the required standard of care. Because of this potential liability, hospitals must make physician credentialing a priority.

### Theories and Trends in Liability

Three legal theories exist on which a hospital may be found liable for the negligence of its medical staff:[1]

- *Respondeat superior.* A principal may be held liable for the actions of its agents.[2] Historically, however, hospitals have not been held accountable for the actions of nonemployee physicians because such physicians are independent contractors, not agents of the hospital.
- *Apparent agency.* A hospital may be held liable for the actions of a nonemployee physician if it permitted the physician to function in such a fashion that a reasonable person would conclude that he or she was in fact a hospital employee or agent. This situation arises most frequently in a hospital emergency room.[3]
- *Corporate negligence.* A hospital may be held liable for the negligence of its medical staff if the hospital fails to exercise reasonable care in the selection and retention of its medical staff, and this negligence is the proximate cause of the patient's injury. *Darling v. Charleston Community Memorial Hospital*[4] first established the notion that a hospital could be found liable in a medical malpractice action if it permitted a staff physician to perform surgical procedures for which he or she was not qualified. Corporate negligence is the most sweeping of the three theories.[5]

As an Arizona trial court has noted, "The emerging trend is to hold the hospital responsible where it failed to monitor and review medical services being provided within its walls."[6] In *Elam v. College Park Hospital,*[7] three malpractice lawsuits had been filed against a practitioner who was a member of the hospital's podiatric staff. Although the hospital's Medical Care

Evaluation Committee had been aware of these earlier lawsuits for nearly five months before the surgery in question, it took no action with respect to the practitioner's clinical privileges. The court found the hospital subject to liability under the doctrine of corporate negligence for the negligent conduct of an independent podiatrist who was neither an employed nor an agent of the hospital, but who simply used the hospital's facilities as a member of its medical staff. The court turned the Elam case into a warning to all hospitals: "We hold a hospital is accountable for negligently screening the competence of its medical staff to insure the adequacy of medical care rendered to patients at its facility."[8]

## The Importance of Credentialing

The potential liability for allowing an unqualified physician to become or remain a member of a medical staff makes the credentialing process especially critical to hospitals. Most hospital governing boards are not qualified to judge a physician's professional skills. Therefore the board delegates to the medical staff the responsibility and authority to evaluate all matters relating to medical staff membership status, clinical privileges, and disciplinary and corrective action. But if the medical staff fails to do its job, the board must act independently. The duty to take action is a nondelegable function that rests with the hospital's governing body.

In *Purcell v. Zimbelman*[9] a patient suffered complications as a result of surgery negligently performed by a general surgeon. The patient sued the physician and the hospital where the surgery took place, contending that the hospital had a duty to the public to allow only professionally competent physicians to use its facilities.

The hospital countered that it should not be held liable for its department of surgery's failure to act on the department's knowledge that several malpractice actions were pending against the physician. The court disagreed, stating that if the medical staff does not take action, the hospital's governing board must act on its own initiative.

### Misericordia

An important case on the investigation of medical staff applicant qualifications is *Johnson v. Misericordia Community Hospital*.[10] *Misericordia* involved a physician's negligence in attempting to remove a pin fragment from a patient's hip. The principal issue on appeal was whether a hospital owed its patients a duty of due care in the selection of its medical staff and in the granting of specialized surgical privileges. The court held that such a duty exists and that the hospital had breached that duty.

Because the hospital appeared to have done little right in its credentialing process, *Misericordia* teaches many lessons. The hospital did not have a functioning credentials committee and did not even try to verify the physician's credentials. It did not investigate any of the statements in his application or contact any of his references. Also, it did not investigate why the physician had failed to complete the portion of the application regarding malpractice insurance. Any investigation would have raised serious doubts about the physician's competence and veracity.

The court stated, "The failure to investigate a medical staff applicant's qualifications for the privileges requested gives rise to a foreseeable risk of unreasonable harm and we hold that a hospital has a duty to exercise due care in the selection of its medical staff."[11]

The court held that the standard of "ordinary care under the circumstances" in the selection of medical staff was applicable to the hospital, and the plaintiff *"was only obliged to prove that Misericordia did not make a reasonable effort to determine whether [the physician] was qualified to perform orthopedic surgery."*[12] The hospital was charged with constructive knowledge of information that it could have readily obtained by contacting the hospitals referred to by the physician in his application.

## Reapplication

These important principles apply to customary periodic reapplications for staff membership and clinical privileges, as well. In *Bell v. Sharp Cabrillo Hospital*,[13] a physician was reappointed to the staff even though his reappointment application disclosed that one hospital had refused to renew his clinical privileges and another had revoked them. Key medical staff officers failed to determine the reasons for the adverse actions, even though the physician had signed a release allowing verification of the information. As a consequence, the hospital was found liable for failing to exercise reasonable care in reexamining the professional competence of a long-time member of the medical staff.

## Effective Credentialing

A hospital can minimize its exposure to liability in several practical ways. First, it can ensure that its medical staff's application forms, bylaws, rules, and regulations are framed to protect the staff and the hospital. Appropriate application and reapplication forms ask the correct questions; the answers to such questions will disclose telltale information regarding professional

**Table 1. Effective Credentialing: The Questions to Ask**

**The Application Form**
- Education, training, and professional experience?
- Physical or mental impairments?
- Disciplinary actions elsewhere?
- Denials of staff membership?
- Status of liability insurance?
- Malpractice claims and payments?
- Credentials verified?
- Application complete?

**Professional References**
- In writing?
- Supportive or lukewarm?
- Hints of professional inadequacy or unacceptable behavior? (If yes, inquire further.)
- From former teachers or instructors?
- From know practice partners?
- From well-regarded professionals?
- From those who really know?
- From all those who should be listed as references?
- Telephone conversation indicated?

**The Reappointment Process**
- Information meaningfully updated?
- Intervening denials of staff membership?
- Clinical privileges adversely affected elsewhere?
- Performance indicators in other settings?
- Liability insurance status?
- Pending or concluded malpractice claims? Unfavorable indicators
- Controversy about the candidate? Why?
- Objective unfavorable recommendations?
- Clinically supportable objections?
- Requested privileges consistent with competence?
- Consistent with the hospital's needs?
- Reasons for unfavorable staff committee reports?
- Proposed action consistent with that for other physicians? If not, why?

    **If Adverse Findings are Suggested**
- Supported by substantive, objective evidence?

---

**Table 1. Effective Credentialing: The Questions to Ask (Cont'd.)**

- Specific cases or clinical procedures targeted?
- Supported by clinical audits?
- Complaints from competitors?
- Personal or business reasons involved?
- Other practitioners supportive while only competitors criticize?

**If Adverse Action Is Proposed**
- Termination of membership?
- Suspension or restriction of privileges?
- Probation?
- Further training and experience?
- Mandatory consultation or professional assistance?
- Remedy commensurate with the deficiency?
- Least intrusive imposition?
- Enhance the quality of clinical work?

---

training, skills, and demeanor. The Box lists some practical questions for effective credentialing.

The hospital board cannot be timid about inquiring into these matters, however sensitive they might be. Both the chief executive officer and the medical staff representative delivering the recommendation must be prepared to respond to the board's probing. At the conclusion of the discussion, all concerned should be comfortable with the objectivity, fairness, and consistency in the application of reasonable standards when reviewing a candidate.

## Clinical Privileges

The candidate should seek only clinical privileges reasonably consistent with his or her training and competence. If doubts exist about the privileges requested, the hospital board should ask the appropriate staff committee or clinical department to reexamine the applicant's credentials and offer more complete documentation or support for the recommendation. It is not unusual for the medical staff or the board to require additional clinical training or education, offer standby assistance or personal participation with another physician for a number of the specific procedures, or require mandatory consultations and monitoring by a professional colleague on a probationary basis.

### Reappointments

Hospital should avoid automatic, unverified reappointments. Reappointment applications should update the application with respect to disciplinary actions in other settings, denials of staff membership in other facilities, liability insurance coverage, and the status of malpractice suits.

The medical staff credentials committee should make certain that all the application questions are fully answered. Evasive answers or questions left blank are red flags that suggest the possibility of important information deliberately withheld. As demonstrated in *Misericordia,* failure to inquire further may well be grounds for liability if the information could have prevented an incompetent or unqualified practitioner from being granted the privileges in question.

### Adverse Information

Adverse information should be supported with substantive findings or rationale. If the complaints are focused on professional skill, a trained and experienced director of medical staff services or medical coordinator should cite specific cases or procedures supported by clinical audits or department-specific reviews. In smaller facilities this responsibility may be delegated to a member of the management team who works closely with the medical staff and is responsible for coordinating its activities. Also, in handling problem files or questionable entries on applications, it is important to involve medical staff leaders in the information review and reference verification processes. Telephone conferences between professional colleagues often lead to disclosure of important, reliable information.

If a remedy, such as further training or mandatory consultation, is proposed, it should be consistent with the claimed deficiency; that is, the remedy should be the least intrusive imposition consistent with the concern for high-quality work. For example, a physician may not have sufficient experience in the specific clinical procedure for which he or she has requested privileges. To ensure competency, the privilege may be granted subject to carefully framed conditions of proctorship, consultations, attendance, or other assistance by another qualified practitioner who holds such privileges.

### Healthcare Entity's Values

For a healthcare entity to credential effectively, it must associate the credentialing process with its prevailing concern for high-quality patient care and document that ideal. It is extremely important to associate the process (both favorable and unfavorable actions) with the need to ensure high-quality patient care. Thus, if the medical staff and board take unfavorable action against a practitioner, the focus of the inquiry, the documentation, or any conditions imposed on the practitioner's clinical activities should reflect an abiding interest in quality assurance and correct clinical practice.

Preservation of market share and elimination of competition must never enter into the credentialing process. The focus must be on high-quality patient care. Preventing a competent and qualified physician from treating patients to protect the patient base or other physicians' incomes smacks of anticompetitive conduct and is a violation of antitrust laws. Although medical staffs and governing boards generally enjoy qualified protection from antitrust liability in peer review and quality assurance activities, that immunity may be jeopardized when commercial or business reasons creep into the process.[14]

## Medical Staff Bylaws

The only thing worse than not having good, well-framed bylaws is having them but not following them. If a hospital deviates from its own medical staff bylaws when processing an application or granting clinical privileges, it invites liability from a variety of quarters, such as an aggrieved physician whose reputation has been damaged, a physician who has been deprived privileges because the application process is inconsistent with the bylaw requirements, or a patient who claims to have been injured because the hospital ignored quality assessment or departmental protocols described in the bylaws.

Bylaws constitute self-imposed standards of procedural due process and, in some instances, even self-imposed standards of care. Executive and medical staff leaders should carefully frame bylaws so they do not create impossible levels of performance and compliance. The law measures professional skill, clinical performance, and quality assessments against standards of reasonableness and adequacy, so through its bylaws a hospital should not impose on itself a higher standard.

Executive and medical staff leaders must work closely with well-informed legal counsel in writing bylaws. The bylaws are a key document that will provide the basic road map for the credentialing process-from receipt of the application through granting of privileges or hearings and appeals. Case law is replete with instances in which unskillfully written bylaws spawned needless litigation.

**Health Care Act**

Congress has passed an act to help protect hospitals, care givers, and patients—the Health Care Quality Improvement Act of 1986.[15] Moreover, the act is supportive of all the concepts and strategies needed for effective credentialing. The act is an attempt to provide qualified immunity against civil liability in the case of an adverse peer review that is conducted in good faith with the reasonable belief that such action is taken to promote high-quality healthcare. In the first case decided under the act, a court held that the act provided immunity from federal antitrust liability to a hospital and certain of its staff doctors for their peer review activities.[16]

The act established the National Practitioner Data Bank[17] to encourage peer review activities and to help hospitals check physicians' credentials. Information available in the data bank may prevent unqualified doctors from moving to another state in an attempt to conceal their incompetencies.

The data bank, which opened in September 1990, will serve as a national clearinghouse for healthcare entities to report and request information about any physician who has been subject to an adverse action concerning clinical privileges or a malpractice suit.[18]

## Requesting Information

The act requires that a hospital request information from the data bank about every physician who applies for admission to the medical staff or for clinical privileges. In addition, at least every two years, a hospital must ask the data bank for an update concerning each physician who is on its medical staff or who has been granted clinical privileges. If a hospital fails to request such information, it is deemed by law to have knowledge of all information it could have learned had it made the request.

## Reporting

To ensure that the data bank includes comprehensive, up-to-date information, healthcare entities are required to report certain information about physicians and other practitioners within a specified period after an action. In general, the act requires reports of medical malpractice payments, sanctions by boards of medical examiners, and adverse actions taken by a professional review body of a healthcare entity. Any healthcare entity that fails to meet the reporting requirements may (for a period of three years) lose the immunity from liability granted under the act. By the same token, the reversal of a healthcare entity's professional review action or an agency's reinstatement of a license must be reported in the same time frame and in the same manner as other reportable actions.

Under the act, any organization or individual (including an insurance company, hospital, or self-insurance program) that makes even a nominal payment in settlement or partial settlement of a malpractice claim must report the payment to the data bank within 30 days of payment. Failure to report such a payment may result in a fine of up to $10,000. The waiver of a hospital's or practitioner's outstanding debt in settlement of a claim is not considered a payment on a malpractice claim and need not be reported.

If a healthcare entity takes action that adversely affects a physician's clinical privileges for more than 30 days, the entity must report that action to the appropriate state licensing board. The healthcare entity must also report the physician's surrender of clinical privileges in the course of an investigation or in an exchange for the cancellation or the discontinuance of an investigation. A practitioner's decision to voluntarily reduce privileges for reasons of personal preference is not a reportable event.

Healthcare entities must submit reports of this kind to the appropriate state board or agency within 15 days after the date the adverse action is formally adopted. State licensing boards, in turn, are required to pass along such information to the data bank no more than 15 days after they receive it.

## Importance of Compliance

The data bank is an important new information clearinghouse for a hospital's credentialing, peer review, and quality assurance functions. The data bank enhances a hospital's ability to verify a physician's credentials, hence enhancing its ability to deliver high-quality care. Severe sanctions will be levied on hospitals that fail to comply with the requirements to provide information to and seek information from the data bank. Hospitals must therefore take steps to comply with the data bank's information requesting and reporting requirements.

**References**

1. Diane M. Janulis and Alan D. Hornstein, "Damned If You Do, Damned If You Don't: Hospitals' Liability for Physician's Malpractice," *Nebraska Law Review*, vol. 64, 1985, p. 689.
2. See *Carranza v. Tucson Medical Center*, 135 Ariz. 490, 662 P.2d 455 (1983).

3. See *Mehlman v. Powell*, 281 Md. 269, 378 A.2d 1121 (1977).

4. *Darling v. Charleston Community Memorial Hospital*, 50 Ill. App.2d 253, 200 N.E.2d 149 (1964), aff'd., 33 Ill.2d 326, 211 N.E.2d 253 (1965), cert. den., 383 U.S. 946 (1966).

5. For a listing of states whose courts have expressly adopted the corporate negligence doctrine, see *Insinga v. Labelle*, _________ Fla. _________, 543 So.2d 209, 213-214 (1989).

6. *Fridena v. Evans*, 127 Ariz. 516, 622 P.2d 463, 466 (1980).

7. *Elam v. College Park Hospital*, 132 Cal. App.3d 332, 183 Cal. Rptr. 156 (1982).

8. *Elam*, p. 165 (emphasis added).

9. *Purcell v. Zimbelman*, 18 Ariz. App. 75, 500 P.2d 335 (1972).

10. *Johnson v. Misericordia Community Hospital*, 99 Wis.2d 708, 301 N.W.2d 156 (1981).

11. *Misericordia*, p. 164.

12. *Misericordia*, p. 172 (emphasis in original).

13. *Bell v. Sharp Cabrillo Hospital*, 212 Cal. App. 3d 1034, 260 Cal. Rptr. 886 (1989).

14. For a discussion of the scope of immunity and loss of protection because of a violation of antitrust precepts, see *Patrick v. Burget*, 108 S.Ct. 1658 (1988). This case was based on facts arising before the enactment of the Health Care Quality Improvement Act (discussed below). Because of the egregious anticompetitive nature of the defendants' actions in this case, they probably would not have been entitled to immunity under the act even if it had been applicable.

15. Public Law 99-660, 100 Statute 3784; as amended by Public Law 100-77, 101 Statute 986.

16. *Austin v. McNamara*, 731 F. Supp. 934 (C.D. Cal 1990); see also Mark A. Kadzielski, "Court Upholds Law's Immunities in Peer Review Cases," *Health Progress*, July-August 1990, pp. 21, 31.

17. Mark A. Kadzielski, "Practitioner Data Bank to Open Soon," Health Progress, March 1990, pp. 87-88.

18. 54 Fed. Reg. 42722, 45 C.F.R. 60 et seq.

# Current Legal Developments in Medical Staff Credentialing Disputes


Michael R. Callahan
Damon N. Vocke


In the past decade, the granting of privileges to practice in hospital settings, once virtually the sole province of the medical profession, has come under increased scrutiny by the courts. Physicians and other health professionals whose privileges have been denied or suspended have argued that they have been denied due process in the decision making or that the hospital staff has rejected them for reasons other than their professional competence. As access to hospitals is essential for many types of medical practice and typically provides the greatest economic benefits, courts have been increasingly willing to consider such cases on the basis of the economic and property rights involved and also as part of growing social concern about the quality and cost of medical care. This chapter discusses legal developments in these areas, utilizing a number of examples from Illinois as well as from other jurisdictions. In addition, recommendations for methods of approaching credentialing decisions will be made based on current legal trends. While many of the cases cited refer to nonpsychiatric practice, the principles involved are equally applicable to mental health professionals.

## Applications for Privileges

In order for hospital credentials committees to ensure that sufficient information is available from which to make appropriate decisions concerning membership in their medical staff organization, these committees should specifically inquire of applicants about the limits, if any, of their malpractice coverage; the names of other hospitals where they have had staff privileges and whether their privileges have been adversely affected; whether their licenses to practice or medical staff privileges have ever been revoked or suspended or whether they have been subjected to supervision because of deviations from appropriate practice; the number, if any, of malpractice suits filed against them, the nature of the suits, and their disposition; whether their participation in Medicare, Medicaid, or any other third-party payer program has ever been suspended; whether their application for staff privileges at any hospital has ever been denied or withdrawn; and other similar questions. Hospitals are also beginning to ask these important questions one at a time, and using reappointment as a means of fulfilling its quality assurance, licensing, and accreditation requirements.

Many hospitals are now including waiver clauses in their application forms; through such clauses, the physician applicant agrees to release any materials other hospitals or other parties possess that are relevant to a decision on his or her application and agrees to hold the hospital and other parties blameless for the release of such information should he or she subsequently file a lawsuit. Such clauses also apply in the event that the hospital denies the application or suspends, reduces, or terminates the physician's privileges. It has also become common to include statements that the medical staff bylaws do not constitute a contract in order to preclude later charges by physicians that the hospital has breached its contract with them through disciplinary actions.

Since many malpractice suits filed against hospitals involve charges that the physician was not competent to perform the particular procedures in question, credentials committees must pay more careful attention to the specific privileges they grant. Hospital medical staffs and boards have an obligation to ensure that physicians perform only procedures for which they are qualified and formally credentialed.

Many hospital bylaws do not provide for hearings for applicants denied staff privileges. There is currently no Illinois case law requiring such hearings; but there are federal regulations (Code of Federal Regulations, volume 42, Section 405.102 (e)(7)), and professional standards (Joint Commission on Accreditation of Hospitals, n.d. Section I.B.9) require or recommend that rejected applicants receive a fair hearing.

Hospitals have been receiving increased applications for privileges from nonphysicians and have been subject to litigation for refusing to grant such privileges (see Chapter Five). As courts have differed in their decisions in these cases, hospitals should determine their needs for nonphysicians and allied health professionals before receiving applications for privileges from these practitioners. This determination should be initiated and the final decisions should be made by the hospital's board of directors, with consultation by its medical staff.

## Corrective Action for Current Medical Staff Members

Corrective action includes any action taken by the medical staff, hospital administration, and/or board of trustees that reduces, suspends, terminates, or otherwise adversely affects the medical staff privileges of a physician already on that staff. Decisions leading to reprimands, censure, or requirements for supervision are not legally considered to be corrective actions unless otherwise stated in the bylaws. It is important that the hospital board review and make the final decisions on all such corrective measures.

One different approach to the corrective action process arises out of concerns within the medical profession that the process is overly legalistic and adversarial. This approach calls for an "intraprofessional conference and review" to serve as a forum for the resolution of issues involving professional conduct and competence. The purpose of such conferences is to promote the resolution of differences on an intraprofessional basis while still giving the adversely affected physician all of the rights he or she has under current bylaw procedures. The conference is not a formal courtroom proceeding, and rules of law governing the questioning of witnesses or the presentation of evidence do not apply. In addition, an adversarial confrontation is not contemplated. The role, if any, of legal counsel is usually limited to advising clients. Counsel are not permitted to "examine" or "cross-examine" witnesses. Many medical staffs have recently adopted these procedures as a substitute for more legalistic ones.

Traditional grounds for corrective action include suspension or revocation of the physician's license to practice by the state licensing board; failure to obtain malpractice insurance (*Kelly v. St. Vincent Hospital*, 1984; *Renforth v. Fayette Memorial Hospital Association*, 1979) even if the physician cannot afford such insurance or it is unavailable (*Holmes v. Hoemako Hospital*, 1977); the physician's disruptive behavior or inability to work with colleagues (*Bricker v. Crane*, 1978; *Miller v. Indiana Hospital*, 1980; overutilization of the hospital resources (*Anton v. San Antonio Community Hospital*, 1977; *Knapp v. Palos Community Hospital*, 1984; *Spencer v. Community Hospital of Evanston*, 1980); and violation of hospital rules, such as failure to follow medical records policies (*Peterson v. Tucson General Hospital, Inc*, 1976) or failure to pay library assessments (*Chapman v. People Community Hospital*, 1984). More recent grounds for corrective action including failure to abide by diagnostic related group (DRG) policies; failure to obtain specialty board certification; failure to utilize the hospital's services; moving one's practice beyond certain geographical boundaries (Joint Commission on Accreditation of Hospitals, n.d., Section IV.B.2(c)); and removal or denial of privileges based on the existence of exclusive contracts (*Hyde v. Jefferson Parish Hospital District No.2*, 1984; *Mays v. Hospital Authority of Henry County*, 1984).

## Procedural Considerations in Corrective Action

In Illinois and most other jurisdictions, physicians have no constitutional rights to hospital privileges (*Settler v. Hopedale Medical Foundation*, 1980). Moreover, the doctrine of state action is not applicable to private hospitals, and therefore physicians are not entitled to due process or equal protection when their privileges are reduced, suspended, or terminated (*Jain v. Northwest Community Hospital*, 1978). Hospitals are permitted to adopt reasonable rules for their own governance and internal management, including the granting or removal of privileges, as long as the rules are neither arbitrary nor capricious (*Fahey v. Holy Family Hospital*, 1975).

Under the public policy in Illinois, courts will not review a private hospital's initial medical staff appointment decisions (*Barrows v. Northwest Community Hospital*, 1988). It is, however, unsettled whether the rule of nonreview applies when an initial applicant claims state antitrust violations, fraud, or tortious interference with an existing business relationship (*Barrows v. Northwest Community Hospital*, 1988). Where a physician has been denied medical staff privileges or has his or her privileges adversely affected, courts are usually concerned only with whether or not the hospital has substantially complied with its own medical staff bylaws (*Maimon v. Sisters of the Third Order of St. Francis*, 1983; *Siquiera v. Northwestern Memorial Hospital*, 1985).

If, however, the plaintiff physician is able to sufficiently establish the existence of bias or prejudice on the part of the voting members of the medical staff, courts may reverse the hospital's denial or revocation of privileges (*Ladenheim v. Union County Hospital District*, 1979; *Van Daele v. Vinci*, 1972). Depending on the evidence, the physician may be able to assert an antitrust claim under a group boycott or conspiracy theory.

In order to avoid liability when making decisions to take corrective action, hospitals should make sure that their bylaws, standards, rules, and regulations are carefully crafted to provide procedural protections for staff facing disciplinary actions. Sufficient documentation, including medical records, incident reports, patient complaints, utilization reviews, quality assurance reports, audits, committee minutes, and past statements by the physician under investigation, should be assembled, both to document the bases for the ultimate decision and to demonstrate that a thorough investigation has taken place. It should be remembered that hospitals may be held liable for failure to take corrective action against physicians who practice below the acceptable standards of care; if the decision is made to take little or no corrective action, the hospital must be prepared to justify its decision. Careful thought should also be given to the type of corrective action taken to ensure that it is appropriate to and commensurate with the deviation from professional standards revealed by the investigation, although courts will generally defer to a hospital's decision. Sanctions may include summary suspension, required supervision, reduction or termination of privileges, or reprimand. Appropriateness of the action taken may be supported by demonstration that persons involved in the alleged misconduct have been interviewed, that the action is linked to the provision of quality care, that all relevant information has been gathered, and that the medical staff as a whole is supportive of the action taken.

## Notice of Hearing

Physicians facing corrective action should be provided with written notice of the proposed action. The letter should cite the relevant bylaw provisions and the basis for the recommended action or actions, including references to specific incident reports, charts, and audits. The letter should be tied to the bylaw language and should set for the physician's rights under the bylaws. All relevant documents and the relevant parts of the bylaws should be attached to the letter, which should be sent by registered or certified mail or delivered by personal messenger. The hospital should be sure to adhere to the time requirements specified in the bylaws but should be flexible regarding the physician's response. Applicable court decisions regarding notice should be observed. Note that the charges need not be drawn with the same precision as required in a judicial action (*Kelly v. Police Board of Chicago*, 1975). For example, in *Kaplan v. Carney* (1975), the physician had received notice that physician records showed "evidence of exaggerated diagnoses, inappropriate treatment, and errors of medical judgment," but the notice did not refer to specific patient charts, and the physician was not given the charts in question until the day before the hearing; the court found that these procedures complied with due process requirements.

## Use of Outside Consultants

If proposed consultants are not covered by the hospital's insurance policy, be prepared to enter into an indemnification agreement in order to treat the consultant as the hospital's agent for quality assurance purposes. If consultants are to be used, the physician should be notified, and his or her agreement to the selection of the consultant should be sought in order to prevent subsequent claims of bias or prejudice. The consultant should have a good reputation and should practice in the same specialty as the physician under investigation. Consultants should be familiarized with the applicable standards and regulations, but should be given only that information on which the hospital relied in making its recommendation for corrective action. The hospital should define the scope of the consultant's task and the form (but not the content) of the opinion sought, which should be as objective as possible. The consultant's report should be given to the physician, but only if corrective action is ultimately recommended. While outside consultants may be useful in countering claims of in-house discrimination, the hospital may feel compelled to accept recommendations with which it disagrees. For this reason, the use of multiple consultants may be advisable.

## Hearing Panel

Panel members should be chosen who have not been involved with previous corrective actions themselves and who are not actual or perceived competitors in order to avoid charges of bias or discrimination. Backup panel members should also be chosen in case of disqualifications. The panel should represent a cross-section of physicians with regard to temperament and sympathies toward the physician facing the hearing and should represent a balance of various medical specialties; it should always contain one or more members from the same specialty as the physician facing the hearing. When it has been difficult to use a peer who is not a competitor, some hospitals are beginning to bring in nonstaff physicians to serve on the panel. Emphasis should be placed on characterizing the hearing as an intraprofessional conference rather than as an adversarial hearing. The appointment of a representative from the hospital's medical staff may be specified in the bylaws; if not, seek guidance from the chief of staff and other administrative staff. The physician most familiar with the grounds for corrective action may be a logical choice. In any event, someone should be chosen who is of the same specialty and who commands respect. The representative should spend a significant amount of time with the hospital counsel. The physician should be notified in advance of the proposed panel members and asked if he or she has objections to any. If so, the physician should respond in writing, stating the basis for any objections. An alternative would be to provide a list of proposed panel members and to permit the physician to choose from the list.

## Representation by Legal Counsel

There is no legal requirement in Illinois that the physician be represented by legal counsel; the trend in the case law, however, is to permit representation (*Garrow v. Elizabeth General Hospital and Dispensary*, 1979). Hospitals should request that the physician inform the panel in a timely fashion if he or she intends to be represented by legal counsel; if legal representation is permitted, the hospital should also secure legal counsel. If the physician is not permitted legal representation, representation by another physician should be allowed. Where representation is allowed, the attorney's role should be limited to that of adviser. Counsel should be permitted to make opening statements, to raise procedural and other objections to the panel, and to present written objections or presentation on behalf of the physician, but direct or cross-examination should not be allowed.

The role of counsel for the medical staff should parallel that for the physician's counsel; he or she should properly prepare the presenters. Counsel for the hearing panel should meet with the panel members prior to the hearing in order to familiarize them with the purpose of the hearing, the medical staff bylaws and their role under those bylaws, and the procedures to be followed. He or she should inform the panel members of their protections under the relevant state laws and should make sure that they seek advice of counsel on procedural matters before issuing a final ruling.

## The Hearing

At the outset of the hearing, the panel should read from a statement prepared by counsel regarding the nature of the case, its procedural history, the role of the hearing panel and legal counsel, the order of presentation, and the type of recommendations the panel is authorized to make. The affected physician should be asked if he or she has any objections to the rules, any of the actions of the panel to date, or any claimed bylaw violations. The panel should suggest that any such objections be presented in writing prior to the hearing so that the panel can cure any defects (*Even v. Longmont United Hospital Association*, 1981; *Ritter v. Board of Commissioners*, 1981). The panel should inquire of both sides as to how they wish to proceed and the number of witnesses to be called. The panel may itself call witnesses, request relevant documents not entered by either party, and ask questions of any party during the hearing.

The panel should not require adherence to strict rules of evidence, committee minutes, medical records, consultations, reports, and other relevant material should be readily accepted. Evidence of the practice of other physicians should not be admissible in defense of the physician whose case is being heard. All evidence that is accepted should be secured to assure confidentiality.

The burden of proof may properly be imposed on the charged physician (*Anton v. San Antonio Community Hospital*, 1977; *Pinsker v. Pacific Coast Society of Orthodontists*, 1974). Where due process applies, only adequate notice of charges and a reasonable opportunity to respond (*Duffield v. Charleston Area Medical Center, Inc*, 1974; *Kaplan v. Carney*, 1975) are required. The right to cross-examine is not mandated (*Woodbury v. McKinnon*, 1971). Courts typically defer to medical judgments and avoid individual review of the evidence presented (*Jain v. Northwest Community Hospital*, 1978; *Ritter v. Board of Commissioners*, 1981; *Sosa v. Board of Managers of Val Verde Memorial Hospital*, 1971), but some courts have begun to move toward a substantial evidence rule (*Silver v. Castle Memorial Hospital*, 1972). To be legally relevant, bias or prejudice alleged against medical staff members must have arisen from an extrajudicial source unrelated to the peer review proceedings (*Ladenheim v. Union County Hospital District*, 1979). Generalized, as opposed to specific, findings are acceptable if in compliance with the hospital bylaws (*Knapp v. Palos Community Hospital*, 1984).

Counsel should assist the panel in drafting findings and recommendations. The hearing panel usually has great flexibility in fashioning a remedy to deviations from accepted practice, as long as it conforms to the hospital bylaws. Specific findings based on evidence reviewed should be put in writing, and evidence should be cited to support the decision, together with specific reference to violations of the applicable bylaws, rules, or regulations. If corrective action is recommended, it should be tied to the nature of the problems that were uncovered by the peer review process.

## Appellate Hearing

Neither the Joint Commission on Accreditation of Healthcare Organizations (JCAHO) nor the courts have required the establishment of an appeals process from an ad hoc hearing recommendation. A request for an appeal by either party, if allowed, should be to the hospital board of directors or to a committee appointed by the board. If the physician is permitted to appear before the appeals panel, he or she should be permitted to raise any objections with respect either to the procedures followed or to the decision. The appellant should be encouraged to submit the reasons for the appeal in writing to the appeals panel prior to the appeal hearing. Usually no evidence may be presented at the appeal that was not otherwise available to the original hearing panel. The burden of the appeal falls on the appellant.

## Role of the Board of Directors

The Joint Commission on Accreditation of Hospitals, case law, and Illinois statutes require that the hospital governing board make all final decisions regarding credentialing. These requirements serve to insulate the medical staff from liability and to satisfy fiduciary responsibilities to the hospital (*Darling v. Charleston Community Memorial Hospital*, 1966; *Pickle v. Carns*, 1982). The board should engage in thorough discussion of corrective action proceedings in order to avoid claims that it is simply a rubber stamp for the medical staff (*Weiss v. York Hospital*, 1985). The discussions should be carefully detailed in the board's minutes and in its final report. Courts have upheld board decisions despite the fact that the board's decision disagreed with the recommendations of the medical staff (*Siquiera v. Northwestern Memorial Hospital*, 1985).

## Reporting Decisions to Other Agencies

Illinois and most other states now require hospitals to report all final decisions regarding suspension, termination, or reduction of medical staff privileges of a physician who engages in unprofessional conduct to the state agency that controls professional licensure. Although these agencies also seek the underlying peer review material that supported the corrective action decision, a hospital should make sure that it is not violating any confidentiality statutes. It is also important to recognize that material given to the state may become available to the public and therefore to the plaintiff's attorneys; for this reason, discretion must be used.

## Litigation Arising out of Corrective Action

Physicians who have received adverse decisions concerning their privileges have sought relief in court based on a variety of grounds, including violation of medical staff bylaws, violation of constitutional guarantees of due process and equal protection, defamation (*Green v. Silver Cross Hospital*, 1984; *Matview v. Johnson*, 1982; *Spencer v. Community Hospital of Evanston*, 1980), conspiracy (*Maimon v. Sisters of the Third Order of St. Francis*, 1983), tortious interference with a contract or a business relationship (*Buckner v. Lower Florida Keys Hospital District*, 1981; *Murray v. Bridgeport Hospital*, 1984) state or federal antitrust violations (*Patrick v. Burget*, 1988), and intentional infliction of emotional distress (*Gordon v. Lancaster Osteopathic Hospital Association*, 1985). While Illinois has not held that medical staff bylaws constitute a contract, other state courts are divided on the issue. Physicians have also sought injunctive relief from corrective action, but typically without much success (*Curle v. Evangelical Hospital Association*, 1980; *Dos Santos v. Columbus-Cuneo-Cabrini Medical Center*, 1982; *Early v. Bristol Memorial Hospital, Inc*, 1980; *Rutledge v. St. Vincent Memorial Hospital*, 1966).

Federal antitrust claims against physicians participating on peer review committees are usually based on charges of group boycott under Section 1 of the Sherman Antitrust Act when the committee in question is denying, revoking, or restricting staff privileges. This claim alleges that some or all of the peer review participants are competition for the excluded physician and that these members acted to restrict or eliminate competition. Until the recent Supreme Court discussion in *Patrick v. Burget* (1988), a defendant-physician could successfully invoke the state-action doctrine; this doctrine attempts to apply federal commitment laws to peer review participants who are performing their duties under a state law that is clearly articulated and actively supervised by the state. Since *Patrick v. Burget*, the state-action doctrine cannot be satisfied unless the appropriate state agency has the ultimate authority in credentialing decisions, determining whether hospital credentialing decisions comport with state regulatory policy and correcting abuses. Frequently, there are no state statutes that grant this authority to the state; hence, the state-action doctrine is not applicable.

The Health Care Quality Improvement Act of 1986 was enacted in response to the restrictive approach to antitrust immunity and is concerned with the prevalence of medical malpractice and the reluctance of physicians to participate in the peer review process. The act is intended to restrict the ability of physicians to move from state to state without discovery of their incompetence. To foster participation in peer review, the act provides physicians who engage in peer review with qualified immunity from liability for their participation as long as the hospital complies with certain notice, hearing and mandatory reporting requirements.

A physician denied privileges, or whose privileges have been restricted or revoked, may also claim a violation of his or her civil rights. Under Title VII of the Civil Rights Act of 1964, it is unlawful for an employer to discriminate on the basis of race, religion, sex, or national origin. The trend in case law has been to consider physicians as "employees" with standing to sue hospitals for unlawful discrimination under Title VII despite the fact that they are usually independent contractors. An "employer" under Title VII may be any party who significantly affects access to any individual's employment opportunities. Thus, although physicians may not technically be employed by a hospital but are actually employed by their patients, the loss of staff privileges may significantly affect their employment so that they have standing to sue under Title VII.

Litigation has also arisen from interpretation of the Illinois Medical Studies Act. The act states that any information obtained in the course of internal quality control shall be privileged and confidential; such information can only be used for medical research, the improvement of quality of care, or for granting, limiting, or revoking staff privileges. Typically, the provision bars disclosure of documents compiled in the course of granting, restricting, or suspending a doctor's staff privileges. But in situations in which information was obtained independently of such procedures, discovery may be permitted. For example, a recent medical malpractice decision held that the results of polygraph tests administered to nurses to determine whether they altered patients' records were not privileged under the state's Medical Studies Act (*Marsh v. Lake Forest Hospital*, 1988). In addition, the claim of confidentiality cannot be invoked to deny a physician access to or use of the information on which a decision is based in a proceeding to decide his or her staff privileges or in a judicial review of such proceedings.

Protections for the peer review process included in the act have been found constitutional (*Jenkins v. Wu*, 1984), and the evidence presented in corrective action hearings is also protected (*Mennes v. South Chicago Community Hospital*, 1981). But hospitals may not use the protections of the act to deny access to relevant evidence to physician under review (*Gleason v. St. Elizabeth Medical Center*, 1985; *Richter v. Diamond*, 1985). If a court requires discovery of evidence that the hospital wishes to suppress, the hospital may seek to be held in contempt in order to appeal directly to the state supreme court (*Jenkins v. Wu*, 1984; *Niven v. Siquiera*, 1985; *Richter v. Diamond*, 1985).

Recent amendments to the act (and similar legislation in other jurisdictions) have provided increased protections for the peer review process to encourage appropriate and effective internal professional review of medical conduct without unnecessary interference from the courts.

An additional safeguard found within a Medical Studies Act amendment provides that disclosure of any privileged information, whether proper or improper, shall not waive or have any effect on the confidentiality, nondiscoverability, or nonadmissibility of that information (*Gleason v. St. Elizabeth Medical Center*, 1985; *Richter v. Diamond*, 1985). This amendment has received retroactive application by an Illinois appellate court to prohibit discovery of infection control reports in two medical malpractice cases filed in 1983.

A recent amendment to the Hospital Licensing Act is similarly designed to encourage peer review by health care providers; the amendment provides immunity from civil liability to any hospital or individual that participates in the peer review process for the purpose of internal quality control, improving patient care, or professional discipline (Illinois Revised Statutes, Chapter 111-1/2, Section 151.2). However, this amendment does not relieve any individual or hospital from liability arising from the treatment of a patient.

## References

*Anton v. San Antonio Community Hospital*, 19 Cal. 3d 802, 567 P.2d 1162 (1977).

*Barrows v. Northwest Community Hospital*, No. 65055 (Ill. S.C., May 1988).

*Bricker v. Crane*, 118 N.H. 249, 387 A.2d 321 (1978).

*Buckner v. Lower Florida Keys Hospital District*, 403 So.2d 1025 (Fla. App. Ct. 1981).

*Chapman v. People Community Hospital*, 362 N.W.2d 755 (Mich. App. 1984).

*Curle v. Evangelical Hospital Association*, 89 Ill. App. 3d 45, 411 N.E.2d 326 (2nd Dist. 1980).

*Darling v. Charleston Community Memorial Hospital*, 33 Ill. 2d 236, 211 N.E. 2d 253 (1965); cert. denied, sub nom *Charleston Community Hospital v. Darling*, 383 U.S. 946 (1966).

*Dos Santos v. Columbus-Cuneo-Cabrini Medical Center*, 684 E.2d 1346 (7th Cir. 1982).

*Duffield v. Charleston Area Medical Center, Inc.*, 503 F.2d 512 (4th Cir. 1974).

*Early v. Bristol Memorial Hospital, Inc,* 508 F. Supp. 35 (E.D. Tenn. 1980).

*Even v. Longmont United Hospital Association,* 629 P.2d 1100 (Co.App.1981).

*Fahey v. Holy Family Hospital,* 32 Ill. App.3d 537 336 N.E.2s (1st Dist. 1975).

*Garrow v. Elizabeth General Hospital and Dispensary,* 79 N.J. 549, 401 A.2d 533 (1979).

*Gleason v. St. Elizabeth Medical Center,* 135 Ill. App.3d 92 (1985).

*Gordon v. Lancaster Osteopathic Hospital Association,* 489 A.2d 1364 (Pa. Super. Ct. 1985).

*Green v. Silver Cross Hospital,* 606 F. Supp. 87 (N.D. Ill. 1984).

*Holmes v. Hoemako Hospital,* 117 Ariz. 403, 573 P.2d 477 (1977).

*Hyde v. Jefferson Parish Hospital District No.2,* 80 L.Ed. 2, 104 S. Ct. 1551 (1984).

*Jain v. Northwest Community Hospital,* 67 Ill. App. 3d 850, 385 N.E. 2d 109 (1st Dist. 1978).

*Jenkins v. Wu,* 102 Ill. 2d 468, 468 N.E. 2d 1162 (Ill. 1984).

Joint Commission on Accreditation of Hospitals, *Revised Standards for Accreditation of Hospitals.* Chicago: Joint Commission on Accreditation of Hospitals, n.d.

*Kaplan v. Carney,* 404 F. Supp. 161 (E.D. Mo.1975).

*Kelly v. Police Board of Chicago,* 25 Ill. App.3d 559, 323 N.E.2d 624 (1st Dist. 1975).

*Kelly v. St. Vincent Hospital,* (N.M. App. Ct. 1984).

*Knapp v. Palos Community Hospital,* 125 Ill. App. 3d 244, 465 N.E.2d 554 (1st Dist. 1984).

*Ladenheim v. Union County Hospital District,* 76 Ill. App.3d 394, 394 N.E.2d 770 (5th Dist. 1979).

*Maimon v. Sisters of the Third Order of St. Francis,* 20 Ill. App. 3d 1090, 458 N.E.. 2d 1317 (4th Dist. 1983).

*Marsh v. Lake Forest Hospital,* 166 Ill. App.3d 70, 519 N.E.2d 504 (1988).

*Matview v. Johnson,* 111 Ill. App.3d 639, 444 N.E.2d 606 (1st Dist. 1982).

*Mays v. Hospital Authority of Henry County,* 582 F. Supp. 425 (N.D. Ga. 1984).

*Mennes v. South Chicago Community Hospital,* 100 Ill. App. 3d 1029 (1st Dist. 1981).

*Miller v. Indiana Hospital,* 277 Pa. Super. 370, 419 A.2d 1191 (1980).

*Murray v. Bridgeport Hospital,* 480 A. 2d 610 (1984).

*Niven v. Siqueira,* 109 Ill.2d 357, 487 N.E.2d 937 (1985).

*Patrick v. Burget,* 56 U.S.L.W. 4430 (U.S., May 17, 1988).

*Peterson v. Tucson General Hospital., Inc* 114 Ariz. 66, 559 P.2d 186 (Ariz.

App. 1976).

*Pickle v. Carns*, 106 Ill. App. 3d 734, 435 N.E.2d 877 (2nd Dist. 1982).

*Pinsker v. Pacific Coast Society of Orthodontists*, 12 Cal. 3d 541, 526 P.2d 253 (1974).

*Renforth v. Fayette Memorial Hospital Association*, 178 Ind. App. 475, 383 N.E.2d 368 (1978); cert. denied, 444 U.S. 930 (1979).

*Richter v. Diamond*, 108 Ill.2d 265 (1985).

*Ritter v. Board of Commissioners*, 96 Wash.2d 503, 637 P.2d 940 (1981).

*Rutledge v. St. Vincent Memorial Hospital*, 67 Ill. App.2d 156, 214 N.E.2d 131 (5th Dist. 1966).

*Settler v. Hopedale Medical Foundation*, 88 Ill. App. 3d 850, 400 N.E.2d 577 (3rd Dist. 1980).

*Silver v. Castle Memorial Hospital*, 53 Hawaii 475, 497 P.2d 564 (1972); cert. denied, 409 U.S. 1048 (1972).

*Siquiera v. Northwestern Memorial Hospital*, 1985.

*Sosa v. Board of Managers of Val Verde Memorial Hospital*, 437 F.2d 173 (5th Cir. 1971).

*Spencer v. Community Hospital of Evanston*, 87 Ill. App. 3d 214, 408 N.E.2d 1981 (1st Dist. 1980).

*Van Daele v. Vinci*, 51 Ill. 2d 389, 282 N.E. 2d 728 (1972).

*Weiss v. York Hospital*, 745 F. 2d 786 (2nd Cir. 1984); cert. denied, 105 S. Ct. 1777 (1985).

*Woodbury v. McKinnon*, 447 F.2d 839 (5th Cir. 1971).

# Hospital Privileges: Speak Softly, But Carry A Big Lawyer

Arthur R. Chenen, JD

Diplomacy is often more effective than firepower. Here's expert advice on when to be cooperative and when to be combative.

A physician recently came to me terribly upset. He'd been ill and out of practice for a year, and now was well enough to resume work. However, his hospital wanted proof that he still had all his medical skills.

"That not only impugns my integrity and reputation," he declared, "it's an intrusion on my privacy. I've been on that staff for 15 years without one black mark against me. I'll fight this in court if necessary."

I tried to calm the doctor by clarifying two important points for him:

First, I noted, during the year he'd been out of practice, courts repeatedly had emphasized that hospitals have a corporate responsibility to assure the competence of their medical staff members. "So if something did go wrong on one of your cases, and you and the hospital had to go to court," I said, "the plaintiff's attorney could say to the hospital, 'Hey, this guy was gone for a year, and you let him come back without proper check on his competence and his health.' The hospital wouldn't stand a chance—and neither would you."

Second, I pointed out, the hospital had a primary duty to protect patients from harm. "You also have that duty, and your record shows you've lived up to it," I reminded the doctor. "By going along with the hospital, you'll be protecting that record and acting in your own best interest."

The doctor finally agreed, and we worked out with the hospital a temporary monitoring program—which, incidentally, has just ended satisfactorily for all concerned.

The moral: Don't overreact if your privileges are threatened. Many doctors, I've found, react with anger or fear. As a result, they tackle the problem irrationally, rather than reasonably. Take the time—and seek the necessary advice—to evaluate and deal with the problem.


## Don't Underreact

Many doctors submit to what they think is a minor restriction on their privileges without questioning it, figuring, "No big deal."

Don't be too sure. There may be repercussions you can't anticipate. Example:

An ophthalmologist was informed that the complication rate in some of his cases was slightly high, and it was suggested that his next three procedures be monitored. He didn't object.

Months later, two other hospitals where he had privileges notified him that renewal was being held up because he'd been "disciplined" at hospital *x*. He also found out that the "disciplinary" action had been reported to the state agency responsible for policing doctors—the first blot on his record. On top of that, his referrals and income were dropping drastically because word of the action against him had gotten around.

Only then did the doctor come to me, wanting to know what to do. At that point, there was nothing that could be done about the primary problem, the restriction on his privileges. He had complied with it, and the time for appeal was long past.

I did find out, though, that the disciplinary action should *not* have been reported by the hospital. It was not a significant action that had lasted more than 45 days and so, under California law, it wasn't reportable. Consequently, I was able to have the report expunged from the state disciplinary agency's files. On behalf of the ophthalmologist, I've also filed suit for damages against the reporting hospital.

All this probably could have been averted if the ophthalmologist had questioned the restriction in the beginning, thus clarifying the matter for himself and the hospital.

## Know Your Hospital's Bylaws

Many doctors don't bother to read their hospitals' bylaws—or, if they do, they don't understand them. So when trouble crops up, they don't know their rights.*

A cardiologist contacted me because he was threatened with dismissal from his hospital staff. After studying the problem, I saw it was basically a personality clash with his department head. Yet, because the cardiologist hadn't read the staff bylaws, which spelled out very specifically the reasons for which a doctor could be thrown off the staff, he feared he was in big trouble.

The whole thing was straightened out in a simple staff conference. In essence, the cardiologist and the department chief agreed to stop provoking each other.

Lesson: Staff bylaws are your first line of defense in any privileges battle. Make sure you understand them.

## If You've Made a Mistake, Admit It

It was a serious case. An internist had left a hospitalized patient to attend a basketball playoff game out of town. During his absence, the patient took a turn for the worse. The chief of the department had to take over, and he was hampered by a lack of up-to-date progress notes. It looked as if the attending physician would, at the very least, lose his privileges.

However, he made exactly the right move. He immediately presented himself before the peer review committee and stated: "I made a mistake. Please let me explain."

It then became clear that (1) the internist, a popular doctor who couldn't say No to a new patient, had overloaded himself; (2) because his chief office assistant was ill, he'd fallen behind in his record-keeping; (3) he'd spent five straight hours in the hospital with the patient in question, and had left only when it appeared the medical problem was under control; (4) he'd arranged for coverage, but that doctor unfortunately was busy with a patient of his own when the call from the hospital came in; (5) the internist had never before been disciplined; and (6) the patient had suffered no lasting harm.

Result: The physician was let off with relatively light sanctions. He was ordered to keep his records up to date, and to hold his patient load to a reasonable level.

---

*See "Your Surprising Ally in a Privileges Fight," *Medical Economics*, June 10, 1985.

Admitting a mistake usually relieves the tension between the accused physician and the peer reviewers. They understand mistakes; they've made a few themselves.

## Get an Objective Opinion

I learned about this the hard way. One of my earliest doctor clients was an older general practitioner who retained me to represent him in a privileges fight. He had an excellent reputation, the only GP in his hospital to hold OBG privileges. Now the hospital wanted to revoke them and turn them over to a board-certified obstetrician.

The GP had a very authoritative manner, and he convinced me he was absolutely in the right. During the peer review proceedings, however, the hospital called in outside medical experts who identified cases where he'd waited too long before calling in consultants.

The GP resigned before the reviewers could pass judgment on him. If I'd known of the basic flaw in his defense, I might have gotten him off with a stipulation that he call in consultants promptly under certain circumstances.

More recently, an internist came to me after he'd been accused of faulty reading of X-rays. I brought in two radiology experts who agreed there were some mistakes, but they were within the acceptable range.

Moreover, I discovered, the cases against the internist had been picked out selectively rather than randomly by the hospital radiologist, who'd had some disagreement with the internist and investigated the basic charge against him. When I suggested to the radiologist that we be allowed to select some of his cases and see how they compared with the internist's, the charge disappeared.

## Know When to Compromise

Very often staff physicians get into trouble because they try to do more than they're really able to do. A case in point:

A family practitioner had been practicing in a northern California hospital for 35 years when, partly because of his advancing age, questions were raised about his general capabilities. Peer reviewers found he was doing fine except in obstetrics, where a report stated, "He really is not performing at community standards today."

On behalf of the doctor, I worked out a compromise with the hospital: He voluntarily relinquished his privileges to deliver babies and was allowed to retain all others.

In another case, a general surgeon was performing 15 different procedures at a certain hospital. A review of his work showed that he was having trouble with two of them, and he was given notice that his privileges were under scrutiny.

At first, he wanted to fight. 'They'll probably want to monitor me," he said, "but I won't put up with that."

I asked him how often he performed the two procedures in question. "A few times a year."

Then, I pointed out, he didn't really need those particular privileges. Wouldn't it make sense to give them up and hold on to the ones he did most often? He agreed it would, and that was the basis for a compromise we reached the hospital: He wouldn't do the two procedures, and they wouldn't monitor the rest of his work.

Peer reviewers don't like confrontations. The anger takes a lot out of everybody, and usually aggravates rather than eases problems. Seek compromise.


## Consult a Lawyer Early

A phone call I received not long ago is typical of many I get from doctors: "They're throwing me off the staff of my hospital."

"You mean you've received notice they intend to initiate action against you?"

"No, the governing board has acted and I'm off the staff. What can I do?"

The only answer at that point is: Sue, if you can. The damage has been done.

Let me clarify a particular point here. If you're trying to obtain hospital privileges, don't immediately bring in a lawyer—that can turn the application process into an adversarial one.* But if you're trying to retain your privileges, the situation is adversarial from the start. Points of law are involved, so get legal advice as soon as you receive notice of possible action. And go to a lawyer who's knowledgeable in hospital law. Your local bar association or medical society can probably give you a referral.

Another good reason not to wait too long for legal advice: You might be trapped into summary suspension. Hospitals are becoming increasingly aggressive in their disciplinary actions, not only against incompetent doctors but also those who simply displease them. Rather than spend a lot of time and money in getting rid of an unwanted doctor, they summarily suspend him.

---

*See "Ways You Can Win the Privileges Game," *Medical Economics*, Sept. 23, 1985.

In doing that, though, they may be acting illegally. Basically, a medical staff member can be summarily suspended only if his presence in the hospital constitutes an immediate threat to patients. A good lawyer can tell you at once whether a summary suspension is justified—and possibly save you from having to battle your way back in.


## Don't Start a Fight You Can't Finish

If you're unable to resolve a privileges dispute through compromise or negotiation, you face a big question: Shall I mount a full-scale war?

If you know you're in the wrong, you'd probably be better off to cut your losses and make the best of it. If you're right, of course, and you have a good case, gird for combat.

Before you do, though, make sure you're willing and able to go the whole route. Consider these four points: (1) The process can be long and arduous, both in the hospital and in the courts. (2) It can be emotionally and financially exhausting. (3) At some point, the records may become public, bringing unwanted attention. (4) Under most bylaws and in most courts, the accused doctor has the burden of proving he's right—unlike a criminal trial, where you're presumed innocent until proved guilty. I've seen more than a few doctors give up.

Some of those doctors made the mistake of relying on the medical staff for help. As one surgeon told me, "They're my friends—they'll support me."

Maybe they were his friends, but they didn't support him—for two reasons: They were in competition with him for referrals, and they were unwilling to antagonize a powerful department chief who wanted the accused doctor off the staff.

As I always caution my doctor clients: "Medical staff support may be a mile wide, but it's usually only an inch deep. Don't count on it."

# Hospital Privileges


Sarah Dillian Cohn, CNM, MSN, JD



**Abstract**

This article describes the process of obtaining hospital privileges and the legal and practical ways of challenging a denial of privileges to a certified nurse midwife. In general, the political and practical means have been more effective than other challenges; but in the future, threats of legal action may be more common and more effective.


For the majority of nurse-midwives, access to hospital privileges is of critical importance. As illustrated in the 1982 survey *Nurse-Midwifery in the United States*, 88% of all responding nurse-midwives were managing intrapartum patients and performing deliveries, and 80% were doing so in a traditional hospital setting.[1] For such certified nurse-midwives (CNM), denial of hospital privileges would mean that they could no longer admit patients, attend patients in labor and delivery, nor make post-partum rounds within the given institution. Practice, as a practical matter, thus would become limited to office work.

## Obtaining Hospital Privileges

The hospital privilege mechanism is defined in the bylaws of the institu-


Reprinted by permission of JOURNAL OF NURSE-MIDWIFERY, Volume 31, Page 42, 1986. Copyright American College of Nurse Midwives.

tion. A copy of the bylaws plus application materials usually are available from the medical staff office. In some institutions, the CNM also may need to apply to the nursing service; but the same application may suffice.

Careful reading of the bylaws is important. Both the CNM and the institution must follow every step in the procedure, or actions taken may be subject to later challenge.

In hospitals, where nonphysicians have been credentialed, bylaws may have separate procedures for physicians and for nonphysician providers. In all cases, an application must be completed and references are required. The application then is submitted to the first committee specified in the bylaws—usually the obstetrics/gynecology department. Its recommendation then is forwarded to the Medical Staff Credentials Committee or its equivalent and finally to the Board of Trustees of the hospital or some other Board charged officially with the final decision.

A recommendation made by the obstetrics/gynecology department can be approved or disapproved at any step of the process. However, the initial recommendation, especially if opposing privileges, rarely is overturned by other committees, although the power to do so exists. Other physicians and hospital personnel are reluctant to force the department to accept personnel to which it is opposed unless there is a firm legal or political reason to do so. Bylaws may allow for appeal of an adverse decision.

A challenge to denial of privileges on procedural grounds is possible. It may, however, be an exercise in futility because the hospital may reconsider the application carefully following its procedures and again may reject the application.

Hospital privileges, once granted, are limited for all physicians and nonphysicians. For example, even though a physician has an unlimited state license to practice medicine and surgery, the institution granting privileges does so only in a practice area for which the physician has produced credentials. A hospital also may require that a new physician be supervised in the operating room by another attending physician for a period of time or may require a second opinion before a forceps delivery is undertaken. The CNM is subject to similar controls. The institution has the right to limit CNM practice, for example, to certain functions delineated in approved standing orders. It also may specifically exclude certain functions. For example, standing orders for CNMs may state that the nurse-midwife may not perform a paracervical block or may not repair a fourth-degree laceration without physician consultation.

Some hospitals that grant admitting privileges to nurse-midwives require that the admissions be jointly in the name of the nurse-midwife and her consulting physician; in some places, this is called coadmission. This may be required by a local law or regulation or may be viewed by the hospital as a necessary safeguard for patient protection. Even when this is not done, it is common for the hospital to require that the CNM name the consulting physician for purposes of the medical record. Current Joint Commission on Accreditation of Hospitals (JCAH) Standards, which are discussed later in this article, make the problem more complicated by requiring that certain aspects of the care provided by an admitting nonphysician be confirmed or endorsed by a qualified physician.

The above constraints may be matters for negotiation during or after the privileges application, but many CNMs do not even get that far. The outright denial of privileges to a CNM is not uncommon. The denial may be one of two types: 1) Denial of privileges to an individual CNM on grounds of inadequate credentials; or 2) Denial of privileges to a CNM because the institution does not want CNMs working in the institution despite credentials.

## Denial of Privileges Due to Inadequate Credentials

A hospital has the right and probably the legal duty to deny privileges to any applicant who fails to demonstrate the required credentials, although bylaws may permit an appeal within the hospital of an adverse decision. There have been many court cases that have tried to clarify which credentials requirements are reasonable and which are not; nearly all the cases have involved physicians. Among those requirements that have been held as reasonable are the following: 1) evidence of adequate professional liability insurance held by the applicant; 2) documentation of complete hospital records maintained by the applicant; and 3) references from other hospitals where the applicant has practiced. It would not be permissible for a hospital to refuse privileges solely on the basis of the race of the applicant, however.

There apparently has been no legal challenge by a CNM whose application for privileges has been denied on the basis of inadequate credentials. A case of this type, even though it has potential for a positive outcome, has certain disadvantages. First, the CNM's credentials would be made very public, exposing a lack of demonstrated expertise for example. Second, unreasonable credentialing practice by the hospital may be difficult to prove, especially if the hospital has granted privileges to other, better qualified CNMs. In this case, there is no pattern of discrimination but, instead, a hospital that can defend itself by pointing to its high standards for those who provide patient care. The CNM, in turn, must prove that the hospital's standards for denying privileges were not reasonably related to hospital function—a difficult and perhaps impossible task.

Overall, assuming that the hospital has patient-care-related criteria that it applies in a reasonable manner, a challenge by one who is not recognized as qualified is unlikely to be successful. When, on the other hand, the hospital refuses privileges to a CNM solely because she is a CNM, regardless of her credentials, other legal pressures may be applied.

## Group Exclusion

The discussion of this category of denial of hospital privileges assumes that all possible administrative solutions have failed. That is, an appeal to the hospital board or other body has failed, all procedures in bylaws were carefully followed by the hospital when it denied privileges, and the denial is final.

There are practical and political alternatives that should be considered before instituting legal action. First, one way to attempt to change the denial is to wait and try again. While this may not be financially and/or emotionally feasible, it should be considered if, for example, the obstetrics department has a few members close to retirement age. A short wait, combined with whatever pressure can be brought to bear by medical colleagues and the public, might result in a favorable vote by the department after a CNM has reapplied for hospital privileges.

A hospital that denies privileges to all CNMs may face antitrust challenge, particularly if all other hospitals in town do not permit CNM practice. The Federal Trade Commission (FTC) Bureau of Competition may investigate a complaint of anticompetitive hospital practices made by a CNM or other person. As a practical matter, however, the FTC has limited resources and, in its discretion, may refuse to pursue a complaint. The threat of a complaint to the FTC along with information about the consent decree against an insurer,[2] and the pending legal action against three hospitals in Tennessee for anticompetitive practices,[3] may be sufficient to encourage a hospital to reconsider its denial.

A CNM also may choose to sue in Federal Court alleging violation of the Sherman Act (the antitrust law). Allegations in the Tennessee case mentioned above are of this nature. A case of this kind is costly (many thousands of dollars) and lengthy (many years from institution of suit to trial or settlement); during its pendency the CNM still will be unable to practice at the target institution unless it changes its policies. Victory in a case of this kind is not assured and likely will depend in part upon the competitive characteristics of the local community and the circumstances of the denial of the privileges. A significant loss by the hospital, furthermore, is likely to result in appeals through the Federal Court System and those courts may reverse the initial CNM victory; in any case, years will pass during which the CNM waits for privileges. In addition to the above considerations, a CNM who considers suing for privileges should carefully consider the interpersonal ramifications; that is, while a case may be won, if the community is a small one, practice may be isolated and lonely when virtually the entire medical community has been polarized. For some CNMs (in some communities this may not be an important consideration) these implications may influence greatly the final decision. Local legal counsel is critical in making the decision to sue.

## Relevant Statutes

Because some nurse-midwives and other health care professionals have had difficulties in obtaining hospital privileges and legal remedies are uncertain, expensive, and time consuming, legislatures are becoming involved in changing the law. Two jurisdictions currently have laws addressing nondiscrimination in granting hospital privileges.

The first was passed in the District of Columbia in February, 1984, and is part of a statute that licenses health care facilities. It provides that: "(a) The accordance and delineation of clinical privileges shall be determined on an individual basis and commensurate with an applicant's education, training, experience, and demonstrated current competence ... (T)he governing body, or designated persons so functioning, shall ensure that decisions on clinical privileges and staff membership are based on an objective evaluation of an applicant's credentials, free of anticompetitive intent or purpose."

After a section that lists factors not considered valid for consideration in making hospital privileges decisions, the act states that: "(c) No provision of District of Columbia law, institutional or staff bylaw of a facility or agency, rule, regulation, or practice shall prohibit qualified certified registered nurse anesthetists, certified nurse-midwives, certified nurse practitioners, podiatrists, or psychologists from being accorded clinical privileges and appointed to all categories of staff membership at those facilities and agencies that offer the kinds of services that can be performed by either members of these health professions or physicians."[4]

Procedures for processing of privileges applications and for due process on rejection also are provided.

At least one hospital that had not previously granted privileges to nurse-midwives did so, but made the privileges quite restrictive. A request for an opinion from the District of Columbia Corporation Counsel regarding the legality of this action is now pending.[5]

Ohio became the second jurisdiction to legislate nondiscrimination in privileges in an act that became effective in December 1984. It is much less broad and detailed than the District of Columbia legislation. With regard to nurse-midwives, the law states that a hospital that provides maternity services may not discriminate against a person "solely on the basis that the person is certified to practice (as a) nurse-midwife. An application from a nurse-midwife shall contain the name of a physician member of the hospital's medical staff who holds clinical privileges in obstetrics at that hospital and who has agreed to direct and supervise the applicant (in accordance with other provisions of Ohio law)."[6]

Passing legislation of this kind elsewhere can be time consuming, expensive, and perhaps difficult, but is an alternative for which the entire local chapter and supporters can work. As the problem in the District of Columbia points out, however, even a statute may not provide the final answer.

## Other Solutions

Pressure is being applied, both legal and political, to the Joint Commission on Accreditation of Hospitals to require instead of simply permit their accredited hospitals to grant privileges to nonphysicians. The 1984 JCAH Standards require that the medical staff be made of licensed physicians and dentists; other provisions are made for podiatrists and nurse-anesthetists. The 1985 Standards state that the medical staff includes licensed physicians and, for the first time, "may include other licensed individuals permitted by law and by the hospital to provide patient care services independently in the hospital."[7]

"When the non-physician members of the medical staff are granted privileges to admit patients to inpatient services, provision is made for prompt medical evaluation of these patients by a qualified physician."[8]

Persons other than physicians, "who are permitted to provide patient care services independently may perform the history and physical examination, if granted such privileges and if the findings, conclusions, and assessment of risk are confirmed or endorsed by a qualified physician."[8] These standards are somewhat restrictive but nevertheless are a change from the 1984 Standards; however, they merely permit rather than require hospitals that are JCAH accredited to grant medical staff privileges to nonphysicians. A change in these Standards will be extremely useful because the JCAH accredits thousands of hospitals across the country and does so at least every 3 years.

## References

1. American College of Nurse-Midwives: Nurse-Midwifery in the United States. Washington, DC, American College of Nurse-Midwives, 1982, p. 29.
2. See 48 *Federal Register* 27089 (June 13, 1983) for the proposed consent decree.
3. *Nurse Midwifery Associates v. Hibbitt.* Civ. A. No. 82-3208; See 549 F. Supp. 1185 (1982).
4. District of Columbia Code, Section 32-1307 (a), (c) (1984).
5. American College of Nurse-Midwives: Quickening, March/April 1985, p. 15.
6. Page's Ohio Revised Code Annotated, Section 3701.351 (1984).
7. Joint Commission on Accreditation of Hospitals Standards. 1985, p. 1.
8. Ibid, p. 10.

# Considering Economic Factors in Hospital Privilege Decisions

John J. Eller and Sanford V. Teplitzky

Of the myriad problems facing hospitals today, the most important one is economic survival. Hospitals in the next decade will be facing the serious problem of capital scarcity. Most hospitals are nonprofit and do not have access to equity financing, so debt capacity takes on special significance. Creditworthiness is an essential element of qualifying and gaining access to debt financing, which requires a consistent excess of revenues over expenses (i.e., profit), plus some significant capital on hand for major capital projects. It will be most difficult to be truly profitable in the current climate, which is characterized by cost containment initiatives and restrictive reimbursement practices.

Though there is an important relationship between these institutional concerns and the medical staff, the opportunity to use the medical staff privileging process to achieve or maintain solvency has been ignored. Most criteria presently used in the appointment process (including both initial appointments and reappointments) relate to clinical competence and the quality of medical care, but not to fiscal concerns. Nevertheless, even under applicable legal limitations, criteria that add the dimension of business and economic considerations may be developed. Since hospitals have a fiduciary duty to remain solvent through good business decisions, it is legitimate to deal with medical staff appointments in terms of both professional



**245**

(medical) criteria concerned with patient care and business and economic criteria concerned with hospital solvency. Hospitals can and should consciously appoint the right "mix" of physicians who will be economic assets to the hospital instead of liabilities.

Few hospitals are operating at capacity today. Presumably only "full" hospitals might need to find defensible ways of controlling growth and monitoring economic performance of the existing medical staff; most hospitals would be delighted to maintain or expand the staff with virtually any clinically qualified practitioners. However, the key is not the size of the medical staff, but rather the economic performance characteristics of the staff, which are important to both fully utilized and under-utilized hospitals.

First, it could do more harm than good to maintain or expand the staff with physicians whose economic performance profile is so deviant from DRG payment levels, and Professional Review Organization (PRO) and third-party payer norms, that the hospital would suffer an incremental loss for each admission by those physicians. Second, a hospital may need to protect itself from being "swallowed up" or inappropriately dominated by one or more types of practitioners, or from other imbalances in services or resource consumption that could result from an unchecked privileging system. Third, the new criteria to be developed could allow delineation of privileges to be more targeted, and performance standards to be specified, to ensure that new staff members perform appropriately, subject to nonrenewal of privileges or other sanctions. Fourth, the criteria could be applied in the reappointment process for the existing medical staff to similarly ensure adherence to performance that is in the hospital's fiscal interests, tied to sanctions such as the reduction or termination of privileges.

## The Legal Basis for Economically Based Privileges

Existing law concerning the criteria for medical staff appointments, which is primarily case law rather than statutes, reflects the common conception of hospitals as service institutions rather than businesses. It focuses primarily on qualitative considerations of physicians and the care they render. "Quality of care" to a large extent defies adequate definition, yet courts have treated it as the standard by which most medical staff appointments are judged, probably because there have been few other grounds that hospitals have considered in the privileging process.

In the absence of clear standards of "quality of care", courts have deferred to the discretion of hospital boards in discharging their duty to appoint and reappoint competent medical staff members. Judicial intervention occurs only when the criteria set by the hospital are either not reasonable or not fairly administered. Courts will substitute their judgment only where there has been an unreasonable exercise of board discretion. A hospital board's decision will be upheld if it is not arbitrary, capricious, unreasonable, or discriminatory, and is rationally related to documented, legitimate institutional objectives concerning patient welfare, community needs, and institutional operations. However, privileging decisions have not been elevated to the status of a science. There need be no rigid, formalistic systems of criteria with numerical weights and priorities that might obscure substance with form.

Present law thus does contain elements that allow for expansion of acceptable substantive criteria for medical staff appointments to include business and economic criteria. Viewing hospitals as corporations with a responsibility to remain solvent, and utilizing data on the financial consequences to hospitals of physicians' patterns of practice, it is now possible and legitimate to justify medical staff appointment decisions with business and economic analyses.

The following model focuses on the process for initial privileging decisions. With relatively little modification, the model may be adapted to deal with medical staff reappointments, delineation of privileges, and questions of termination, reduction, or suspension of privileges.

## A Model for Incorporating Concerns for Hospital Solvency Into the Privileging Process

A number of building blocks must be in place before any physician applications are considered. The model which follows will of course need to be tailored to fit the circumstances of a given hospital, and should be used only for guidance.

### Health and Hospital Planning

Institutional goals and objectives (both qualitative and quantitative) must be established and fully documented in a formal board approved master plan, with a clear statement of how those goals and objectives will be met, specifically indicating medical staff needs to accomplish and maximize desired ends. The plan must address numerous areas of institutional need, including considerations of patient care and business aspects of hospital operations. It may be based on detailed analyses of the hospital's mission, quality of care, patient and community needs, hospital admissions, operating room utilization, utilization of other hospital services and facilities, operating and capital budget projections, regulatory requirements, teaching programs, existing medical staff analyses (by individual physician, specialty, and department, concerning age, revenue generated, admission patterns, utilization of services and facilities, patient length of stay, consultations given, location of office and residence, patient days, etc.), need for additional medical staff and special expertise, and the ideal mix of patients and physicians identified through analysis of DRGs and case mix planning. The master plan should address the institutional need for financial viability, with specific reference to such needs as using hospital resources efficiently, increasing ambulatory surgery volumes, increasing patient days, decreasing average length of stay, or increasing revenues.

Based on this master plan, criteria that relate to the institutional need for financial viability may then be developed for use in the appointment process. One of the factors that may be specified in this regard is average length of stay (ALOS) norms. DRG data available from PROs allow hospitals to ascertain the actual patterns of practice and resource consumption of applicant physicians and the financial consequences of their utilization profile on the hospital. It may be decided that privileges will not be granted to any physicians who have historically demonstrated inappropriate utilization, whose ALOS experience exceeds the statewide norm (case mix adjusted) by, for example, more than 10 percent. As an alternative, if the hospital badly needs physicians and is confident that its utilization review program is effective, it may state that physicians whose ALOS experience is between 10 percent and 50 percent over the state norm will be admitted with the proviso—to be a condition of reappointment—that their patterns of practice at the hospital must change so as to have an ALOS within 10 percent of the state norm within one year.

Alternatively, the hospital could decide that any applicant who has been the subject of adverse PRO or third-party payer action should not be granted privileges if partial or total reimbursement of a certain frequency or magnitude had previously been denied to affected hospitals. A "clean record" might be a threshold criterion in the privileging process. For existing medical staff, a physician's performance in this area could result in reduction, termination, or non-renewal of privileges. Where negative action is contemplated based on differential utilization, the hospital should afford the physician an opportunity to explain his performance. There may be justifiable reasons for the apparently aberrant behavior, involving factors such as his/her patients' unusual severity of illness.

It is reasonable for the hospital to use privileging sanctions for anyone who will cause the hospital to fail to meet its financial needs because of poor practices relative to DRG norms. The actual figures or standards used could vary, since it may be better to recoup some fixed costs for a filled bed and supporting services and forfeit the profit than to lose all income by denying privileges and keeping beds empty. For hospitals in the desirable position of having full occupancy and a scarcity of beds, a hospital may well have a legitimate objective to exclude or sanction physicians who are financial "losers."

A study of inpatient operating room (O.R.) capacity and utilization may indicate that there is unused capacity in the O.R. suite, and that the maximum level of efficiency and hospital profitability requires increased usage. Hours of usage can be translated into numbers of cases needed and physicians needed to bring those cases to the hospital. This would be a legitimate business reason for granting privileges to surgeons in preference to physicians seeking privileges in the department of medicine, assuming that there were legitimate reasons why only a limited number of applicants could be approved. A range in the number of needed surgeons, rather than a specific number, may be specified. Thus, three plastic surgeons may be equivalent to one orthopod in terms of average surgical minutes per case. By analogy, medical cases needed to fill beds may similarly be analyzed in terms of ALOS by specialty, to assure balanced utilization of the dedicated and general medical units.

As an example of legitimate discrimination among surgeons, consider an underutilized ambulatory surgery facility (ASF) within a hospital that is discrete from the inpatient surgery service. Again, given the assumption that there are legitimate reasons for not allowing unlimited appointments to the medical staff for qualified applicants, analyses of existing medical staff practices may show that the ASF is most appropriately, fully and profitably (for the hospital) used by general, GYN, plastic and otolaryngology surgeons. "Other" surgeons (e.g., neurosurgeons or orthopods) may then be excluded.

Similar analyses may be conducted concerning under- or over-utilized ancillary services. Under cost-reimbursement methods, heavy ancillary usage is most profitable for the hospital; under DRG reimbursement the reverse is true. It is possible to specify those types of inpatient and outpatient cases that use ancillary services in the manner best for the hospital and establish a profile of needed physicians who will treat those patients.

An age profile of the medical staff may indicate an aging medical staff in certain specialties, with no younger physicians in that area to guarantee a stream of similar cases. It would be in the hospital's best financial interests to have a more even age spread for physicians in a specialty to assure continuity in the source of future patients.

Study of physicians by age may also reveal that physicians "peak out" in hospital usage in a certain age range, and then begin to phase out their practice. This also may be useful information in planning for a continuous flow of patients (and revenue) in a given specialty. Needs for medical staff in that specialty would then be specified so as to fill the gaps that could otherwise be detrimental to the hospital's business interests. It should be noted that age discrimination is illegal only in employment contexts, not in medical staff appointments cases concerning routine attending physicians.

Analysis of available data also may indicate that a physician's admissions are directly correlated with office proximity to the hospital. That would be a sufficient basis for giving preference to applicants with offices in the hospital's primary service area.

A final example is the application by a new partner of an existing medical staff member who is a big user of the hospital. In many instances the source, nature and volume of patients of the partnership are important to the financial well-being of the hospital. Granting privileges to the new partner will assure the hospital of the continued flow of patients from the practice. Though there is economic benefit to the partnership, this would not be the primary purpose of granting privileges; it is the hospital's financial needs that are paramount and justify the decision.

These are only a few examples of economic factors in staff decisions that relate to legitimate institutional financial objectives.


### Revision of Procedures and Bylaws

The second prerequisite for a valid privileging process incorporating business and economic criteria is the establishment of formal procedures, as documented in medical staff and board of trustees bylaws, and other hospital documentation of privileging procedures. Any conditions to be placed on new appointments, sanctions for existing staff, or sanctions to be enforced through the reappointment process, must be provided for. To accomplish this will require a good deal of education and cooperation of all involved parties. These changes must be accomplished before any applications or privileges are considered, in order to obviate due process concerns of specific physicians who may feel they have been singled out for ad hoc treatment.

Among the principal new elements of a revised procedure that must be folded into a typical existing privileging process are the following:

- **Privileging committee of the board of trustees.** The board of trustees institutes a permanent, multidisciplinary Medical Staff Privileging Committee (hereafter "MSPC"). Voting members of the committee include non-physician members of the board of trustees; the president of the medical staff; the chairman of the medical staff credentials committee; and representatives of administration.

- **Board approval of statement needs and factors in the privileging process.** At least annually, the MSPC makes recommendations to the board concerning medical staff needs based on the master plan, updated data analyses, and appropriate consultation with medical staff committees. Recommendations include the list of factors to be used in judging applicants with values assigned to each factor. The board has final authority to accept, modify or reject the recommendations. Medical staff needs thus recognized by the board serve as goals to be achieved during the next round of privileging.

  Figure 1 (page 252) provides a sample of some medical staff goals and privileging factors the MSPC might recommend, and the board might adopt, for use in the privileging process to ascertain whether an applicant will enhance the hospital's viability and solvency.

  Figure 2 (page 254) provides a shorthand "Applicant Rating System" to be adopted by the board that assigns values to the various items. In this example, ratings on each of the principal variables have been categorized as "desirable" (+), "acceptable" (A), and "undesirable" (−). When reviewing a large number of variables or applicants, shorthand representation of "+", "A", or "−" on summary sheets provides a quick visual overview to assess an individual applicant's merits, or to compare one individual to another. As such a system becomes refined and developed at a hospital, it would be possible to quantify various factors and assign numerical weights to each category.

- **Modify medical staff application form.** The application form for medical staff privileges is modified as necessary. The most important modification is the request for the physician's PRO identification number at other hospitals at which he has privileges, and an authorization for the hospital to secure patient data (preserving patient anonymity) from the PRO concerning that physician's caseload at each hospital. This requires no consent by the patients as long as their identities are not divulged. Other modifications to the application form would depend on the factors deemed important to the hospital, such as the number of admissions the physician expects to bring to the hospital in each of his first three years of practice there (e.g., the "committed admissions" factor).

  The hospital should ascertain the costs of obtaining and processing the PRO data, as well as any other substantial additional costs that may be necessitated by these revisions in the privileging process. Application fees may legitimately increase accordingly to cover such

**Figure 1. Statement of Medical Staff Needs and Factors to be Evaluated in The Medical Staff Privileging Process**

1. Medical Staff needs are as follows:

MEDICINE

Additions are needed in Internal Medicine, which includes the sub-specialties of Endocrinology and Rheumatology (8-10), Pulmonary Medicine (1-2), Cardiology (2-5), Gastroenterology (2-3), and Hematology (1).

OB/GYN

No restrictions on privileging; recruit approximately five per year with emphasis on younger physicians. Special consideration should be given to those practicing in our catchment area and to sub-specialists (e.g., Maternal-Fetal Medicine, Reproductive Endocrinology, and Oncology).

EMERGENCY MEDICINE

When additions are needed, full-time physicians should be considered.

SURGERY

Additions are needed in Thoracic Surgery (1), Vascular Surgery (one young, exclusively vascular surgeon), Plastic Surgery (outpatient surgery privileges only: 2-4), ENT (2-4), Ophthalmology (1-2), and Open-Heart Surgery (1).

Additions of outstanding candidates may be considered in the following categories: General Surgery (outpatient surgery privileges only), Colon and Rectal Surgery, Neurosurgery, Urology, and Oral Surgery (outpatient surgery privileges only).

No need for additional medical staff is found in the following categories: Orthopedic Surgery, Surgical Oncology.

ANESTHESIA

No need.

RADIOLOGY

No need.

PEDIATRICS

No restrictions on privileging for fully credentialed physicians. Subspecialty consultant staff needed in Cardiology, Nephrology, Hematology, Gastroenterology, Allergy and Developmental Pediatrics. Need full-time Neonatologist.

---

**Figure 1—continued**

1. PSYCHIATRY
   No restrictions on privileging for fully credentialed physicians unless or until the Board of Trustees directs otherwise.
   PATHOLOGY
   No need.
2. Physicians with outstanding credentials will be given preference for privileges over those with acceptable credentials. Those with unsatisfactory credentials will not be admitted to the staff.
3. An applicant whose pattern of practice is below the state average, as reflected in his case mix adjusted DRG/ALOS profile, will be given first preference for privileges. Second preference will be given to an applicant whose profile is no greater than 10 percent above the state average.
4. Younger physicians (55 years of age or younger) are to be given preference for privileges.
5. Physicians proposing to admit 50 or more patients annually will be given first preference. Second preference will be given to those proposing to admit between 25 and 49 patients annually.
6. First preference will be given to applicants with offices in the Hospital's primary service area. Second preference will be given to those with offices in the Hospital's secondary service area.
7. Any other factors that have not been anticipated but which the applicant proves to be germane will be evaluated as part of the privileging process.
8. There is no formula or numerical ranking system to be used to derive the MSPC recommendation for privileges; the recommendation must be a judgment of the MSPC taking the various enumerated factors into account. An applicant whose credentials are unsatisfactory will not be granted privileges. An applicant whose credentials are at least acceptable may or may not be recommended for privileges, depending on the MSPC evaluation of all relevant factors.

---

costs. Not only will this be of obvious financial benefit to the hospital, but it is likely to discourage applications from physicians who do not intend to have a significant practice at the hospital and who would only be an administrative burden to maintain on the staff.

- **Batch-process applications by clinical department.** Applications for medical staff privileges are processed by batching them within departments, with no preference given according to date of applications. That is, applications of all surgeons are batched and considered to be in competition with one another; applications of all physicians applying for privileges in the department of medicine are batched in competition with one another, etc.

For example, one orthopod applying for privileges would not only be competing against other orthopods seeking privileges (of which there might be none, one, or several) but also against all other surgeons, including urologists, thoracic surgeons, etc. The reasoning here is that it is frequently difficult to say with confidence that one additional specialist in any given category is truly necessary or not necessary. Analysis of trend data for each specialty, or trend data on community morbidity and mortality for a disease category, usually cannot compel a conclusion one way or the other in any individual applicant's case.

- **Process applications semiannually.** Rather than processing applications as they are submitted, semiannual processing allows for economy of committee action, and economy of staff action in updating data used as a basis for credentialing physicians. It may also permit a wider choice within any given specialty if there are competing applications submitted within the six-month period.

---

### Figure 2. Applicant Rating System

|  | Desirable (+) | Acceptable (A) | Undesirable (−) |
|---|---|---|---|
| Specialty | Recognized that additions are needed | No special recognition that additions are needed or not needed | Recognized that additions are not needed |
| Credentials | Outstanding | Satisfactory | Unsatisfactory |
| DRG/ALOS | Below average | Average to 10% above average | Greater than 10% above average |
| Age | 55 and under | N/A | 56 or older |
| Committed Admissions | 50 or more annually | 25-49 | Under 250 |
| Office Location | Primary service area | Secondary service area | Tertiary service area |
| Other Factors | Desirable | Acceptable | Undesirable |
| Privileging Recommendation | Privileges granted, credentials satisfactory | Privileges not granted, credentials satisfactory | Privileges not granted, credentials unsatisfactory |

- **Clinical competence of specific applicants.** The credentials committee of the medical staff continues to review applications and made recommendations to the medical executive committee, which in turn makes recommendations to the MSPC concerning applicants whom it considers clinically qualified or unqualified. Medical staff review of specific applicants is thus limited to an assessment of professional competence, as it historically has been.
- **MSPC makes recommendations to the board of trustees.** The MSPC reviews recommendations and makes its own recommendations to the board of trustees.
- **Board of trustees takes action.** The board of trustees makes one of three possible decisions concerning each applicant:

  1. Privileges not granted, credentials unsatisfactory. This decision is communicated to the applicant and may be appealed.
  2. Privileges not granted, credentials satisfactory. This decision asserts that the applicant is qualified, but is not needed at this time. The applicant will be permitted to remain in the unprioritized "pool" of applicants to be batched in the next round of privileging.
  3. Privileges granted, credentials satisfactory. This may include minimum and maximum performance requirements.

  In addition to the normal options of approval or disapproval, a new category of decision asserts that the applicant's credentials are satisfactory relying on the medical staff recommendation, but that privileges will not be granted for reasons grounded in the process described above. The board of trustees thereby takes account of the medical staff opinion regarding competence, but reserves to itself the final privileging decision, which rests on both clinical *and* economic grounds. For the first time, an otherwise clinically qualified physician may be refused appointment or reappointment to the medical staff because of business needs of the institution as determined exclusively by the board. The applicant is not disapproved; he remains in the pool of applicants and may be reconsidered in the next batch of applications to be processed. If the hospital subsequently finds a need for a physician with his background and pattern of performance, he may be admitted to the medical staff.

  Figure 3 (page 256) provides a flow chart of the privileging process described above.
- **Implementing the revised privileging process.** Once the criteria concerning business and economic needs of the hospital have been established, and necessary revisions in hospital procedures have been made,

## Figure 3. Privileging Process

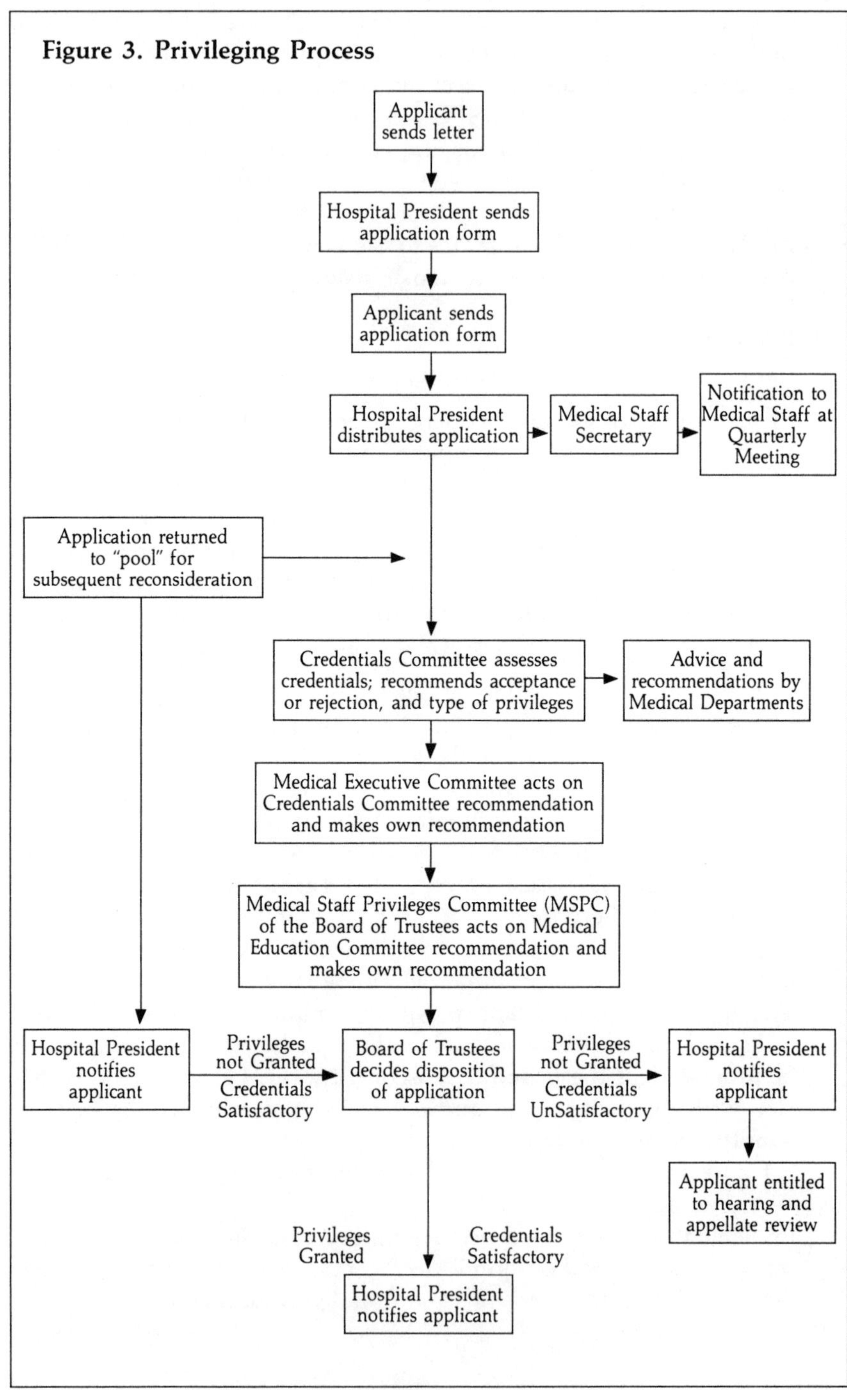

**Figure 4. Screening Criteria**

COMPLETION OF APPLICATION

1. If an applicant fails to provide PRO identification numbers at hospitals at which he has privileges, or fails to authorize release of PRO data to the hospitals, or the numbers so provided fail to yield 25 cases on which to base a judgment of his pattern of practice, the applicant will be informed that his application is incomplete and will not be processed. If the applicant provides an acceptable justification for the incompleteness, the application may be considered for further processing at the MSPC's discretion. If the applicant provides the needed information, the application will be considered complete in that respect and will continue to be processed.

2. If an applicant fails to provide an expected number of admissions to the hospital, the applicant will be informed that his application is incomplete and will not be processed. If the applicant provides an acceptable justification for the incompleteness, the application may be considered for further processing at the MSPC's discretion. If the applicant provides the needed information, the application will be considered complete in that respect and will continue to be processed.

PRIORITIES IN REVIEW OF COMPLETED APPLICATIONS

1. If an applicant's credentials are deemed to be unsatisfactory by the MSPC, the recommendation to the Board of Trustees will be that privileges should not be granted, regardless of other factors to be considered in the privileging process.

2. If an applicant is applying for privileges in a specialty in which it is recognized that staff additions are not needed, the recommendation to the Board of Trustees will be that privileges should not be granted, regardless of other factors to be considered in the privileging process.

3. If an applicant's pattern of practice shows that his ALOS is within 10 percent of the average in the state, or below the average, the recommendation to the Board of Trustees will be that privileges should be granted, unless the MSPC determines that any other factor(s) ought to be given priority consideration for the applicant.

4. If an applicant indicates that he expects to admit fewer than 25 patients annually to the hospital by the third year in which he has privileges, the recommendation to the Board of Trustees will be that privileges should not be granted, unless the MSPC determines that any other factor(s) ought to be given priority consideration for the applicant.

5. All remaining factors on the grid will be considered and given weight depending on the degree of importance as determined by the MSPC.

the hospital is at last ready to deal with applicants for medical staff privileges. It is essential to have these building blocks in place so that the hospital will not be subject to substantive or procedural challenges.

Figure 4 (page 257) illustrates "Screening Criteria" that may be adopted by the MSPC and Board of Trustees to be used by the MSPC staff in reviewing an application for completeness and in making threshold determinations as to the ultimate approvability of the application.

A "Pattern of Practice Worksheet" can then be developed by the MSPC staff to compile data relevant to the process and to provide the MSPC with pattern of practice information of the applicant at specific hospitals (if it desires to review this level of detail). Data from the form are later summarized and graphically displayed to the MSPC. This worksheet is first used to determine the physician's overall average length of stay (ALOS) as compared to state averages. Data are accessed through use of the physician's PRO identification number at each hospital at which the physician has privileges, as listed on the application for privileges. PRO computer runs can provide the level of detail desired by the hospital. Additional calculations are made by the hospital as necessary to determine the physician's overall ALOS and to complete the worksheet. Included on the worksheet is the physician's expected number of admissions during his third year on staff at the hospital, which is also found on the application for privileges.

After the pattern of practice worksheet has been completed for all physicians slated for review, the physicians are grouped according to specialty and identified by number so that total anonymity will be preserved throughout the process. This procedure ensures a high degree of objectivity during the MSPC's review process, thereby strengthening the process against challenge. During the earlier stage of medical staff review of the applicant's credentials, his identity would of course be known to the credentials committee.

Finally, an overall evaluation "grid" is completed for each specialty represented and presented to the MSPC. A non-voting individual such as the vice president for medical affairs would be present at the MSPC meeting with each applicant's file to respond to questions at whatever level of depth is required, while maintaining the applicant's anonymity.

Information found on the grid includes the specialty being considered, hospital identified needs in that specialty, the findings of the medical executive committee regarding the physician's credentials, information transferred from the pattern of practice worksheet for each physician in that specialty, a privileging recommendation by the MSPC staff, and other relevant comments. This grouping of information affords a comparative review of physicians by specialty. Specialty grids are grouped by department to afford comparison on a departmental level.

Each applicant is considered individually by the MSPC, and each MSPC member casts his vote on his copy of the grid. Individual rating of applicants by individual MSPC members strengthens the process and helps insulate it from challenge.

The final privileging decision is that of the board of trustees, based on a review of a grid summarizing the MSPC votes.

Though numerous factors are considered in the process, and some are threshold factors that dictate disapproval, the MSPC and the board usually must use their judgment in weighing the various factors for each applicant. A rigid numerical system would make committee review of individual applicants practically unnecessary and would be more easily challenged as formalistic and unable to deal fairly and reasonably on a case by case basis.

The medical staff privileging model presented in this article integrates quality of care and hospital solvency considerations into a legally viable framework. It adds numerous advantages to existing privileging procedures, allowing a balancing of qualitative and quantitative considerations in a flexible system. It provides for appropriate participation by the medical staff, administration, and the board of trustees. Through use of this model, hospitals can more confidently make necessary decisions in all questions of medical staff privileges, while simultaneously enhancing their financial viability through the judicious selection and retention of physicians who will be economic assets, rather than liabilities.

# Physicians' Rights as Hospital Staff Members

Henry R. Fenton

Physicians may be denied appointment to the staff of a hospital or may find themselves threatened by removal or limitation of their staff privileges for reasons that have nothing to do with their competence. This article reviews the conditions under which physicians can or cannot be legally denied staff membership or reappointment, as well as the legal precedents for fair procedure if a hospital tries to remove a physician from its staff. All physicians should be aware of their rights in these areas to protect themselves from unjust denial of staff privileges, which could result in adverse career consequences.

It is important for physicians to be aware of their legal rights when they are being considered for staff membership in a public or private hospital, or when their membership is threatened by charges of misconduct or inadequate performance. Staff physicians are independent contractors, not employees, and their employment rights are more limited than those of workers in the private and public sectors. They must therefore be more vigilant in exercising their rights to ensure protection against the arbitrary or unfair denial of staff privileges.

Some physicians may be under the impression that they have no reason to be concerned, or even informed, about their rights because revocation or denial of staff privileges is something that happens only to incompe-



**261**

tent physicians. Or they may believe that denial or revocation of staff privileges, while somewhat inhibiting one's practice, does not pose a real threat to one's career. These views are incorrect.

First, a capable physician and skillful surgeon may be denied admission to the staff of a hospital or steps may be taken to remove him or her from the staff by competitors who will gain economically by such a move. Personality conflicts, strong disagreements with other staff members, or any number of other arbitrary reasons can be the basis of false accusations unrelated to the physician's ability to function effectively as a member of a hospital staff.

Second, denial of an application for staff privileges or removal from a hospital staff can have various adverse consequences. Because of the reporting requirement of Business and Professions Code S805, denial or revocation of staff membership can lead to a disciplinary proceeding before the Board of Medical Quality Assurance (BMQA). It can also lead to the denial of staff privileges at other hospitals.

Third, hospitals are far more disposed to take disciplinary action against staff physicians at the slightest indication of negligence, error, or omission as a result of a recent court decision[1] maintaining that a hospital may be liable for the negligent conduct of a staff physician if the physician was imprudently selected or retained.

Finally, recent changes in the law permitting the rapid growth of preferred provider organizations (PPOs) have been accompanied by a system of utilization review for the purpose of cutting medical costs. Decisions made by reviewers about the necessity of particular services—whether that review occurs before or after hospital admission—can lead to disagreements and, ultimately, to efforts to impose discipline on recalcitrant members of a hospital's staff.


## The Right to Fair Treatment

A hospital's bylaws set forth the conditions under which physicians become members of the staff; they also regulate physicians' relationships with their colleagues on the staff and with other personnel in the hospital. Any action to discipline a staff member or to remove him or her from the staff must be pursuant to the hospital bylaws. In fact, Business & Professions Code S2282 prohibits physicians from practicing in private hospitals with five or more physicians without bylaws that require, at a minimum, that there be (1) a formal, self-governing medical staff, (2) review of all staff appointments at least biennially, (3) staff appointments only of physicians and surgeons competent in their respective fields and worthy in professional ethics, and (4) periodic peer review.

In addition to bylaw provisions, laws have evolved concerning physicians' rights to be appointed or retained on a hospital staff. Due to various court cases, it is now well established that justification must be given for rejection or removal from the staff of a public or private hospital. Some courts have required that the basis for removal be rational, not arbitrary, capricious, or discriminatory.

According to a decision by the California Supreme Court,[2*] rejection of a physician from a hospital staff is prohibited unless it can be shown that a real and substantial danger exists for the patients treated by the physician in question—that is, it must be shown that these patients receive other than a high quality of medical care at the hospital if the physician is admitted to or retained on the staff.

Other laws affecting conditions under which staff membership can or cannot be denied include the following:

- Hospital bylaws may include a requirement of malpractice insurance for membership on the staff. In one California case,[3] the court upheld a hospital's refusal to reappoint a doctor to the medical staff because he failed to maintain malpractice insurance with a "recognized insurance company." The court held that any insurance requirement proposed by a hospital as a condition for membership on the staff was allowable, as long as it was not arbitrary, irrational, or discriminatory. In the case in question, the physician had obtained insurance for $1 million per occurrence; however, the insurance carrier was based in Central America and was not admitted in California to conduct a malpractice insurance business. Thus, held the court, the hospital properly interpreted its own rule to require insurance in the minimum amount of $500,000 with an insurance company admitted to transact insurance business in California.
- Hospitals cannot use overly vague bylaws to exclude a physician from staff membership because this might allow discriminatory or nonuniform application.
- A physician cannot be excluded from the staff of a hospital on the basis of failure to include references from active members of the hospital staff. Such a rule, held one court of appeals,[4] would pose too great a danger that necessary endorsements would be arbitrarily or discriminatorily withheld.

---

*The references cited here pertain to California court decisions and statutes. Such rulings are analogous to other states' statutory provisions. Moreover, California has set precedents that traditionally guide and influence legal actions in other courts. Nonetheless, the law varies from state to state and should therefore be reviewed carefully.

- A hospital cannot deny a physician the right to staff privileges because of past disciplinary action by the BMQA.[5] If, however, the hospital bases its decision on the circumstances that led to the BMQA proceeding, and if those circumstances currently constitute a rational basis for denial of staff privileges, the exclusion might be upheld.
- A physician cannot be denied staff membership exclusively on the basis that he or she has been denied privileges at some other hospital.[5]
- A physician cannot be denied staff membership on the basis of nonmembership in a medical society.
- A hospital cannot condition staff membership on a physician's participation or nonparticipation in a PPO.

### The Right to Fair Procedure

With some important exceptions, which will be noted, the procedural requirements that apply to staff application or revocation are the same for public and private hospitals.

The courts have held that physicians who are rejected for admission to the hospital staff, or who are removed from the staff for a reason related to their performance or qualifications as a physician or surgeon, are entitled to have the decision made against them in accordance with a fair procedure.[6] The basic components of that fair procedure are the following:

- The physician is entitled to adequate notice of the charges that are the basis for rejection or removal. The notice must be provided sufficiently in advance of the hearing so that a defense may be prepared. The charges must be sufficiently specific that the physician can understand what he or she is being accused of. Moreover, the charges must make it clear that removal from the staff is being contemplated.
- In the case of staff removal, the physician is entitled to present his or her defense at a hearing prior to the effective date of removal.[7]
- At the hearing, physicians must be given an opportunity to confront and cross-examine the witnesses testifying against them and to present witnesses and evidence in their defense. In the case of a private hospital, however, neither hospital nor the accused physician has subpoena power. Nonetheless, "fundamental fairness" requires that witnesses against the physician be made available by the hospital and that the evidence relied on also be made available.[8] Public hospitals, on the other hand, have subpoena power in such cases, and physicians must be careful to request that their witnesses be subpoenaed.

- The accused physician is entitled to an impartial hearing panel. Therefore, he or she is entitled to a "voir dire"—that is, a preliminary examination—of the members of the hearing panel or the appeals panel to ensure that the panel is impartial.[8] Thus, if a business competitor of the accused or someone else who has a direct pecuniary interest in the outcome of the proceeding is on the panel, the accused can challenge the panel member on that basis. Fair procedure also requires that any physician who participated in the investigation of the charges as a member of the investigatory committee cannot sit as a member of the hearing committee or the review committee.[9]

- To date, the California courts have rejected the argument that physicians are entitled in all cases to be represented by an attorney. Generally, unless the hospital is represented by an attorney or unless the bylaws provide for the right to be represented by an attorney at the hearing, the accused physician may not be represented by counsel at either the initial hearing or the appeals hearing.

  Although accused physicians may, if permissible under the bylaws, represent themselves at the hearing or be represented by another member of the staff, they would be well advised to retain competent counsel to assist in the preparation of their defense, even if they are not allowed to be represented by an attorney in the hearing. A qualified attorney will ensure that the correct procedural points are raised, that the correct questions are asked on direct examination and cross-examination, that the appropriate objections are made, that the appropriate voir dire is conducted of the hearing panel, that the evidence necessary for the presentation of the accused's case is made available, and that a timely and proper request is made for the presence of those witnesses who may be necessary to the defense of the case.

- The accused physician is also entitled to obtain fair disclosure of the basis of the charges against him or her. Although formal disclosure such as is normally provided in the court system (consisting of depositions, interrogatories, and notices to produce documents) is unavailable, the requirement of fair procedure demands that the accused physician have an adequate opportunity to respond to the charges and to prepare a defense. This contemplates disclosure of the evidence against him.

- Formal court rules of evidence are not followed in these cases. If the case is ultimately appealed in the court system, however, it is required that any finding made against the physician be supported by competent, non-hearsay evidence.

- Although the courts have upheld bylaws, placing the burden of going forward with the evidence and the burden of proof on the physician, they have so held only on the basis that the hospital was required to make a "substantial showing" in support of its recommendation of removal or nonreappointment.[10] If the bylaws do not assign the burden of proof, it is generally on the hospital.

- Hospital bylaws generally provide for review of a decision by the governing body of the hospital or an appeals committee. Although it is required by the Joint Commission on Accreditation of Hospitals, it is not necessarily required as a matter of fair procedure.
- The physician is entitled to a written decision from the hospital including the bases for the decision.[6]
- The physician is entitled to a complete record of the proceedings, whether that record is transcribed by a court reporter, tape recorder, or some other form, so that he or she can obtain review of the decision in the courts.[6]

## The Right to Court Review

Physicians can challenge exclusion or removal from the staff of a hospital in court only after they have exhausted the administrative remedies available to them under the hospital bylaws. Moreover, any points that they wish to raise in court or any evidence that they want to present must first be presented in the hearings at the hospital level under the doctrine of the exhaustion of administrative remedies.

Physicians in public hospitals are entitled to have the hospital's decision against them reviewed by a judge under the independent judgment rule. However, their counterparts who are denied staff privileges in private hospitals may obtain review in court, but the court is required to sustain the decision of the hospital if there is substantial evidence to support that decision.

The difference between the independent judgment rule and the substantial evidence rule is very significant. Under the independent judgment rule the court is required to determine independently whether or not the findings made by the hospital in support of its decision to remove the physician from the staff are supported by the evidence. If not, the staff removal may be set aside. In contrast, when the court applies the substantial evidence rule, it must view the evidence presented in the hearing at the hospital level in a light most favorable to the hospital's findings, and it must interpret the evidence, if it can do so, to support those findings. Thus, it is far more difficult to obtain a reversal of a private hospital's decision to remove from the staff or not reappoint a physician, than a public hospital's decision to take the same action.

In a recent case, the California Supreme Court held that physicians who are denied admission to the staff of a public hospital are not entitled to have a court review of the hospital's decision under the independent judgment rule and that the substantial evidence rule applies. Although the court held that the physician's interest in obtaining staff privileges was fundamental and conceivably crucial to his livelihood, the applicant, held the court, did not have a vested right to those privileges. Hence, he was entitled only to have the court review the denial of privileges under the substantial evidence rule.

## The Consequences of Denial or Restriction of Staff Privileges

Physicians who face denial or restriction of staff privileges must bear in mind that their immediate situation may affect their right to practice medicine and their chances of obtaining staff privileges at other hospitals. As mentioned above, California Business and Professions Code S805 requires hospitals to report to the BMQA when any physician, psychologist, podiatrist, or dentist "is denied staff privileges, removed from the medical staff of such institution, or if his staff privileges are restricted for a cumulative total of 45 days in any calendar year for any medical disciplinary cause or reason."

The threat posed to the physician's privileges in other hospitals for the remainder of his or her career derives from Business and Professions Code S805.5. This requires that every hospital request a report from the BMQA before appointing a new staff member to determine whether any report on the physician has ever been made by a hospital under S805.

Resignation in the face of threatened disciplinary action or after a suspension will not necessarily prevent a report to the BMQA. In fact, S805 states that if removal from the staff or restriction of staff privileges is by resignation as a result of a bargain in lieu of medical disciplinary action, the hospital is required to report this to the BMQA. Under S805.5, this report will subsequently be made available to all other hospitals where the physician may apply for staff privileges or for a renewal of staff privileges.

Therefore, any physician who faces restriction or denial of staff privileges must act quickly not only to resolve the immediate situation, but to avoid, if possible, a report to the BMQA. Although it may be possible to resolve a situation where suspension, restriction, or removal is threatened or has occurred, action must be taken as soon as possible and the advice of a competent attorney in this area should be obtained. In many cases, the physician may decide to vigorously contest the attempt to restrict or deny staff privileges. This decision must be made before staff privileges are restricted for a total of 45 days in any calendar year to avoid a report to the BMQA.

Finally, it is important to understand how seriously hospitals take the reporting requirement. Section 805 provides that failure to make a report pursuant to this section is a misdemeanor. But more importantly, based on a 1982 court decision,[1] some hospitals maintain that any failure to comply strictly with S805 of the Business and Professions Code would increase their potential liability for any future acts of malpractice by physicians whose staff privileges were previously denied or restricted.

### Looking Ahead: The Effect of PPOs

As more hospitals contract with PPOs and more physicians participate as providers in such organizations through economic necessity, conflicts may arise between the independent physician, exercising professional responsibility to his or her patients, and the economic self-interest of the insurance company or other entity that operates the PPO.

In a case in California,[13] a patient was admitted to a hospital for an aortic graft insert. Although the treating physician requested an eight-day extension of the patient's hospitalization after the operation, a Medi-Cal consultant for the state of California authorized only four extra days. The patient subsequently developed complications that resulted in the amputation of a portion of his leg. A lawsuit against the state of California ensued, and a judgment was rendered in favor of the patient in the sum of $500,000. However, the Court of Appeals reversed the judgment against the state of California on the basis that the treating physician was ultimately responsible for discharging the patient.

The nature of utilization review presents the danger that similar disagreements may result between the PPO and the provider physician about whether or not a particular procedure or course of treatment is medically necessary. Physicians have an obligation to their patients to provide whatever treatment they deem necessary in their professional judgment. They may not compromise that judgment, even if the PPO disagrees with them.

When such disagreements occur, they may result in steps to remove the physician from the PPO. At the same time, or shortly thereafter, the hospital may take steps to dismiss the physician from its staff. Although to date there are no published decisions concerning these issues, some possible defenses for physicians confronted with such cases are the following:

- First, and perhaps foremost, is the protection provided by California Health and Safety Code S1322, which prohibits conditioning hospital staff membership on participation in a PPO or exclusive provider organization. To the extent that removal from the staff is based on the events that resulted in dismissal from the PPO, physicians may well be able to rely on this code in their defense.

- Another basis for a defense in such cases may be Business and Professions Code S2400, which prohibits the corporate practice of law. If it can be shown that the attempted removal is a result of a disagreement between the PPO and a physician about whether or not certain treatment was medically necessary, it may be argued that PPOs do not have a right to make medical judgments.

- The law clearly provides that in public and private hospitals the staff of the hospital must exist separately from the hospital, must be formally organized with appropriate officers and bylaws, and must be self-governing. To the extent that PPOs attempt to dictate to physicians on the staffs of hospitals what treatment should be provided or the manner in which treatment should be provided, they interfere with the independence of the medical staff and violate these provisions.

- Physicians facing removal in such cases can argue that they exercised their professional responsibility to ensure that their patients received a high quality of medical care at the hospital. The courts have held that a physician is entitled to retain staff membership unless it can be shown that retention may present a danger that patients treated by the physician would receive other than a high quality of medical care. Physicians threatened with removal from the staff can rely on these cases in their defense.

- Physicians who are excluded from a PPO may, in some instances, be able to cite a cause of action under the anti-trust laws. This can only be determined on a case-by-case basis, depending on the size and nature of the PPO and the contractual arrangements among the PPO, the hospital, other hospitals, and the provider physicians.

## Conclusion

The right of physicians to be members of hospital staffs is integral to their right to practice medicine. For this reason, it is essential that all physicians have at least a rudimentary understanding of the nature of their rights for fair treatment and fair procedure when applying for staff membership or when faced with the threat of removal from a hospital staff.

## References


1. *Elam v College Park Hospital*, 132 Cal App3d 322 (1982).
2. *Miller v Eisenhower Medical Center*, 27 Cal3d 614 (1980).

3. *Wilkinson v Madera Community Hospital*, 144 Cal App3d 436 (1983).

4. *Ascherman v St Francis Memorial Hospital*, 45 Cal App3d 623 (1975).

5. *Ascherman v San Francisco Medical Society*, 34 Cal App3d 623 (1974).

6. *Anton v San Antonio Community Hospital*, 19 Cal3d 802 (1977).

7. *Ezekial v Winkley*, 20 Cal3d 267 (1977).

8. *Hackenthal v California Medical Association*, 138 Cal App3d 435 (1982).

9. *Applebaum v Board of Directors*, 104 Cal App3d 648 (1980).

10. *Pick v Santa Ana-Tustin Community Hospital*, 130 Cal App3d 970 (1982).

11. *Unterthiner v Desert Hospital District*, 33 Cal3d 285 (1983).

12. *Marmion v Mercy Hospital [ Medical Center*, 145 Cal App3d 72 (1983).

13. *Wickline v State of California*, 228 Cal Rptr 681 (1981).

# Hospital Privileges for Family Physicians

## Patterns of Recent Residency Graduates, Residency Director Perceptions, and Resident Expectations

Kevin Scott Ferentz, MD, Jeffery Sobal, PhD
Richard Colgan, MD

A national mail survey was performed that examined reports of recent residency graduates about hospital privileges for family physicians, perceptions of residency program directors about the percentage of their graduates who obtain privileges, and plans of third year residents for seeking privileges. Privileges in medicine, pediatrics, surgery, obstetrics, and coronary care/intensive care units (CCU/ICU) were examined. Questionnaires were mailed to a random sample of 308 residency graduates aged 30 to 35 years, all 383 family practice residency directors, and a random sample of 319 third-year residents. Two mailings produced an 82 percent response rate. Most recent graduates had privileges in medicine (97 percent), pediatrics (95 percent), and CCU/ICU (87 percent). A majority (64 percent) had obstetric privileges, and a minority (36 percent) had surgical privileges. Directors were accurate in their perceptions of privileges attained by graduates in medicine, pediatrics, and CCU/ICU, but underestimated the percentage who had privileges in surgery and overestimated the percentage who had privileges in obstetrics. Residents planned on seeking privileges in medicine, pediatrics, and obstetrics at a rate similar to recent graduates, with lower percentages planning on seeking them in surgery and CCU/ICU. Privileges in surgery and obstetrics were more prevalent in the Midwest and West.

Baltimore, Maryland Reprinted by permission, J. FAMILY PRACTICE. Volume 27, Page 297, 1988. Copyright Appleton & Lange.

Past studies have described hospital privileges of family physicians in groups,[1] states,[2,3] regions,[4,5] and nationally.[6] These reports show that most family physicians have privileges in at least one hospital. Earlier research[7] noted that few family physicians were dissatisfied with their privileges. In the 1980s, however, there has been rising concern about the difficulty of obtaining hospital privileges by family physicians. Many reports document problems in obtaining privileges for general adult inpatient care,[8] surgery,[9] critical care,[10] and obstetrics.[11]

With this increasing concern about obtaining privileges arises the question as to the role of residency training in obtaining privileges. Past investigations focus upon practicing physicians and do not consider the expectations about obtaining privileges held by residents or the perceptions of residency directors about attainment of privileges by graduates of their programs. This study compares recent graduate experiences, residency director perceptions, and residents' expectations regarding obtaining hospital privileges in five areas.

## Methods

A questionnaire was developed to examine hospital privileges for family physicians and was pretested on a small sample of family physicians and family practice residents. Three parallel versions were developed, asking similar questions modified to fit the situations of (1) recent residency graduates, (2) program directors, and (3) third-year residents. Recent graduates were asked whether they had privileges in medicine, pediatrics, surgery, obstetrics, and CCU/ICU. Program directors were asked to estimate the percentage of their graduates that had privileges in these areas: most (more than 75 percent), some 25 to 75 percent, few (less than 25 percent), or none. Residents were asked whether they would seek privileges in these areas.

All three groups provided their sex, age, state where their residency program was located, and type of residency program (university, community [university administered, university affiliated, or nonaffiliated], or military). Program directors indicated how long they had directed the program. Recent graduates were asked the year they completed their residency, the state where they currently practiced, and the size of the community they served. States were grouped for analysis into the four US Census Bureau geographical regions: Northeast, South, Midwest, and West.[12]

The sample included three groups of family physicians. The first group was a random national sample of 308 residency program graduates aged 30 to 35 years who graduated from their residencies from 1977 through

| Characteristic | Recent Graduates (n=242) Percent | Program Directors (n=342) Percent | Residents (n=240) Percent |
|---|---|---|---|
| Sex | | | |
| Male | 88.4 | 94.7 | 77.9 |
| Age (mean years) | 32.7 | 46.8 | 30.3 |
| Residency region* | | | |
| Northeast | 16.8 | 21.3 (20)** | 17.2 (18) |
| South | 40.6 | 31.5 (33) | 33.1 (33) |
| Midwest | 29.5 | 31.5 (31) | 35.1 (32) |
| West | 13.1 | 15.7 (16) | 14.6 (17) |
| Type of program | | | |
| University | 18.9 | 15.3 (17) | 14.3 (21) |
| Community-university administered | 14.3 | 17.9 (15) | 11.3 (15) |
| Community-university affiliated | 51.7 | 55.6 (54) | 57.1 (51) |
| Community-unaffiliated | 10.1 | 7.1 (10) | 13.9 (8) |
| Military | 5.0 | 4.1 (4) | 3.5 (5) |
| Practice region* | | | |
| Northeast | 13.6 | | |
| South | 40.5 | | |
| Midwest | 25.2 | | |
| West | 20.7 | | |
| Practice location | | | |
| Rural | 21.7 | | |
| Small town | 32.1 | | |
| Suburban | 22.9 | | |
| Urban | 23.3 | | |

** Grouped by state into Census Bureau Regions*
*** Numbers in parentheses indicate the national percentages as calculated from the 1986 Directory of Family Practice Residencies*

1985. The second group included all 383 family practice residency program directors in the United States. The third group was a random national sample of 319 third-year family practice residents (class of 1985-86), who represent 13.2 percent of all third-year residents of that year. All samples were drawn from the master database of the American Academy of Family Physicians (AAFP). One follow-up mailing to nonrespondents was done. The final response rates were recent graduates 79 percent, residency directors 89 percent, and third-year residents 75 percent, for an overall response rate of 82 percent. Data were analyzed using chi-square as a measure of significance.[13]

## Results

The demographics of the groups (Table 1) are representative of recent graduates of family practice residencies, program directors of family practice residencies, and third-year residents in family practice in terms of sex, residency region, and type of program.[14]

Hospital privilege comparisons between the groups are presented for five different areas in Table 2. Hospital privileges for recent graduates represent those who have privileges in the above areas. Hospital privileges for program directors represent their estimate of the percentage of their graduates who obtain privileges in these areas. Hospital privileges for residents represent those who plan on applying for privileges in these areas.

In medicine, hospital privileges are almost universally obtained by recent graduates, nearly all program directors believe more than 75 percent of their graduates obtain these privileges, and almost all third-year residents plan on applying for them. In pediatrics the situation is similar.

In surgery, over one third of recent graduates have hospital privileges and more than one quarter of third-year residents plan on applying for privileges in this area. This difference between recent graduates and third-year residents was significant ($P < .04$). The majority of directors believe few ($<25$ percent) or none of their graduates obtain these privileges.

Regarding obstetrics, almost two thirds of recent graduates have privileges, and 56 percent of graduating residents planned on applying for these privileges. This difference in percentage was not significant. About one half of the program directors felt that most ($>75$ percent) of their residents obtain obstetrical privileges.

Concerning CCU/ICU, 87 percent of recent graduates had privileges, but only 78 percent of residents planned to apply for privileges. This difference was significant ($P < .01$). Two thirds (66 percent) of directors believed that most ($>75$ percent) of their graduates get CCU/ICU privileges.

When graduates were divided into two groups, those finishing their residencies from 1977 to 1981 and those completing their residencies from 1982 to 1985, there was a significant decrease in the percentage of those with privileges in surgery for the most recent graduates ($P < .05$). The hospital privileges of these two groups of graduates were compared with

| Table 2. Percentage of Respondents with Hospital Privileges by Group | | | |
|---|---|---|---|
| Privileges | Recent Graduates* (n=246) | Program Directors* (n=344) | Residents*** (n=240) |
| Medicine | 97.1 | 99.1 | 97.5 |
| Pediatrics | 94.9 | 95.7 | 96.2 |
| Surgery | 36.4 | 25.1 | 26.9 |
| Obstetrics | 63.7 | 48.2 | 56.2 |
| CCU/ICU | 87.3 | 66.2 | 78.5 |

** For recent graduates, hospital privileges represents those who have privileges in the above areas*
*** For program directors, hospital privileges represents those who believe more than 75% of their graduates obtain privileges in the above areas*
**** For residents, hospital privileges represents those who plan on applying for privileges in the above areas*
*CCU/ICU—coronary care unit/intensive care unit*

| Table 3. Percentage of Hospital Privileges Gained or Sought by Survey Respondents | | | |
|---|---|---|---|
| Privileges | Graduates* 1977-1981 (n=75) | Graduates 1982-1985 (n=153) | Residents** (n=240) |
| Medicine | 98.6 | 96.1 | 97.5 |
| Pediatrics | 98.6 | 94.0 | 96.2 |
| Surgery*** | 48.6 | 31.5 | 26.9 |
| Obstetrics | 58.3 | 67.6 | 56.2 |
| CCU/ICU† | 90.3 | 86.7 | 78.5 |

** For recent graduates, hospital privileges represents those who have privileges in the above areas*
*** For residents, hospital privileges represents those who plan on applying for privileges in the above areas*
**** P<.01, chi-square*
*† P<.05, chi-square*
*CCU/ICU—coronary care unit/intensive care unit*

the privileges the residents planned on applying for (Table 3). Of the first group of graduates, 48.6 percent had privileges in surgery compared with 31.5 percent of the second group. Only 26.9 percent of the residents planned on applying for these privileges. This trend was significant (P < .01). A similar trend was observed in CCU/ICU privileges, where 90.3 percent of the first group and 86.7 percent of the second group of graduates have privileges, and 78.5 percent of the residents planned on applying for them (P < .05).

The only difference by sex was that male third-year residents were more likely to apply for privileges in CCU/ICU (82 percent) compared with female residents (67 percent). This difference was significant (P < .05).

The regions of the country in which the residency was located made no significant difference for privileges in medicine and CCU/ICU for any of the three groups (Table 4). While there were no regional differences in pediatric privileges for recent graduates and residency directors, residents about to complete programs located in the Northeast were significantly less likely to plan on applying for privileges (P < .05). For surgery and obstetrics, recent graduates were less likely to have privileges (P < .05), residents were less likely to plan on applying for privileges (P < .001), and residency directors believed fewer of their graduates had privileges (P < .001) if their residency was in the Northeast and South compared with those in the Midwest and West.

Regarding the type of residency program (university, community, military, etc) where these physicians completed their training, are completing their training, or are the directors, there were no significant privilege differences for medicine or pediatrics. In surgery graduates of military programs were more likely to have privileges (P < .01), while there were no significant differences for directors of residents of military programs. In obstetrics graduates of programs based in community hospitals without university affiliation were significantly less likely to have privileges (P < .05). Similarly in CCU/ICU the residents in university and military programs were less likely to plan on applying for privileges (P < .001).

Recent graduates practicing in the Midwest and West were more likely to have privileges in surgery and obstetrics (P < .01). There were no other significant differences by region of the country in which the graduate practiced. The only difference in privileges regarding urban and rural practice was that those practicing in urban areas were less likely to have surgical privileges (P < .05).

## Discussion

Obtaining hospital privileges for family physicians has become a controversial issue. The findings of this study about the frequency of hospital privileges for graduates of family practice programs are representative of previous studies in this area.[1-6] Almost all recent graduates report having privileges in medicine, pediatrics, and CCU/ICU, while two thirds have privileges in obstetrics, and one third in surgery. The situation in obstetrics

Table 4. Percentage of Hospital Privileges by Region of Country in Which Residency is Located by Group

| | Recent Graduates* | | | | Program Directors** | | | | Residents*** | | | |
| | Region | | | | Region | | | | Region | | | |
| Privileges | NE | S | MW | W | NE | S | MW | W | NE | S | MW | W |
|---|---|---|---|---|---|---|---|---|---|---|---|---|
| Medicine | 98 | 95 | 99 | 100 | 99 | 99 | 99 | 100 | 95 | 98 | 99 | 97 |
| Pediatrics | 93 | 93 | 97 | 100 | 94 | 92 | 98 | 100 | 87† | 97 | 99 | 97 |
| Surgery | 20† | 34† | 44 | 52 | 19† | 15† | 39 | 26 | 17† | 15† | 42 | 31 |
| Obstetrics | 42† | 55† | 83 | 79 | 27† | 37† | 73 | 48 | 38† | 7† | 80 | 64 |
| CCU/ICU | 85 | 88 | 90 | 83 | 65 | 61 | 75 | 58 | 82 | 74 | 84 | 74 |

* For recent graduates hospital privileges represents the percentage who have privileges in the above areas
** For program directors hospital privileges represents the percentage who believe more than 75% of their graduates obtain privileges in the above areas
*** For residents hospital privileges represents the percentage who plan on applying for privileges in the above areas
† P < .05, chi-square
‡ P < .01, chi-square
CCU/ICU—coronary care unit/intensive care unit

is likely to change in the near future because of rising malpractice premiums, and there is recent documentation of declining numbers of family physicians providing obstetrical care.[15]

Program directors perceive that the vast majority of their graduates will obtain privileges in medicine, pediatrics and CCU/ICU similar to the actual percentage of graduates who have these privileges. Their estimates, however, do not coincide with the data obtained from recent graduates in two areas. Directors underestimated the percentage of graduates who obtain privileges in surgery and overestimated the percentage with privileges in obstetrics. These misperceptions may influence directors' emphasis on training residents in these areas. A number of family practice programs have published follow-up studies of their graduates, obtaining data concerning hospital privileges obtained by their graduates.[16-20] It would be beneficial for all program directors to survey their graduates periodically regarding type of practice, hospital privileges, and so on, as such a survey would enable them to alter their curriculum to best suit the training needs of their graduates in practice.

Almost all the residents intend to apply for privileges in medicine and pediatrics. The percentage who plan on seeking privileges in surgery and CCU/ICU is significantly less than the percentage of recent graduates who have privileges in these areas. When graduates were divided into two groups based on how recently they completed their residencies, a significant decrease in the percentage of those with privileges in surgery was observed. When the percentage of residents planning on seeking privileges in surgery and CCU/ICU was compared with the percentage of the two groups of recent graduates who have privileges in these areas, a significant trend was seen regarding privileges in surgery and CCU/ICU. The data in this study suggest that residents will follow in the footsteps of their counterparts from previous resident cohorts in applying for medicine, pediatric, and obstetrical privileges, with a possible decline in the number of family physicians seeking privileges in surgery and CCU/ICU.

Regional patterns in privileges that have been discussed in other studies[6] also emerge from these data. An emphasis on both obstetrical and surgical privileges clearly existed for programs and physicians in the Midwest and West. Medical students applying for family practice residencies who are interested in obstetrics and surgery might do well to enter a program in the Midwest or West or later practice in those areas.

The lack of differences in privileges by type of program was surprising. Graduates of military programs were more likely to have privileges in surgery and graduates of programs at community hospitals without university affiliation were less likely to do obstetrics, but otherwise all types of programs were similar in the proportion of privileges attained by their graduates and the perception of their directors about their graduates. Residents completing military and university programs were less likely to plan on seeking privileges in CCU/ICU, which may have to do with their relative lack of role models in intensive care units.[10]

This study has several limitations. Only recent graduates were examined, and those in practice longer may have different privileges, as may older non-residency-trained general practitioners. The apparent misperceptions of the directors might be due to their basing their estimates on the experience of graduates from all years, while only graduates from 1977 through 1985 were sampled in this study. Data on graduates' privileges were self-reported and may be subject to reporting bias. Another confounding factor may be variations in the level of privileges, ie, a hospital may grant surgical privileges to surgeons only, but family physicians may first assist, so privileges in surgery may have meant different things to different respondents. The 82 percent response rate, although better than most mail surveys of physicians,[21] still leaves some physicians unrepresented.

Because of the significance of the topic to medical practice, there is sure to be a great deal of research in the future on privileges for family physicians. In light of the differences between the perceptions of directors and experiences of recent graduates, it would be valuable to see how that issue influences curriculum in residency programs. Only third-year residents were examined in this study, and the changing perceptions of residents over the course of their training regarding privileges and plans for obtaining them should be explored. Additionally, as more family physicians begin to work for health maintenance organizations, it will be interesting to see whether greater emphasis is placed on family physicians as providers of outpatient care only. Attempts to limit family physicians' presence in hospitals must be carefully documented.

In conclusion, most recent residency graduates in this study had privileges in medicine, pediatrics, and CCU/ICU, with a majority in obstetrics, and a minority in surgery. Residency program directors were accurate in their perceptions of privileges held by their graduates in medicine, pediatrics, and CCU/ICU, but they underestimated the percentage who had privileges in surgery and overestimated the percentage in obstetrics. Third-year residents planned on seeking privileges at a rate similar to that recent graduates in medicine, pediatrics, and obstetrics, with lower percentages planning on seeking them in the surgery and CCU/ICU. The programs in the Midwest and West were more likely to produce residents with privileges in surgery and obstetrics, but there were few other consistent demographic patterns.

These findings should encourage residency directors to examine more actively the privilege patterns of their graduates and to consider that information in curriculum planning. Additional research on hospital privileges for family physicians is definitely needed.

**References**


1. Slabaugh RC, Gingiewicz M, Babineau RA: The hospital work of a family practice group in a medium size community in New England. *J Fam Pract* 1980; 11:287-297
2. Warburton SW Jr, Sadler GR: Family physician hospital privileges in New Jersey. *J Fam Pract* 1978; 7:1019-1026
3. Warburton SW, Bobula JA, Wolff GT: Hospital privileges of family physicians in North Carolina. *J Fam Pract* 1981; 12:725-728
4. Hansen DV, Sundwall DN, Kane RL: Hospital privileges for family physicians. *J Fam Pract* 1977; 5:805-809
5. Sundwall DN, Hansen DV: Hospital privileges for family physicians: A comparative study between the New England states and the Intermountain states. *J Fam Pract* 1979; 9:885-894
6. Clinton C, Schmittling G, Stern TL, Black RR: Hospital privileges for family physicians: A national study of office based members of the American Academy of Family Physicians. *J Fam Pract* 1981; 13:361-371
7. Mechanic D: The organization of medical practice and practice orientations among physicians in prepaid and nonprepaid primary care settings. *Med Care* 1975; 13:189-204
8. Weiss BD: Hospital privileges for family physicians at university hospitals. *J Fam Pract* 1984; 18:747-753
9. Marien MW: The surgical role of family physicians. *Am J Public Health* 1982; 72:1359-1363
10. Weiss BD: Family physicians in university hospital intensive care units. *J Fam Pract* 1983; 17:693-696
11. Stern TL, Schmittling G, Clinton C, Black RR; Hospital privileges for graduates of family practice residency programs. *J Fam Pract* 1981; 13:1013-1020
12. Statistical Abstract of the United States 1986, ed 106. *Bureau of the Census.* Government Printing Office, 1986
13. Norusis MJ: SPSS PC+. Chicago, SPSS, 1986
14. 1986 Directory of Family Practice Residency Programs. Kansas City, Mo, American Academy of Family Physicians, 1986
15. Weiss BD: The effect of malpractice insurance costs on family physicians' hospital practices. *J Fam Pract* 1986; 23:55-58

16. Ciriacy EW, Bland CJ, Stoller JE, Prestwood JS: Graduate follow-up in the University of Minnesota affiliated hospitals residency training program in family practice and community health. *J Fam Pract* 1980; 11:719-730

17. Mayo F, Wood M, Marsland DW, et al: Graduate follow-up in the Medical College of Virginia/Virginia Commonwealth University family practice residency system. *J Fam Pract* 1980; 11:731-742

18. Geyman JP, Cherkin DC, Deisher JB, Gordon MJ: Graduate follow-up in the University of Washington family practice residency network. *J Fam Pract* 1980; 11:743-752

19. Hecht RC, Farrell JG: Graduate follow-up in the University of Wisconsin family practice residency programs. *J Fam Pract* 1982; 14:549-555

20. Gaede GL, Brownlee HJ Jr, Gayson RS, Bryant EE: Graduate follow-up in the US Air Force family practice residency programs. *J Fam Pract* 1984; 17:1057-1063

21. Shostek H, Fairweather WR: Physician response rates to mail and personal interview surveys. *Public Opinion Q* 1979; 43:206-217

# Physicians' Hospital Privileges— The Business of Practicing Medicine

Harold L. Hirsh


**Abstract**

The relationship between hospitals and the attending physicians with privileges to have their patients admitted to the hospitals for treatment has changed significantly in the last 10 years. One of the reasons for this change is the new attitude to the practice of medicine, which is now considered a branch of business just as much as any other commercial or industrial enterprise. The author reviews the legal aspects of the changing relationship.


Membership on a hospital staff has become critical to the great majority of physicians in this country. Hospitals invariably require staff membership as a prerequisite for rendition of medical services by a physician to a hospitalized patient. Nowadays, a physician who is not allowed to practice in a hospital is, for all practical purposes, denied the opportunity to practice his profession. Some consider physicians' hospital privileges to be at risk. The structure of our health care delivery system is such that there are situations in which a physician may wrongfully be denied the right to practice in a hospital. In a previous article, we have reviewed the duty of any hospital under the judicial doctrine of "corporate liability" and by congressional and state legislation to control the demeanor of attend-


Reprinted by permission MEDICINE & LAW, Volume 6, Page 227, 1987. Copyright Medicine and Law

ing physicians. On the other hand, it has the obligation to render them "due process" and "equal protection."

In the process of obtaining or maintaining hospital privileges, the attending physician may be the victim of unfair business practices even though these are proscribed by state and/or federal laws, or of tortious interference with his relationships with his patients. In some instances, hospitals have misunderstood their role in interpreting and implementing their legal duties: in other circumstances, they have deliberately abused and oppressed physicians because of their administrative zeal and greed.

Until recently, the courts were generally unwilling to interfere with a hospital board's decision and substitute their judgment for that of the board vis-à-vis physicians' privileges. This is no longer viable. In the last two decades the courts have generally recognized how ominous the situation is and have become sensitive to the omnipotence of hospitals in this area. To that end, they have provided forums for disenfranchised physicians who have been denied or deprived of staff appointments, and invoked appropriate remedies. In response to these transgressions the courts have intervened on the physicians' behalf, protecting their status in the hospital. Many times, a physician may have no way to remedy the situation other than to seek redress in the courts.

## Medical Staff

As to the protection and preservation of the independence of the medical staff, the courts have held that only the medical staff may promulgate and adopt the rules, regulations and by-laws under which they operate, and hospital boards of trustees are restricted to approving these by-laws.[1] Any insoluble conflicts are properly brought before the courts.

## Civil Rights

Where appropriate, some courts have come to the aid of physicians with grievances by holding that any hospital that receives federal funds under the Hill-Burton legislation, Medicare, Medicaid, and/or other grants, cannot discriminate on the basis of race, color or national origin in its medical staff appointments under the Civil Rights Act of 1964.[2-4] Under these circumstances some courts have invoked the Fifth and Fourteenth Amendments and deemed that the receipt of these funds cloaked the hospital with the mantle of state action requiring due process and equal protection to be extended to physicians with regard to their hospital staff appointments.

Most courts have been willing to invoke this protection for physicians only in public, and not in private, hospitals.[5-7]


## Civil Conspiracy

The courts, in recent times, have generally provided adequate remedies for capricious, discriminatory or arbitrary treatment of a physician in matters concerned with staff appointments.[8-10] But judicial relief often cannot be obtained in other situations, where the harm to the physician, although perhaps just as devastating, is more subtle in nature and cannot be easily classified as capricious. These cases often involve situations where for economic or personal reasons various staff physicians, without any opposition from the governing board of a hospital, or even with their acquiescence, conspire to prevent another physician from pursuing his profession in a hospital. Legally this is termed a "civil conspiracy." Civil conspiracy is defined as a combination of two or more persons who by concerted action accomplish an unlawful purpose, or accomplish some purpose not in itself unlawful, by unlawful means. In essence, the courts have said that everyone has the right to establish, engage in, and conduct a lawful business or profession. To that end, everyone is entitled to the protection of organized society through its courts whenever that right is unlawfully violated. An actionable wrong is established against anyone who is said to have intentionally interfered with that right, without justifiable cause or excuse. It is, therefore, an actionable wrong for two or more persons to conspire maliciously to injure and damage another in the conduct of that lawful business or profession. That includes preventing a physician from being granted hospital privileges[11,12] and depriving a physician from practicing medicine by the unlawful withholding of necessary medical assistance.[13]

The evolution of this philosophy undoubtedly has been assisted by the courts' recognition that for these purposes health care professionals and deliverers of services are involved in commerce as a business or trade, as well as a profession.[14-17]

Recovery under this theory, however, is often fraught with difficulty, principally because it is necessary for the plaintiff to show that the defendants actually entered into a conspiracy agreement or combination among themselves. In fact, this requirement has blocked various attempts by physicians to seek recovery under this doctrine.[18-21] Faced with the situation of a legal wrong inflicted on a physician, which would otherwise remain unremedied, the courts have begun to recognize the need for judicial relief, and are invoking the doctrine of civil conspiracy.[11-13]

If a physician-plaintiff is able to prove that the defendants did act in concert to injure him, the civil conspiracy charge is broad enough to encompass a variety of wrongs actionable under common law. In a California case[22] the court stated that a cause of action was valid for common law restraint of trade when it was shown that the defendants, members of the governing board of a hospital and various staff physicians, entered into a conspiracy intentionally to interfere with the plaintiff-osteopath's business by arbitrarily denying him staff privileges.

Similarly, in a Missouri case[11] the court employed a civil conspiracy theory to uphold a complaint that denying hospital privileges constituted interference with the contractual rights between the plaintiff and his patients. The physician was able to prove that several physicians and the hospital's governing board had conspired to prevent him from acquiring membership of the hospital staff.

The flexibility of the legal theory of civil conspiracy in hospital staff cases is demonstrated by a recent Florida case.[12] The surgeon-plaintiff brought suit, on behalf of the patients, against a hospital and all the staff anesthesiologists, alleging a conspiracy to refuse to provide him with anesthesiological services. This resulted in his financial ruin. The court recognized the dilemma of the surgeon and certified the civil conspiracy charge as a valid theory of recovery. It emphasized that civil conspiracy may entitle an individual to relief by virtue of the defendant's concerted action even though the same activity by one of the defendants alone would not be actionable. The court reasoned that even though an anesthesiologist has the legitimate right to refuse to render his services to a surgeon, where all anesthesiologists of a hospital agreed to refuse their services to a competent staff surgeon this conduct amounted to an effective deprivation of the surgeon's practice at the hospital. This gives rise to an independent wrong under the concept of civil conspiracy.

The rights of a physician to practice his profession in a hospital without being molested financially was succinctly stated in another recent case.[14] The court held that everyone has the right to establish and conduct a lawful business or engage in a lawful profession, and is entitled to the protection of the courts and a remedy whenever that right is unlawfully violated.

A review of these cases reveals that the conspiracy is usually cloaked in what appear to be legitimate circumstances. They usually fall into one of two categories; the conspiracy results in the denial or withdrawal of hospital staff privileges, or effectively deprives the physician of the opportunity to practice at his hospital by sequestering available beds for admission or operating room space and time. Now, the physician who is injured by a conspiracy to deprive him of his right to practice his profession may confidently seek relief under the common law principle of civil conspiracy.

## State Unfair Business Practice Acts and Federal Antitrust Laws

Physicians have also attempted to secure relief when denied hospital privileges by relying on federal or state statutory protection (antitrust laws) proscribing unfair business or trade practices. Under these laws it is illegal for individuals or groups to conspire to prevent others from carrying on similar business competitively. These federal antitrust laws and state unfair business trade practice acts which proscribe such activities were enacted in times past and were not available to physicians for several reasons. The complainant had to be involved in a trade or business that was engaged in interstate commerce. He was not able to redress an economic injury unless there had also been a detriment to the general public. A private individual is precluded from obtaining relief if injury to the public in general cannot be demonstrated.[23]

Recent supreme court decisions have emphasized the "trade" aspects of the learned professions; the theory that the medical profession is not a trade is no longer a viable defense.[15-17] The federal antitrust laws no longer make exceptions for the learned professions (medicine, dentistry, law, etc.), although some states still retain the exemption.

Furthermore, private hospitals can no longer afford to rely on protection from suits under federal antitrust laws; Congress has held them to be sufficiently involved in interstate commerce to be governed by the labor relations laws.[25] The Supreme Court has held that local hospital business sufficiently impacts on interstate commerce to place them within the jurisdiction of the federal antitrust laws.[26]

The federal statutes require demonstration of a "substantial impact upon interstate commerce." In a recent case, a federal court ruled[27] that a physician was justified in suing a hospital for violation of the federal antitrust laws in the form of restraint of trade by excluding him from staff membership if he could prove that significant number of his patients received Medicare or Medicaid benefits. The court held that the sending of claims and the receipt of payment through the mail satisfied the interstate commerce requirement, even though both his and the hospital's patients were almost exclusively from a local area of Michigan.

Recovery under these state and federal statutory schemes is still fraught with great obstacles. For a suit to be successful, an injury to the public in general must be demonstrated. The physician whose injury is essentially a personal one in such a situation will still be hard put to overcome this barrier. However, the courts have accepted the premise that not only the physician but also his patients suffer by his deprivation of hospital facilities. They will not be treated by the physician of their choice if he cannot obtain hospital privileges at the facility that they prefer.[28]

## Exclusive Contracts

There have now been a significant number of lawsuits in which exclusive contracts have been challenged as in violation of state and federal antitrust laws and of common law prohibitions against interference with contractual relationships (physician-patient) and restraint of trade. Hospitals' decisions to enter into exclusive contracts for some medical services by granting privileges to only one or a few physicians have almost uniformly been upheld by the courts as good faith attempts to insure competent quality medical care. Antitrust and unfair business practice laws have been held not to have been violated by such contracts granting exclusive rights to practice a medical specialty when the contract was not unreasonable.

When a hospital has decided to operate a particular department through the use of an exclusive contract, justifying its decision on the basis of high-quality patient care, reduced costs, and the facilitation of hospital administration, the decision has invariably been upheld by the courts.[29-43] Such cases have been concerned with various specialties, particularly radiology, emergency room services, pathology and cardiology services, and outpatient referrals.

Furthermore, an attending physician's rights to seek outside professional consultants for his patient's care may be reasonably limited by a hospital's use of exclusive professional service contracts.[44]

## Closed Staffs

As the number of practicing physicians has grown and the available hospital facilities have remained relatively constant, hospitals have attempted to resolve the problem by a "closed staff" policy. Physicians who would otherwise be eligible for hospital privileges have been denied appointment. Physicians faced with this reality have sought assistance and redress from the courts on the basis of antitrust and unfair business practice laws. This has resulted in a challenge to the concept of unwarranted suppression of competition including undue limits that private parties may impose upon the number of competitors in a market and undue limits that private parties may impose upon competing professionals, as well as the unfair exclusion of particular individuals from practice opportunities.

Courts have considered several factors when physicians have challenged the closed staff policy. They have noted that to some reasonable degree hospitals are responsible for providing optimal service to the community and that there is no absolute right to close a staff even though the physician may have access to other hospital beds in the area. The courts have required some balancing of the interests of the surrounding community and of the medical profession, and of the economic implications for the hospital and physicians presently on the medical staff and for those physicians who would be excluded from staff appointments.

Courts have sustained boards of trustees closing their staffs when this has been motivated by a desire to maintain a good quality of patient care. In a New Jersey case,[45] the court held that a hospital may restrict privileges if the services would otherwise be overtaxed. The court noted, however, that privileges could not routinely be denied to physicians moving into the area, and any denial motivated by a desire to exclude newcomers and protect the existing staff would not be tolerated.

In another New Jersey case,[46] a hospital imposed a moratorium on granting new staff privileges except to physicians who had no other hospital affiliation and who practiced certain designated limited specialties. In the previous 10 years, despite several expansions, the occupancy rate was greater than recommended by appropriate agencies. Continued over-utilization would be dangerous to patients, because it would result in a tendency to discharge them prematurely. In order to avoid further overcrowding, the Board of Trustees adopted the moratorium. After 5 years there was still no improvement. When the policy was challenged by several surgeons the court held that the policy could not be 'judicially tolerated' because of its ineffectiveness, noting that it had enhanced the economic interest of some physicians at the expense of other practitioners.

In a third New Jersey case,[47] the court reviewed the denial of staff appointments to two obstetricians based upon a moratorium policy which resulted from an excessive occupancy in the maternity unit. After an extensive review of the evidence the court upheld the moratorium. It did not, however, approve an open-ended moratorium, stating that as soon as additional obstetrics beds became available, occupancy was reduced to manageable proportions, or there were staff vacancies, the failure to admit qualified physicians would not be tolerated.

In a California case,[48] a physician challenged the hospital's closed staff policy with reference to operation of the hospital's chronic renal hemodialysis facility. The court ruled that the alleged hospital's interference with the physician's right to practice his profession in the hospital was justified and that its conduct was privileged, since the decision was not arbitrary, capricious, or wholly lacking in evidentiary support.

Teaching hospitals' actions have been uniformly upheld by the courts when they have denied hospital privileges to nonfaculty members.[49,50]

While the foregoing cases may not be completely comparable, they do indicate that courts will carefully scrutinize any record established by a hospital to justify closure of its staff. Where that record does not clearly indicate that closure is directly related to patient care and the quality of medical practice, courts may be unwilling to condone closure or of a moratorium. Those staff closures found to be unreasonable may then become the basis for antitrust litigation instituted by the excluded physicians. Furthermore, a hospital's governing board has the power to require consultation even of a specialist in the interest of quality care,[47] or the use of the hospital diagnostic equipment rather than outside facilities.[51] An Ohio court has held that certification or eligibility, or membership in the specialty association, or a minimum period of experience may be required before major surgical privileges are granted in a private hospital, and that this is not unreasonable or arbitrary.[52] The same was not true for a public hospital, however.[53]

## Conclusions

Life need not always be unfair for the physician vis-à-vis his right to practice in the hospital. The law has imposed upon hospitals the duty of properly selecting and monitoring its attending physicians—"corporate liability." On the other hand, the law has also protected the practitioner by requiring the hospital to adhere to constitutional fair play and equal protection under the civil rights laws, to procedural and substantive due process, and adherence to the federal and state antitrust and unfair business practice acts. Relief under the common law doctrine of civil conspiracy is also appropriately available.

Physicians who are disenfranchised by hospitals and members of its medical staff now have a spectrum of remedies to right the wrongs, they have sustained. This is the product of courts' sensitivity to the dilemma of a troubled physician whose injury is subtle and the product of action which seems legitimate but is nonetheless intentional and devastating. It recognized the pivotal economic nature of a physician's hospital practice.

Hospital health care has become a triangular arrangement between patient, physician, and hospital. It can become an illicit love triangle. The courts are now willing to intervene because health care delivery may be considered a "business" or "trade," it does impact on interstate commerce, and the inability of a physician to have hospital privileges affects his patients as well as himself. The courts have recognized that a physician without hospital privileges is like a fish out of water.

## References


1. *St John's Regional Hospital Medical Staff v St John's Regional Medical Center* (SD Cir CT Beadle Co. Civ # 73-102 March 3, 1975)
2. *Cypress v Newport New General and Hospital Association*, 357 F 2d 648 (CA 4, 1967)
3. *Eaton v Grubbs*, 329F 2d 710 (CA 4, 1964)
4. *Citta v Delaware Valley Hospital*, 313 F Supp 301 (CA 4, 1970)
5. *Greisman v Newcomb Hospital*, 197 A 2d 817 (NJ 1963)
6. *State ex rel Bronaugh v City of Parkersburg*, 148 W Wa 568 136 SE 2d 783 (1964)
7. *Bello v South Shore Hospital*,—NE2d—(Mass Cap Ind Ct 1981)
   7a. *Foster v Mobile County Hospital Board*, 298, F 2d 227 (CA 5, 1968)
8. *Sosa v Board of Managers of the Val verde Memorial Hospital*, 437 F 2d 173( CA 5, 1971)
9. *Ascherman v St Francis Memorial Hospital*, 45 Cal App 3d 507 119 Cal Rptr 507 (1975)
10. *Suckle v Madison General Hospital*, 326 F Supp 1196; affirmed 499 F 2a 136 (CA 7, 1974)
11. *Cowan v Gibson*, 392 SW 2d 307 (Mo, 1965)
12. *Margolin v Morton F Plant Hospital Association*, 340 So 2d 1090 (Fla App 1977)
13. *Nashville Memorial Hospital v Binkley*, 534 SW 2d 318 (Tenn 1976)
14. *American Medical Association v United States*, 317 US 519 (1943)
15. *United States v College of Pathologists*, Civil Action 66 C-1253 (ND Ill July 1966)
16. *United States v American Society of Anesthesiologists*, 473 F Supp 147 (SD NY, 1975)
17. *United States v Illinois Pediatry Society*, 4 Trade Case 153, 681 (ND Ill February 14, 1977)
18. *Sokol v University Hospital*, 402 F Supp, 1029, (Mass, 1975)
19. *Wolf v Jane Phillips Episcopal Memorial Center*, 593 F 2d 684 (CA 10, 1975)
20. *Crane v International Health Care, Inc.*,—F2d—, (CA 10, 1980; rehearing en banc, 1981)
21. *Riggal v Washington County Medical Society*, 249 F 2d 266 (CA 8, 1957)
22. *Willis v Santa Ana Community Hospital Association*, 58 Cal 2d 806 (1962)
23. *Moles v White* 336 So 2d 427 (Fla App, 1976)
24. *Robinson v Magovern*,—F 2d—(CA3 1981)

25. *The Labor Management Relations Act,* 1974 as amended by Public Laws 86-259, and 93-360, 1974

26. *Hospital Building Co v Trustees of the Rex Hospital,* 48 Ed 2d 338 (1976)

27. *Zamiri v William Beaumont Hospital,* 430 F Supp 875 (DCED Mich, 1979)

28. *Stone v William Beaumont Hospital,*—F Supp-—(DCED Mich, 1981)

29. *Harron v United Hospital Center, Inc* 522 F 2d 1133 (CA 10, 1975); cert denied 424 US 916 (1976)

30. *Datillo v Tucson General Hospital,* 23, Ariz App 392 533 P 2d 700 (1975)

31. *Nankin v Michigan Hospital Service,* 361 F Supp 1199 (ED Mich, 1976)

32. *Navato v Sletten,* 415 F Supp 312 (DC Mo, 1976)

33. *Adler v Montifiore Hospital Association of Western,* Penn 311 A 2d 634 (Pa 1973); cert denied 94 Ct 870 (1974)

34. *Powsner v St Joseph Mercy Hospital of Detroit,*—NW 2d—(Mich, 1977)

35. *Bennell v Virginia,* 104 NW 2d 633 (Minn, 1960)

36. *Centeno v Roseville Community Hospital* 107 Cal App 3d 62, 1979

37. *Blank v Palo Alto-Stanford Hospital Center,* 234 Cal App 3d 379 (1965)

38. *Letsch v Northern San Diego County Hospital,* 246 Cal App 3d 673 (1966)

39. *Smith v Northern Michigan Hospitals, Inc,*—F Supp—(WD Mich, 1981)

40. *Balhuzin v North Kansas Memorial Hospital,*—F 2d—(CA 8, 1978)

41. *Anne Arundal General Hospital, Inc v O'Brien,* 432 A 2d 483 (Ma Ct, Spec App, 1981)

42. *Sokol v University Hospital, Inc,* 402 F Supp 1025 (D Mass, 1975)

43. *Capili v Shott,* 620 F 2d 438 (CA 4, W Va, 1980)

44. *Radiology Professional Corp v Trinidad Area Health Association, Inc,* 565 P 2d 952 (Colo Sup Ct 1978)

45. *Guerrero v Burlington County Memorial Hospital,* 70 NJ 344, 360 A 2d 334 (1976)

46. *Walsky v Pasack Valley Hospital,* 367 A 2d 1204 (NJ, 1976)

47. *Davis v Morristown Memorial Hospital* 106 NJ Sup 33, 254 A 2d 125 (1969)

48. *Lewin v St Joseph Hospital of Orange,* 82 Cal App 3d 36 (1978)

49. *Haydon v Stanford University Hospital,* Case No P 32039 (Superior Court, Santa Clara County, California Memorandum of Intended Decision, July 8, 1977)

50. *Davidson v Tapley*, 395 NYS 2d 41 (NY Sup Ct, App Div, 1977)
51. *Cobb-County Kennestone Hospital Authority v Prince*,—SE 2d—(Ga Sup Ct, 1978)
52. *Khan v Suburban Community Hospital*, 45 Ohio St 2d 39, 340 NE 2d 398 (1976)
53. *Armstrong v Fayette County General Hospital* 553 SE 2d 77; cert denied July 5, 1977 (Tenn 1977)

# Hospital and Medical Staff Relations in the USA
## II. Criteria for Privileges

Harold L. Hirsh

**Abstract**

A hospital has a primary duty, i.e., "corporate responsibility and liability," to maintain the quality of patient care to its patients. The safety and best interests of the patients must, therefore, take precedence over all other concerns of the hospital. For this reason, hospitals have a duty to screen all applicants for medical staff membership thoroughly and to grant staff appointments only to physicians who have demonstrated a sufficient level of current competence to indicate that they will not present a threat to those patients. Courts generally have upheld as reasonable and nonarbitrary any rule criterion, or standard bearing a rational relationship to professional standards of patient care, which are the objective of the hospital.

A hospital may refuse privileges if the refusal is based upon reasonable criteria that are neither arbitrary nor discriminatory. Factors related to the quality of patient care and the professional competence, character, and ethical behavior of the individual physician may serve as a reasonable basis for denial of privileges.

Health Services Administration and National Law Center, George Washington University, 2801 New Mexico Avenue, Washington, DC 20007, USA
Reprinted by permission of MEDICINE & LAW, Volume 7, page 91, 1988. Copyright *Medicine and Law.*

### Criteria

Hospitals have a duty to screen all applicants for medical staff membership thoroughly and to grant staff appointments only to physicians who have demonstrated a sufficient level of current competence to indicate that they will not present a threat to the hospitals' patients.[5,45,46] A hospital may refuse privileges if the refusal is based upon reasonable criteria which are neither arbitrary nor discriminatory. Factors related to the quality of patient care and the professional competence, character, and ethical behavior of the individual physician may serve as a reasonable basis for denial of privileges if these factors are disclosed to the applicant and are well documented so as to comply with the applicable standard of procedural fairness. Courts have generally upheld as reasonable and nonarbitrary any rule or standard bearing a rational relationship to professional standards of patient care, which are the objective of the hospital.

New applications for privileges and annual applications renewal of privileges must be scrutinized and evaluated carefully. This process has been rigorously enforced by the judiciary in recent years.

### Hospital and Medical Staff Bylaws, Rules, and Regulations

Adherence to and compliance with hospital and medical staff bylaws, rules, and regulations has been equated with professional competence, and failure to adhere to them can be the basis for summary or temporary suspension followed by permanent revocation after a due process hearing.[40] Failure to serve in the emergency room is also considered a form of such failure.[41]

### Physical and Mental Status

Applicants can be asked to disclose any physical or mental problem that might impair their ability to practice their profession.[47] The hospital may require an independent medical opinion concerning any problem in the course of the accreditation process.

### Experience and Training

The courts have upheld a hospital's right to require a physician, as a condition for receiving and maintaining privileges, to document his experience, training, and demonstrated competence with sufficient adequacy to assure the governing body and the medical staff that any patient treated by him in the hospital will receive the appropriate quality of medical care.[48] All states now require postgraduate training before granting a new license, which in turn is an absolute requirement before hospital privileges are granted.

## Hospital Standards

A hospital can set standards higher than the minimum required by law if it can be shown that the standards are for the benefit of the patient. Such a hospital policy, in order to bear a reasonable relationship to the operation of the hospital, must embody a legitimate reason for denying medical staff privileges. However, the reasons for the policy should be set out explicitly at the time it is adopted. Furthermore, the policy must bear a reasonable relationship to sound hospital standards; there should be a well-documented basis for it, which should be detailed in hospital procedures. The courts have viewed such policies as a proper exercise of discretion on the part of the hospital when they have been reasonable in relation to sound hospital standards.

## Up-to-Date Competence

Courts have sustained hospital bylaws in relation to professional standards, requiring evidence that the physician has kept "up-to-date" or "abreast" of developments.[50] Evidence of continuing medical education has been declared not to be an inordinate requirement. A court invalidated a hospital bylaw requiring that applicants be given oral and written, tests as the credentials committee at, its discretion determined.[49]

## Professional Society Membership

A hospital may not require staff applicants to be members of a medical society.[51]

## References and Recommendations

It is permissible to ask for letters of reference from persons knowledgeable about the applicant's competence and behavior and to use such letters in the evaluation of the applicant,[52] and also to refuse to continue processing an application until such letters have been received.[53] An acceptable condition for evaluation of applications for appointment to the medical staff is that the applicant submit references from knowledgeable physicians to be evaluated in conjunction with the information in the application. Such a requirement is legitimate.[54] However, the courts have overturned bylaw requirements that recommendations must come from staff members of the hospital in which the applicant is seeking privileges.[55] The requirement that an applicant furnish references from other hospitals in which he has practiced and/or other doctors who have knowledge of his competence is one reasonably calculated to aid in the investigation of qualifications. A requirement that an applicant submit current references evaluating his performance from the head of the hospital at which he had been employed immediately prior to his application to the defendant hospital has been upheld. It is acceptable to require references when the purpose is clearly to obtain informed opinions as a basis on which to evaluate the applicant's prior medical and hospital performance. If an applicant refuses to furnish references his or her application may be rejected.

The key point is that the references requested must deal with prior behavior or competence, which are concerns central to the proper evaluation of an application. Wrongful conduct in the past alone may not be a sufficient ground for denial of staff privileges.[56]

## Geographic Limitations

Medical staff bylaw provisions that require an applicant to live or practice within a certain distance of the hospital, without setting absolute limits, are generally made with the purpose of assuring that a physician who admits patients to the hospital is located close enough to care for them, if necessary, outside the normal visiting hours in the hospital. A geographic limitation rule is not interdicted; but, it must be reasonable.[57] A requirement that the doctor's office be located in the same county as the hospital has been rejected.[58]

## Specialty Privileges

Hospitals may deny or not renew specialty privileges when the physician is not Board-eligible or Board-certified in that specialty.[50] Thus, a physician who could not progress from being Board-eligible to Board-certified was not allowed to continue to practice major surgery.[51]

## Consultation

A hospital's governing board has the power to require consultation, even in the case of a specialist, in the interests of high-quality care.[52-54]

## Medical Records

A physician may be deprived of privileges if he fails to complete medical records adequately and promptly.[29,42] Failure to compile medical histories has been found to be reasonable grounds for suspension or revocation, but so have other, lesser inadequacies in chart keeping.[43]

## Status in Other Hospitals

A hospital can consider the reasons and evidence upon which an action taken by another hospital was based, but must make the decision itself and not delegate the authority to do so. The court has held that rejection by another hospital does not constitute a substantial reason for denial and that a board's action would, thus, be arbitrary if that were the only basis for rejection.

## Malpractice History

A hospital can also require a physician applying for a staff position to list all malpractice claims, settlements, and judgments involving the applicant and a description of the facts surrounding each incident. A physician is not automatically guilty of malpractice simply because a claim, even a successful one, has been made against him or her. But it is only reasonable that a hospital will require information about applicants' claims history in determining whether they are suitable for medical staff membership.[59] Confirmation must be sought from the carrier.

## Malpractice Insurance as a Condition for Staff Appointment

Judicial decisions have specifically upheld the hospital's right to require malpractice insurance as reasonably related to the operating of the hospital, particularly in order to maintain the fiscal integrity of the hospital.[59]

Since the hospital is likely to be sued along with the physician in instances where the incident giving rise to the complaint occurred wholly or partly within the hospital, the hospital will be at both a tactical and a real disadvantage if it has insurance coverage and its codefendant physician does not. Therefore, the physician cannot complain if the hospital sets a policy requiring each member of the medical staff to have malpractice insurance coverage as a condition of appointment and continued practice in the hospital and requiring evidence of such insurance coverage to be submitted yearly, with rejection of any application or reapplication in support of which such evidence is not forthcoming.

Attending physicians must realize that a hospital board of trustees is exposing the institution and its members to great peril if it does not adopt a policy position; obviously, this could be legal and economic suicide. Therefore, a hospital has the legal right to insist on such a requirement and should take some action, because both the hospital and members of its medical staff have a legitimate business interest and need to know the malpractice insurance status of everyone practicing in the hospital.

### Dedication, Reliability, Responsibility and Loyalty

The hospital must constantly monitor the less tangible qualities, such as dedication and reliability, of each attending staff member as they affect his or her relationship with the hospital. The hospital must also make certain that the physician is responsible, dedicated, and loyal to the patients, professionally ethical and moral, and of good reputation.

### Law Abidance

As part of the initial or renewal appointment process, it is legally permissible, as well as professionally appropriate, for the hospital to make a number of inquires about the physician's current professional standing. Questions may include the physician's Drug Enforcement Agency (DEA) status, whether any disciplinary proceedings have been instituted by a medical society, or whether the physician's staff status at other hospitals has been or is in process of being changed as a result of disciplinary action at the time when the application for appointment is made.

Hospitals should not only seek permission from the physician to obtain or verify this information, but can and should make this permission a condition for privileges.

### Ability to Work with Others: Disruptive versus Controversial

One of the conditions for medical staff appointment can be a commitment on the part of the applicant to work with others in ensuring that the best interests of the patients take precedence over all other concerns. This means that each applicant can be asked to demonstrate a willingness to work with others and an ability to get along in an institutional setting. Physicians are required to get along well with their colleagues—the institution-based physicians and nurses and their associates and affiliates.

With the present complexity of hospital care and with the growing involvement between physicians and other hospital personnel and between different specialists in the care of the same patients, the ability of a medical staff applicant to work harmoniously with other staff physicians and with hospital personnel has become an important criterion that has gained increasing judicial recognition. A series of cases have contributed to defining what constitutes a "personality problem," i.e., the nature of a person who is incompatible with and cannot get on with colleagues and associates or even with patients.[59]

However, the California Supreme Court[30] held that mere adverse personality was not a sufficient basis to deny appointment. Being "controversial" cannot be equated with being "disruptive." On the other hand, in the relationship with the institution staff physician, the person under scrutiny must not be "disruptive."

What constitutes a disruptive physician? What sort of people are these? Most often they have personality, character, or behavior problems. A catalogue of the descriptive terms accepted by the courts to describe such a physician include: argumentative, insulting, rude, vulgar, demoralizing, unavailable, uncooperative, unreasonable, intimidating, antagonistic, harassing, inconsiderate, and thoughtless to fellow workers and/or patients. However, this does not include physicians who are merely eccentric or controversial. A physician's medical staff appointment cannot be rejected or repealed because the applicant is considered outspoken, abrasive, hypercritical, or otherwise personally offensive by some of his colleagues. The decision must not be based on whether he is liked or unpopular, but on whether or not he is a troublemaker.

There should be a provision in the medical staff bylaws defining the disruptive physician; difficulties may ensue if action is instituted and the description in the bylaws is vague and ambiguous, and gives the appearance of being arbitrary and capricious. The proper terminology prescribed by the courts to avoid this pitfall has been detailed.

Courts have upheld boards of trustees when they have terminated the contracts of disruptive, and not only of incompetent, physicians. The rationale here is that upsetting normal hospital function is not conducive to optimum patient care, which it is the board's responsibility to maintain. The hospital is no longer solely the physician's workshop; the physician and the hospital share in the care of the patient.

Denials of privileges or suspension have been upheld for:

1. Intentionally making deceptive or misleading entries on a patient's chart, giving false explanations of professional conduct, and providing inadequate care and medical supervision of a critically ill patient;[39]

2. Screaming and swearing, publicly insulting other medical staff members and surreptitiously examining hospital charts of other doctors, and quarreling with hospital guests.[60]

## Good in Every Way

In order for the physician to maintain hospital staff privileges, he is now required to be "good in every way every day." The institution and the physician must remember that as far as the patient is concerned, the physician now functions on a share-and-share-alike basis with the hospital staff. The hospital staff includes the employed physicians, trainees, and nurses, all of whom are charged legally with being health care providers in their own right. The attending physician must keep in mind that the health care facility is under a legal duty of "corporate responsibility and liability" not only to select medical staff properly, but also to their performance continuously. Once the patient enters the hospital, responsibility extends beyond the provision of room, board, and equipment. It is a total care responsibility shared by the hospital and the attending physician. The requirement that the physician to be "good" everywhere extends to his or her own office.

## Time and Time Again

It should be noted that the same situation exists when a physician is reappointed to the staff; reappointment should occur annually (or at an even shorter interval). At the expiration of one term of appointment and prior to reappointment, the physician is in precisely the same legal position as at the time of the original application for staff appointment—an applicant for reappointment. It is entirely appropriate to ask for disclosure of any changes in status relating to the information given at the time of application since appointment or the last reappointment. There should be no current or past adverse action brought by another institution or by a professional society of the licensing board. The physician must be law-abiding. An applicant can be required to disclose any action that may have been taken by a state licensing authority, professional society, or medical care facility to suspend, limit, or revoke the applicant's license, membership, or clinical privileges.[33,37]

## Epilogue

Regarding the physician, the courts have recognized that a physician without hospital staff privileges is like a fish out of water. The granting of a physician's hospital privileges creates a situation in which each party, hospital and physician, has its legal duties and responsibilities toward the other.

## References


5. *Joiner v Mitchell County Hospital Authority*, 125 Ga App 1, 2 186 SE 2d 307, 308 (1971), aff'd 229 Ga 140, 189 SE 2d 412 (1972)

29. *Rao v Aubern General Hospital*, 10 Wash App 361, 517 P 2d 240 (1973)

30. *Miller v Eisenhower Medical Center*, 27 Cal 3d 614, 614 P 2d 258, 166 Cal Rptr 826 (1980)

33. *Woodard v Porter Hospital*, 125 Vt419, 217 A 2d 37 (1966); *Hagan v Osteopathic General Hospital*, 102 R1 717, 232 A 2d 596 (1967); *Khan v Suburban Hospital*, 45 Ohio St 2d 39, 340 NE 2d 398 (1976); *Bricker v Sceva Speare Memorial Hospital*, 11 NH 276, 281 A 2d 589 (1971); *Hawkins v Kinsie*, 540 P 2d 345 (Colo App 1975); *McElhinney v William Booth Memorial Hospital*, 544 SW 2d 216 (Ky 1977); *Ascherman v St Francis Memorial Hospital*, 45 Cal App 3d 507, 119 Cal Rptr 507; *Storrs v Lutheran Hospitals of America*, 609 P 2d 24 (Alaska, 1980)

37. *Ascherman v San Francisco Medical Society*, 497 P 2d 564; 30 Cal App 3d 623, 114 Cal Rptr 681 (1974); *Ascherman v St Francis Memorial Hospital*, 119 Cal Rptr 507 (Cal App, 1975); *Foster v Mobile County Hospital Board*, 398 F 2d 227 (CA 5, 1968); *Milford v People's Community Hospital Authority*, 380 Mich 49, 155 NW 3d 835 (1968); *Falcone v Middlesex County Medical Society*, 170 A 2d 791 (NJ, 1961); *Ware v Benedikt*, 225 Ark 185, 280 SW 2d 234 (1955); *Hamilton County Hospital v Andrews*, 227 Ind 217, 84 NE 2d 469 (1949)

39. *Koelling v Skiff Memorial Hospital*, 259 Iowa 1185, 146 NW 2d 284 (1966)

40. *Klinge v Lutheran Hospital*, 383 F Supp 287 (D Mo, 1974), modified 523 F 2d 56 (CA 8, 1975); *Citta v Delaware Valley Hospital*, 313 F Supp 301 (ED Pa, 1970); *Duby v Baron*, 369 Mass 614, 314 NE 2d 870 (1976)

41. *Yeargin v Hamilton Memorial Hospital*, 229 Cal 870, 195 SE 2d 8 (1972)

42. *Memorial Hospital v Pratt*, 72 Wyo 120, 262 P 2d 682 (1953); *Armstrong v Fayette County General Hospital*, 553 SE 2d 77; certification denied July 5, 1977 (TN, 1977); *Peterson v Tucson Memorial Hospital*, 559 P 2d 186 (Ariz App, 1976)

43. *Ezekeal v Wenkley*, 2 U Cal 3d 267, 142 Cal Rptr 418, 372 P 2d 32 (1977)

45. *Cypress v Newport New General and Hospital Association*, 357 F 2d 648 (CA 4, 1967); *Eaton v Grubbs*, 329 F 2d 710 (CA 4, 1964); *Citta v Delaware Valley Hospital*, 313 F Supp 301 (CA 4, 1970); *Sussman v Overlook Hospital Association*, 231 A 2d 389 (NJ Super, 1967)

46. *Galvin v Rhode Island Hospital*, 12 RI1 411 (1879); *Ferguson v Gonyaw*, 64 Mich App 685, 236, NW 2d 543, 550 (1975); *Boos v O'Donnell*, 421 P 2d 644 (Okla 1966)

47. *Stripling v Jalley*, 253 SW 2d 516 (Mo 1952)

48. *McCray Memorial Hsopital v Hall*, 266 NE 2d 15 (Ind App 1976); *Porter Memorial Hospital v Harvey*, 279 NE 2d 583 (Ind App 1972)

49. *Armstrong v Board of Directors of Fayette County General Hospital*, 553 ISW 2d 77 (Tenn App 1976)

50. *McCray Memorial Hospital v Hall*, 226 NE 2d 15 (Ind App 1976); *Porter Memorial Hospital v Harvey*, 279 NE 2d 583 (Ind App 1972); *Martino v Concord Community Hospital District*, 43 Cal Rptr 255 (Cal App, 1965)

51. *Kahn v Suburban Community Hospital*, 34 NE 2d 298 (Ohio, 1976)

52. *State ex rel, Bronaugh v City of Parkersburg*, 136 SE 2d 783 (W Va. 1964)

53. *Wyatt v Tahoe Forest Hospital District*, 345 P 2d 93 (Cal App 1959)

54. *Schooler v Navarro County Memorial Hospital*, 375 F Supp 841 (ND Tex, 1973)

55. *Foster v Mobile County Hospital Board*, 398 F 2d 227 (5th Cir. 1968)

56. *Klinge v Lutheran Hospital*, 383 F Supp 287 (D Mo, 1974), modified 523 F 2d 56 (CA 8, 1975); *Citta v Delaware Valley Hospital*, 313 F Supp 301 (ED, Pa, 1970); *Duby v Baron*, 369 Mass 614, 314 NE 2d 870 (1976)

57. *Sosa v Board of Managers of Val Verde Memorial Hospital*, 437 F 2d 173 (CA 5, 1971)

58. *Sams v Ohio General Hospital Association*, 413 F 2d 826 (CA 4, 1969)

59. *Huffaker v Bailey*, 540 P 2d 1398 (Or, 1975); *Theussin v Watonga Municipal Hospital Board*, 550 P 2d 938 (Okla 1976)

60. *Anderson v Board of Trustees*, 10 Mich App 348, 159 NW 2d 347 (1968)

# Delineating Clinical Privileges

William F. Jessee, MD

Delineation of clinical privileges is a critical component of a hospital's quality assurance (QA) program. Unlike credentials verification, which is intended to assure that everyone granted medical staff membership or clinical privileges meets certain minimum criteria, privilege delineation is designed to develop a "job description" for each practitioner. This "job description" specifies the services he or she may provide within the institution. Because this determination is based on the individual practitioner's practice, training, and experience, rarely do any two individuals in a particular institution have exactly the same privileges.

The importance of the privilege delineation process is indicated by the Joint Commission on Accreditation of Hospitals' standards for hospital accreditation and by relevant case law. Standard MS.4 of the *Accreditation Manual for Hospitals (AMH)*[1] addresses privilege delineation and contains a number of important requirements. One of these is that the privilege delineation process should not be applied only to members of the medical staff; all individuals permitted by law and by the hospital to provide patient care services independently must have delineated clinical privileges (Required Characteristic MS.4.1). For example, if state law and a hospital's rules permit dentists, podiatrists, clinical psychologists, or nurse

Vice President for Education, Joint Commission on Accreditation of Hospitals, 875 North Michigan Avenue, Chicago, Illinois 60611; 312/642-6061
Reprinted by permission of QRB, June, 1987, Page 209. Copyright JCAHO

| Table 1. Categorical Designations for Pediatric Privileges | |
|---|---|
| **Category I** | The treatment of illnesses, injuries, or conditions, or the performance of procedures that have low risk for the patient (eg, routine newborn care and treatment of uncomplicated pneumonia).<br><br>*Criterion:*<br>Reasonable experience in care of these conditions. Pediatrics residency training and/or other specialty training not required. |
| **Category II** | The treatment of major illnesses, injuries, or conditions, or the performance of procedures posing no significant risk to life (eg, the treatment of undiagnosed anemia; status asthmaticus; routine preoperative and postoperative care of pediatric patients;lumbar puncture; and arterial blood gases, except in newborns).<br><br>*Criterion:*<br>Significant training or experience in pediatrics. Board certification not necessary. |
| **Category III** | The treatment of major illnesses, injuries, or conditions, or the performance of procedures that carry substantial threat to life (eg, treatment of meningitis, drug overdose, erythroblastosis fetalis, or neonatal resuscitation).<br><br>*Criterion:*<br>Board certification in pediatrics: or completion of three years of residency training in pediatrics (acceptable in lieu of certification only for up to five years after training is completed); or other extensive training and experience in the care of these conditions. |
| **Category IV** | The treatment of unusually complex or critical illnesses, injuries, or conditions, or the performance of procedures that carry a serious threat to life (eg, treatment of leukemia or respiratory failure, neonatal intensive care, and renal dialysis).<br><br>*Criterion:*<br>Extensive relevant subspecialty training or experience beyond board certification in pediatrics. |

midwives to provide patient care independently, then all practitioners in any of these disciplines must also have individually delineated clinical privileges. This is true even when these practitioners are not members of the medical staff. However, any individual granted the privilege to admit patients for inpatient treatment *must* be a member of the medical staff (Required Characteristic MS.4.3.1).

Regardless of the approach to evaluating applications for privileges, the process and criteria used must be applied uniformly to all applicants. Joint Commission standards specify that the same level of quality must be assured "within medical staff departments, across departments or services, and between members and nonmembers of the staff who have delineated clinical privileges" (Required Characteristic MS.3.11). This requirement is intended to assure that a patient seeking a particular service from a hospital receives a consistent level of quality care from all practitioners providing the service, irrespective of the practitioners' medical specialties or professional disciplines. This minimal guarantee to the public is not only an accreditation requirement and a legal standard; it is also part of the institution's responsibility to the patients it serves.

## Alternative Approaches

Institutions should carefully consider their approach to the process of granting clinical privileges. A variety of approaches to privilege delineation have been developed, including

- delineation by practitioner specialty;
- delineation by patient risk categories;
- delineation using lists of procedures; and
- approaches combining the previous three methods, particularly combinations of the categorical and procedure list approaches.

The following discussion outlines the strengths and weaknesses of each of these privilege delineation methods.

*Specialty-based approach.* According to this approach, individuals who have completed specialty training are presumed to be qualified to perform all diagnostic and therapeutic activities within the scope of their specialty. Generally, certification or eligibility for certification by the relevant specialty board provides the basis for privilege delineation by specialty.

While simple in concept, the specialty-based approach has a number of practical difficulties. First, careful definition of the scope of each medical specialty is required. Second, diagnoses and procedures that fall within the scope of several different specialists will invariably be identified. For

| Table 2. Procedure List for Plastic and Reconstructive Surgery | |
| --- | --- |
| **Plastic Surgery** | _____ Split- or full-thickness skin grafts, ear, in staged reconstruction |
| *Cleft lip and palate repair* | _____ Otoplasty |
| _____ Lip adhesions | _____ Other, specify: |
| _____ Primary left lip repair, unilateral | *Eyelid reconstruction* |
| _____ Secondary cleft lip repair, bilateral, one stage | _____ Ptosis repair, levator shortening |
| _____ Primary cleft lip repair, two stages | _____ Ptosis repair, sling method |
| _____ Secondary cleft lip repair, two stages | _____ Coloboma repair |
| _____ Cleft palate repair, one stage | _____ Major eyelid reconstruction, post-trauma or tumor |
| _____ Primary cleft palate repair, two stages | _____ Tear duct repair, primary or secondary |
| _____ Primary fistula repair | _____ Dacryocystorhinostomy |
| _____ Pharyngeal flap or pharyngoplasty | _____ Ectropion repair |
| _____ Pushback, or secondary palatal lengthening | _____ Entropion repair |
| _____ Pharyngeal implant or graft | _____ Tarsorrhaphy or canthoplasty |
| _____ Cross-lip flap | _____ Other, specify: |
| _____ Cleft lip nasal repair | *Neck reconstruction* |
| _____ Tongue flap, palate | _____ Thyroglossal duct cyst or sinus excision |
| _____ Columella lengthening | _____ Branchial cleft cyst or sinus excision |
| _____ Repair of lateral or oblique facial cleft | _____ Torticollis correction |
| _____ Other, specify: | _____ Other, specify: |
| *Ear reconstruction* | *Genitourinary tract reconstruction* |
| _____ Repositioning or revision, auricluar remnants | _____ Hypospadias repair, one stage |
| _____ Costal cartilage graft, ear, autogenous | _____ Hypospadias repair, two stages |
| _____ Banked cartilage or allograft, ear | |

| Table 2. Procedure List for Plastic and Reconstructive Surgery (Cont'd.) | |
|---|---|
| _____ Epispadias repair<br>_____ Exstrophy of the bladder repair<br>_____ Vaginal reconstruction for absence of vagina<br>_____ Phalloplasty<br>_____ Clitoriplasty, vaginoplasty (pseudohermaphroditism)<br>_____ Dermis graft for Peyronie's disease<br>_____ Major trauma repair, including skin grafts<br>_____ Insertion of prosthesis<br>_____ Phalloplasty<br>_____ Neocolporrhaphy<br>_____ Vulvectomy<br>_____ Other, specify:<br><br>_Soft tissue repair_<br>_____ Major facial laceratons<br>_____ Major scar or keloid<br>_____ Z-plasty, W-plasty<br>_____ Delays or transfers of distant flaps<br>_____ Dermabrasion (for scars due to acne, trauma, and so forth<br>Flaps:<br>_____ Random cutaneous flap<br>_____ Composite flaps<br>_____ Free flaps (microvascular repair)<br>_____ Myocutaneous flaps<br>_____ Other, specify<br>_Grafts_<br>_____ Skin (split or full thickness, excluding burns)<br>_____ Bone | _____ Cartilage<br>_____ Fascia<br>_____ Dermis<br>_____ Composite<br>_____ Synthetic material<br>_____ Muscle<br>_____ Other, specify:<br>_Burn repair_<br>Immediate treatment prior to grafting:<br>_____ Thermal<br>_____ Chemical<br>_____ Electrical<br>_____ Escharectomy or major debridement<br>_Skin grafting:_<br>_____ Thermal<br>_____ Chemical<br>_____ Electrical<br>_____ Late reconstruction<br>_____ Other, specify:<br>_Pressure ulcer repair_<br>_____ Sacral<br>_____ Ischial<br>_____ Trochanteric<br>_____ Other, specify:<br>_Facial fracture repair and immobilization_<br>Facial fractures:<br>_____ Closed reduction<br>_____ Open reduction and/or fixation<br>Mandibular fractures:<br>_____ Closed reduction and interdental wiring |

### Table 2. Procedure List for Plastic and Reconstructive Surgery (Cont'd.)

_____ Open reduction, with or without interdental wiring

Zygomatic complex frature:
_____ Closed reduction
_____ Open reduction and/or fixation

Maxillary fracture:
_____ Closed reduction and interdental wiring
_____ Open reduction with or without interdental wiring

Orbital floor or rim fracture:
_____ Closed reduction
_____ Open reduction and/or fixation or graft
_____ Other, specify:

*Facial nerve palsy correction*
_____ Nerve repair
_____ Nerve graft
_____ Muscle transfer or graft
_____ Fascia or tendon sling
_____ Other, specify:

*Hand surgery*
_____ Major skin coverage flap or graft, not to include burns
_____ Primary or secondary tendon repair
_____ Primary or secondary nerve repair
_____ Tendon graft
_____ Tendon transfer
_____ Implantation of Silastic rod

_____ Nerve graft
_____ Tenolysis
_____ Neurolysis
_____ Palmer or digital fasciectomy
_____ Pollicization or digital transposition
_____ Island pedicle grafts
_____ Osteotomy
_____ Bone grafting
_____ Arthrodesis
_____ Tenodesis
_____ Arthroplasty with or without prosthesis
_____ Amputation
_____ Fingertip injuries
_____ Fractures
_____ Local flaps or grafts
_____ Syndactyly repair
_____ Polydactyly correction
_____ Macrodactyly correction
_____ Club hand correction
_____ Pollicization, digit
_____ Microvascular replantation
_____ Other, specify:

*Lower extremity reconstruction*
_____ Excision or debridement, ulcer and skin graft
_____ Free flap repair
_____ Muscle flap
_____ Cross-leg flap
_____ Other, specify:

**Aesthetic and Reconstructive Surgery**
*Facial reconstruction*
_____ Face-lift

| Table 2. Procedure List for Plastic and Reconstructive Surgery (Cont'd.) | |
|---|---|
| _____ Brow lift<br>_____ Chemical peel or dermabrasion<br>_____ Biepharoplasty<br>_____ Rhinoplasty<br>_____ Partial nasal reconstruction<br>_____ Complete nasal reconstruction<br>_____ Septoplasty or septectomy<br>_____ Chin implant<br>_____ Otoplasty<br>_____ Hair transplants<br>_____ Other, specify:<br>*Maxillofacial reconstrutive surgery*<br>_____ Mandibular repositioning for prognathism<br>_____ Mandibular repositioning for micrognathism<br>_____ Maxillary osteotomy<br>_____ Major craniofacial reconstruction<br>_____ Other, specify:<br>*Breast reconstruction*<br>_____ Reduction mammaplasty<br>_____ Augmentation mammaplasty<br>_____ Mastopexy<br>_____ Subcutaneous mastectomy<br>_____ Subcutaneous mastectomy for gynecomastia<br>_____ Release of capsular contraction after augmentation mammaplasty | _____ Breast biopsy<br>_____ Mastectomy and reconstruction<br>_____ Staged breast reconstruction<br>_____ Other, specify:<br>*Body contouring*<br>_____ Abdominal dermolipectomy<br>_____ Arm, thigh, or buttock dermolipectomy<br>_____ Liposuction procedures<br>_____ Other, specify<br>**Benign and Malignant Tumors**<br>*Soft tissue tumor excision*<br>_____ Lymphangioma<br>_____ Hemangioma<br>_____ Neurofibroma<br>_____ Pigmented nevi<br>_____ Cysts<br>_____ Lipomata<br>_____ Other specify:<br>*Skin malignancy excision*<br>Basal cell carcinoma:<br>_____ Primary repair<br>_____ Flap or graft<br>Squamous cell carcinoma:<br>_____ Primary repair<br>_____ Flap or graft<br>_____ Malignant melanoma<br>_____ Lymph node dissecton<br>_____ Inguinal node dissection<br>_____ Other, specify: |

example, gastrointestinal endoscopic procedures are often performed both by physicians with training in gastroenterology and by general surgeons. In such a situation, the institution must assure that all individuals performing the procedure provide the same level of quality care. Those granting privileges must also keep in mind that the extent of training received may differ from one individual to another, even within the same specialty, and that not all board-certified specialists have achieved the same level of competence in all areas of their specialty. Specialty training programs vary in regard to the types of patients physicians are trained to treat and the types of procedures physicians are trained to perform. In addition, individual physicians often limit the scope of their practice voluntarily over the course of time, so that they may no longer maintain current competence in all areas of their specialty.

Finally, many hospitals have become entangled in the issue of board eligibility. Physicians who have completed residency training become "board eligible"—that is, eligible to take the board certification exam. In some instances, however, physicians who have failed the test several times may continue to call themselves "board eligible" without receiving additional training. Thus, if a hospital wishes to stress the importance of certification (ie, passing the exam), the time in which eligibility serves as a criterion for privileges should be limited to a certain number of years following completion of residency training (see, for example, the criterion under Category III in Table 1). If the applicant is unable to achieve board certification within that period, then he or she may no longer be eligible for the same level of privileges in the institution.

*Categorical delineation.* Another approach to delineating privileges, often used in the so-called "cognitive" specialties such as internal medicine and pediatrics, is delineation by categories of patient risk. Figure 1 illustrates a categorical approach to delineation of privileges in pediatrics. Patients are classified according to both their individual risk (eg, age, nutritional status) and severity of illness. A practitioner's degree of training and/or experience determines the category of patients for which he or she receives privileges. This approach has the advantage of closely tying patient needs to the training of the practitioner, but is limited in that it requires specific definition of the types of patients in each category who may be treated, a process which leaves considerable room for disagreement. Also, because the assessment of the patient's risk factors of severity of illness allows for a substantial degree of interpretation, it may be difficult to determine whether or not practitioners[5] are practicing within the scope of privileges granted. Nonetheless this is a very popular approach to privilege delineation and is widely used in many U.S. hospitals.

*Procedure lists.* Using procedure lists to delineate privileges is most popular in surgical specialties. This approach permits the greatest degree of specificity both in delineating privileges and in assuring that the privileges accorded are not exceeded. Such lists are both comprehensive and easy to enforce, although the medical staff may view them as burdensome because of their lengthiness. Difficulties often arise in determining the level of detail that should be used in a list. Also, to assure that a list includes all significant procedures being performed, it must be reviewed and updated constantly.

Table 2 shows a procedure list for one surgical subspecialty. Some efforts have been made to use similar lists for internal medicine and other cognitive specialties by listing the illnesses, injuries, or conditions that may be treated. However, this approach is extremely cumbersome and has proved less viable in these specialties; it has generally been discarded in favor of a categorical or specialty-based approach.

*Combinations.* Many institutions are adopting an approach to privilege delineation that combines both the categorical and procedure list methods. Table 3 contains one example of an application for privileges—again applied to pediatrics—based on the combined approach. As Table 3 indicates, this technique permits the general delineation of privileges by categories, but also allows selected high-volume or high-risk procedures to be specifically delineated based on the practitioner's training or experience. In contrast to other methods, this approach provides a balance between the need for flexibility and the need for specificity, particularly when applied to nonsurgical specialties.

## Use of Criteria

No matter which approach is taken to privilege delineation, it is essential to apply professionally developed criteria specifying practitioners' education, training, and experience along with evidence of their current competence (such as number of procedures performed and results). As specified in medical staff Required Characteristic MS.4.2.2 in the *AMH*, such criteria must be developed, specified in the medical staff bylaws, and applied uniformly to all applicants. The criteria should be as detailed and as specific as possible in order to maximize the uniformity of their application and to minimize the exposure of the institution and its medical staff members to potential liability.

Many national specialty societies are developing criteria for granting specific clinical privileges. The American Society for Gastrointestinal Endoscopy, for example, has developed criteria that specify the training and experience necessary for physicians who are granted privileges to perform gastrointestinal endoscopy.[2] In addition, the American College of Physicians is now developing criteria for granting privileges in the various subspecialty areas of internal medicine.[3] Once finalized, these criteria should be valuable in helping hospitals determine privileging requirements for various practice areas.

## Common Problems in Privilege Delineation

Institutions often encounter difficulty with the privilege delineation process. In fact, privilege delineation is one of the standards areas generating frequent contingencies in the Joint Commission survey process.

*Granting privileges for new procedures.* One problem area concerns the granting of privileges for new procedures or technologies. Chemonucleolysis, flexible endoscopy, and various applications of medical lasers are all examples of relatively new technologies that have generated many practical privilege delineation problems. In anticipation of practitioners' tendency to adopt such technologies, hospitals should, as early as possible, begin to develop criteria for determining who will be granted privileges created by new technologies.

To avoid potential privileging problems resulting from new technologies, hospitals may choose to develop their own training courses for performing a new procedure; such courses could be taught by an in-house or visiting expert. Those completing the course successfully could then be granted the privilege to perform the new procedure. Unfortunately, this solution is not practical for many rural hospitals or for smaller institutions that perform a particular procedure relatively infrequently. Alternative options for criteria may include requiring the practitioner to complete an appropriate continuing education course or to undergo a period of supervised practice under the auspices of a recognized training institution or individual. In any event, it is crucial that such criteria be developed early, before the procedure is performed with any frequency within the institution. In addition, it is vital that these criteria be applied uniformly to all individuals seeking the particular privilege.

*Monitoring compliance with privileges.* A second major difficulty in the privilege delineation process is monitoring compliance with privileges. As specified in Required Characteristic MS.4.1.3 in the *AMH*, there must be mechanisms in the institution to insure that all practitioners provide services within the scope of their privileges. For surgical specialties, this standard is often enforced through the use of privilege cards kept in operating suites, which are checked as each surgical procedure is scheduled. For cognitive specialties, a retrospective review process may be more appropriate, since risk factors and severity of illness in these specialties often cannot be evaluated precisely upon hospitalization. This review, which should be incorporated into each clinical department's quality review activities, is a way of assuring that each individual's practice remains within the scope of delineated clinical privileges. The results of this review are particularly important for the privilege renewal process, which will be discussed later in greater detail.

*Territorial issues.* The issue of "turf" is a sensitive aspect of the privilege delineation process. Procedures that may be performed by members of several different departments, such as flexible gastrointestinal endoscopy, have created serious tensions in some institutions. When departments involved cannot agree on criteria for a certain privilege, the medical staff's executive committee is asked to resolve the differences. In such cases it is most important that one set of criteria be established and applied consistently to all individuals performing the procedure, regardless of whether they are internists, surgeons, or non-physician independent practitioners. When the executive committee feels unable to resolve differences among departments, it may wish to consult an expert from outside the institution. Since he or she has no economic interest in the medical practices in the community, the outside consultant can often provide the unbiased expertise necessary to resolve these difficult issues.


## Renewal of Privileges

Regardless of the mechanisms used for delineating clinical privileges, each practitioner's performance must be comprehensively reviewed and reappraised at least every two years. When considering requests for renewed and additional privileges, careful scrutiny should be given to how the applicant has exercised current privileges. Information concerning the applicant's license, health status, liability experience, and other appropriate qualifications determined by the medical staff should, of course, be taken into account. The most important part of the reappraisal process, however, is a comprehensive reevaluation of each individual's performance, judgment, and clinical/technical skills.

To perform this assessment, hospitals must have a mechanism for gathering ongoing data from various departmental QA activities and medical staff monitoring functions (eg, blood usage review, drug usage evaluation, medical records review, and surgical case review). Information on practitioners' compliance with privileges granted and the extent of their practice during the current period should also be compiled. These data can then

**Table 3. Categorical/Procedural Delineation of Pediatric Privileges**

**Categories:**

*Category I* Privileges in this category allow the physician to diagnose and treat uncomplicated diseases where there is no apparent threat to life.
*Criterion:*
Physicians with limited training and experience in pediatrics.

*Category II* Privileges in this category allow the physician to diagnose and treat more complex or severe pediatric diseases.
*Criterion:*
Physicians with extensive experience and/or training in general pediatrics.

*Category III* Privileges in this category allow physicians with certain areas of expertise to diagnose and treat diseases in one or more of the following indicated areas:
________ Neonatology
________ Cardiology
________ Endocrinology
________ Allergy
________ Pulmonary medicine
________ Infectious diseases
*Criterion:*
Physicians with subspecialty training or similar experience in the indicated area.

**Procedures:**

Procedures requested below may require documentation of training and experience.

*I. Neonatal Care Privileges*
________ Class A: Normal care of newborn infants weighing more than 2,000 grams.
________ Class B: Normal care of newborn infants weighing less than 2,000 grams.
________ Class C: Care of preterm, low-birth-weight infants with non-life-threatening illnesses.
________ Class D: Care of all newborn infants, including those with potentially life-threatening illnesses.

---

**Table 3—continued**

*II. Minor Surgical Procedures*
________ Exchange transfusion
________ Peripheral venous cutdowns
________ Umbilical vessel catheterization
________ Intubation
________ Insertion of chest tube for treatment of pneumothorax
________ Other: ____________________________________

(Note: General surgical procedures, such as nevi excision, laceration repair, and drainage of superficial abscesses, are permitted for all individuals with privileges in procedure group I or higher.)

*III. Diagnostic Procedures*
________ Bladder taps
________ Lumbar punctures
________ Laryngoscopy
________ Peripheral arterial puncture
________ Abdominal paracentesis
________ Thoracentesis
________ Bone marrow aspiration
________ Other: ____________________________________

---

be used to develop physician-specific performance profiles that may be reviewed at the time of reappraisal.

Determining the extent to which delineated privileges are actually used is a difficult but important aspect of the renewal process. Clearly, a skill not often used is not maintained. The literature has adequately demonstrated that surgical mortality and morbidity are inversely related to the volume of procedures performed.[4,5] Institutions should therefore carefully consider whether or not to renew a practitioner's privileges to conduct a procedure that he or she has not performed during the previous one- or two-year period. However it must also be recognized that there may be procedures that a practitioner would not be expected to perform regularly (ie, Whipple procedure, esophagectomy, and so forth).

Compliance with the privileges granted is also an important factor to be considered in the renewal process. If an individual has consistently exceeded the privileges granted, disciplinary action or closer monitoring of future performance may be justified. Identification of a practitioner's potential problem areas may be facilitated through the review of patient care outcome data. Such review leads to more careful monitoring of performance and provides constructive feedback for the practitioner. If performance continues to be less favorable than expected, modification of privileges may then be appropriate.

Any request for privileges to perform new procedures should be considered scrupulously at the time of renewal. Evaluation of such requests should be based on the same criteria used for an initial request for privileges and on a careful and appropriate assessment of the applicant's training and skills.

When conducting the periodic performance reappraisal, it may sometimes be helpful to request information from other hospitals. Physicians often practice in multiple institutions, particularly in urban areas. While a hospital may not be able to adequately assess a practitioner based only on performance within that hospital, the aggregate of information from other institutions may permit a more well-founded judgment. Hospitals should not hesitate to seek such information from other institutions in order to make a comprehensive evaluation of performance. When renewing clinical privileges, one cannot assume that "no news is good news"; rather, a concerted effort must be made to obtain detailed information on the clinical judgment and skills of each individual before privileges are renewed.

## Conclusions

The process of clinical privilege delineation is essential to assuring quality care and for minimizing the liability exposure of an institution and its staff. Although many different methods of delineating privileges may be employed, the key to effective privilege delineation is that specific written criteria be applied uniformly to all individuals. Whenever doubt exists as to an individual's training and experience, it is appropriate to seek additional information, both from within and outside the institution. When disputes arise among members of the medical staff regarding qualifications or training, use of outside experts can often avoid potential antitrust problems while maximizing the effectiveness of efforts to assure high-quality care for all patients.

## References

1. Joint Commission on Accreditation of Hospitals: *Accreditation Manual for Hospitals,* 1987 ed. Chicago: Joint Commission, 1986, pp 108-112.
2. American Society for Gastrointestinal Endoscopy (ASGE): *Appropri-*

*ate Use of Gastrointestinal Endoscopy, Consensus Statement.* Manchester, Mass: ASGE, 1986.

3. ACP clinical guidelines may help with credentialing. *Medical Staff News* 15:2, Nov 1986.

4. Luft HS, Bunker J, Enthoven A: Should operations be regionalized? The empirical relation between surgical volume and mortality. *N Engl J Med:* 301:1364-1369, Dec 20, 1979.

5. Showstack JA, et al: Association of volume with outcome of coronary artery bypass graft surgery: Scheduled versus non-scheduled operations. *JAMA:* 257:785-789, Feb 13, 1987.

# Legal Analysis
## *Romaguera* Refrain: Staff Privileges and Exclusive Hospital Contracts

David Kalifon, MD, JD

In this article, the author analyzes the approach taken in three recent Florida cases dealing with staff privileges and exclusive contracts, discusses their impact on physicians, and recommends that other jurisdictions follow this approach.

## Introduction

It is a common practice for hospitals to grant exclusive management and staffing contracts to such hospital-based physicians as radiologists, pathologists, anesthesiologists, and emergency physicians. When such exclusive contracts are formed, however, problems can arise. By limiting the prior physician contractor's access to equipment, surgical suites, or patients, a new exclusive contract may unilaterally abridge that physician's vested medical staff rights and privileges. In *Hospital Corporation of Lake Worth v. Romaguera*,[1] a Florida District Court of Appeal upheld a medical staff bylaw that permitted "medico-administrative physicians" to continue exercising their staff privileges even after their exclusive contracts were terminated. Two recent trial court cases have refined that holding by adding that such continuing privileges cannot be restricted by limiting access to equipment, facilities, and patient information. This article briefly discusses each of these three cases and analyzes their effect on physicians.

## Exclusivity

Exclusivity is often justified by the following: It assures around-the-clock coverage by competent specialists, permits efficient scheduling, and allows effective administration. Because a hospital wishes to avoid conflict with, and competition from, a prior physician when entering into an exclusive contract with a new physician, the hospital will often insist on inserting in each contract a clause that automatically terminates the contracting physician's medical staff privileges, without medical staff due process rights, on termination of the contract.

## Staff Privileges

The granting of staff privileges forms a contract between the medical staff and the individual physician. Like commercial contracts, the privileges contract may not be abridged without the consent of the contracting parties. Thus, the exclusive hospital-physician contract cannot abridge the medical staff-physician privileges contract without the consent of the medical staff. To comply with the requirement of the Joint Commission on Accreditation of Healthcare Organizations ("JCAHO"), medical staff bylaws must provide due process protections for any physician threatened with restriction, suspension, or revocation of privileges. Unfortunately, however, the JCAHO standards expressly permit bylaws to allow for automatic termination of privileges when a hospital-based physician loses his or her contract with the hospital.[2]

What are staff privileges? To a physician, they are the right to perform certain examinations, evaluations, treatments, and procedures within the hospital. Privileges are delineated in detail—e.g., performing coronary angiography, interpreting smears of bone marrow aspirates, performing coronary bypass surgery, or suturing traumatic wounds of emergency department patients.

The exercise of many privileges requires access to expensive equipment, extensive support personnel, and the flow of patients seeking care at the facility. Such privileges cannot be performed practically or safely outside of the hospital setting. Therefore, a hospital can de facto restrict a physician's privileges by granting an exclusive contract to a new physician, thereby limiting the prior physician's access to the necessary equipment, personnel, and patients. This violates the due process protections provided by medical staff bylaws.[3] When a hospital's board of directors ratifies the granting of privileges by the medical staff, the hospital tacitly agrees— i.e., contracts—to provide the necessary equipment, personnel, and patients to the physician. Once those privileges are granted and exercised, the hospital should not be allowed to unilaterally abridge that agreement.

## The Case Law

### Hospital Corporation of Lake Worth v. Romaguera

Dr. Raul Romaguera had an exclusive, written contract to operate the pathology department at the Hospital Corporation of America facility in Lake Worth, Florida. The contract provided that, upon its termination, Dr. Romaguera would lose all his staff privileges without receiving a hearing or any other procedural rights. Subsequently, the medical staff amended its bylaws to permit contract physicians to exercise their privileges even after termination of their contracts. For economic reasons, the hospital terminated Dr. Romaguera's contract, in accordance with its terms, and granted an exclusive contract to a group of competing pathologists.

After the termination, Dr. Romaguera continued to exercise his privileges at the hospital, in accordance with the revised medical staff bylaws. The hospital responded by withdrawing his intrahospital telephone and withholding billing information on his patients. The hospital also accused him of clinical incompetence because of his decreased workload, an accusation that the trial court later found was not made in good faith.

Dr. Romaguera sued the hospital for tortious interference with his business relationships. The trial court found that the amended bylaws took precedence over the contract terms. It ruled that the hospital had improperly interfered with Dr. Romaguera's privileges, and awarded him $450,000 in compensatory damages. The Florida District Court of Appeal affirmed the decision and the compensatory damage award, but rejected the additional punitive damage award of $5.5 million as excessive and unwarranted.[4]

### Reno v. East Pasco Medical Center, Inc.

In December 1988, a Florida court decided a case in favor of a radiologist who had argued that his privileges were restricted de facto when the hospital granted an exclusive contract to another radiology group.[5] The medical staff did not formally restrict, suspend, or revoke Dr. H. Robert Reno's privileges, and he remained on staff. However, since the exclusive contract directed all of the hospital's radiology business to the new group, Dr. Reno, in practice, could no longer exercise his previously granted privileges.

At trial, the jurors found that the hospital, East Pasco Medical Center, Inc., had violated a provision of its own medical staff bylaws concerning staff privileges and had interfered with Dr. Reno's business relationships. Although awarded $754,000 in compensatory damages by the jury, Dr. Reno subsequently settled for $650,000 and relinquished his staff privileges in order to avoid lengthy appeals.

### *Scheller v. Palm Beach Gardens Community Hospital*

In February 1989, a Florida pathologist, Dr. Zbigniew Scheller, won a case in which he had argued that Palm Beach Gardens Community Hospital had harassed him when he continued to exercise his medical staff privileges after termination of his contract.[6] The hospital's medical staff bylaws were unusual in that they allowed staff physicians to choose their own pathologists. Thus, even after his removal by the hospital from his position as director of pathology, Dr. Scheller—a frequent and vocal critic of the hospital administration—was the designated pathologist of 75% of the medical staff. In his lawsuit, Dr. Scheller argued that the hospital, a subsidiary of American Medical International ("AMI"), had harassed him by withholding access to clinical and billing information and selectively "double billing" patients, thus placing Dr. Scheller at a competitive disadvantage. The jury agreed, finding that AMI had unlawfully interfered with Dr. Scheller's business dealings, and awarded him $99,800 in compensatory damages, plus more than $19 million in punitive damages. Considering the size of AMI, this punitive damage award did not seem excessive, since a smaller monetary award would not have punished the defendant or served as a deterrent to others.

### Analysis

The decisions in *Romaguera*, *Reno*, and *Scheller* support the proposition that hospitals cannot abridge, unilaterally and without the consent of the affected parties, the privileges contracts entered into by a medical staff and its practitioners. *Romaguera* establishes that privileges can continue after termination of an exclusive contract. *Reno* and *Scheller* add teeth to *Romaguera* by adding that the continuing privileges must be truly exercisable and not just a paper grant. Although *Reno* and *Scheller* are trial court decisions without precedential value, they hopefully are accurate predictors of how the Florida District Courts of Appeal will act in future cases.

From the hospital's point of view, the holdings in these three cases create a dilemma: How can a hospital grant an exclusive contract if it is unable to restrict or revoke the privileges of the prior contract holder? The hospital must violate either the prior physician's privileges contract with the medical staff or the new physician's exclusivity. Since either action can result in a damage award against the hospital, the hospital's quest for efficiency seems to be undermined.[7]

This situation raises further questions: Are exclusive contracts really necessary for efficiency? Are the traditional rationales justifying exclusive contracts still relevant? Because of the maldistribution of physicians, increasing numbers of specialists in many markets are vying for relatively fewer contracts to manage and staff hospital services and departments. In these markets, exclusivity is not necessary for efficiency in assuring coverage, scheduling, and administration. Many specialists thirst for additional work opportunities and would willingly work an around-the-clock schedule. Many hospital departments, such as surgery, are traditionally open, yet successfully administered. Moreover, surgery departments are typically able to satisfactorily allocate special equipment and the limited number of operating suites among their physician members.[8]

If a hospital believes granting an exclusive contract is in its best interest, how might it circumvent decisions like *Romaguera*? The hospital might reasonably argue that, if it has no right to abridge the physician-medical staff privileges contract, the medical staff should have no right to promise use of hospital equipment and personnel it neither owns nor controls. Hospitals might notify staff physicians that any implied contractual right to use surgical suites or imaging or other equipment or facilities would end upon conclusion of the current staff appointment. Upon reappointment, rights could be granted directly by the hospital administration, on an exclusive or non-exclusive basis, at its sole discretion. In addition, hospitals might continue pressing for favorable judicial decisions. Although Florida may be pro-physician, most jurisdictions are not. Hospitals are generally viewed as sympathetic parties, trying to serve the public in economically difficult times, while physicians are often viewed unsympathetically as "fat cats," fighting simply to preserve unreasonably high incomes and unwarranted autonomy and control.[9]

All physicians must vigorously resist the curtailment of privileges and waiver of due process rights when *any* exclusive contract terminates, because all physicians are ultimately at risk. The rationale of exclusivity is already being used to eliminate an increasing number of hospital services and departments. Initially, radiology, emergency medicine, anesthesiology, and pathology departments were most likely to be closed. Now, pulmonary and gastroenterology labs, cardiology noninvasive testing, cath labs, and even heart surgery services may be controlled by exclusive contracts. Tomorrow, any and all other hospital services and departments may also be controlled. Moreover, with the establishment of a national data bank to collect information on physicians whose privileges are restricted or revoked because of quality of care issues, and the dissemination of this information to hospitals and medical staffs evaluating new physician applicants, it will be difficult indeed for a physician whose record is blemished in any way to practice in a location or setting of his or her choice. Yet, what better way is there for a hospital to terminate the exclusive contract of a popular physician than to allege that the physician is providing less than adequate quality care? How can the physician exonerate himself or herself without the due process hearing rights provided under the medical staff bylaws?[10]

## Conclusion

The *Romaguera, Reno,* and *Scheller* cases have received widespread attention because of their large damage awards, especially the punitive awards. However, they are also noteworthy because they highlight the way hospitals are undermining the autonomy of practitioners and medical staffs, by seeking to control both the privileges and the rights of contracting physicians and to gradually increase the numbers of physicians under their control. Hopefully, jurisdictions faced with similar cases in the future will understand and agree with the insight provided by the Florida courts in these three cases and will follow their lead in holding hospitals liable for such abuses.

## References


1. 511 So.2d 559 (Fla. Dist. Ct. App. 1986); *see* Legal Analysis, Hospital Corporation of Lake Worth v. Romaguera: *Medical Staff Bylaws Really Mean Something,* MED. STAFF COUNS., Vol. 1, No. 1, Summer 1987, at 64.

2. JOINT COMM'N ON ACCREDITATION OF HOSPS., ACCREDITATION MANUAL FOR HOSPITALS MS.1.2.3.1.14 (1989).

3. In 1985, the American Medical Association's House of Delegates recommended that "medical staff members who have been granted clinical privileges are entitled to full due process in any attempt to abridge those privileges by granting of exclusive contracts by the hospital governing body." 119 Hospital Decision to Grant Exclusive Contracts, A.M.A. House of Delegates 39th Interim Meeting, Dec. 8-11, 1985, at 257.

4. *Romaguera*, 511 So. 2d at 564, 565.
5. Reno v. East Pasco Med. Center, Inc., No. 87-318 (Fla. Cir. Ct. Dec. 14, 1988); *see* Am. Med. News, Feb. 24, 1989, at 13.
6. Scheller v. Palm Beach Gardens Community Hosp. (AMI), No. 80-1650 (Fla. Cir. Ct. Feb. 7, 1989); *see* Am. Med. News, Feb. 24, 1989, at 15.
7. Antitrust law permits exclusive contracts in many medical specialties. However, antitrust law cannot, and does not, permit a hospital to violate a contract between other parties.
8. Perhaps, hospitals are seeking control, as well as efficiency. Hospitals exercise significant economic power over the hospital-based physician, for whom loss of a contract can be an economic catastrophe. Such control makes most medical staffs wary of granting hospital-based physicians voting rights on medical executive committees.
9. In this author's opinion, this view is erroneous; most physicians work much harder than other members of the public, including attorneys and judges, realize.
10. Hospitals have long resisted providing due process to physicians contesting credentials actions. Even now, there is a strong structural bias against the physician who is charged.

# Antitrust Implications of Allied Health Practitioner Privilege Decisions and Hospital-Physician Exclusive Contracts

John J. Miles, Esq.

The Health Care Quality Improvement Act, which often protects hospitals and medical staffs from damages resulting from physician credentialing decisions, offers no protection for (1) credentialing decisions affecting allied health practitioners or (2) challenges to exclusive contracts between physicians and hospitals. Since many antitrust-health care actions have involved those two situations, antitrust litigation in those areas is not likely to decline. This article outlines steps that hospitals and their medical staffs can take to minimize the antitrust risks in awarding exclusive contracts and in decisions regarding the credentialing of allied practitioners.

The initial article in this series examining the antitrust ramifications of medical staff activity focused on the credentialing of physicians by hospitals and their medical staffs.[1] The second article discussed how the Health Care Quality Improvement Act of 1986[2] often protects the hospital and its staff from damages in subsequent litigation brought by a physician whose privileges are affected adversely by a credentialing decision.[3]

This article examines the antitrust ramifications of two related situations: (1) the credentialing of so-called "allied health practitioners" by hospitals and their staffs and (2) exclusive contracts between hospitals and physicians. Both subjects have been the focus of substantial antitrust litigation, and importantly, the protections of the Health Care Quality Improvement Act are not applicable to either.[4] These may be the two areas in which staff privilege antitrust litigation continues to flourish.


## I. Problems in Credentialing Allied Health Practitioners

The Joint Commission on Accreditation of Hospitals (JCAH) now permits its accredited facilities to admit "independent" allied health practitioners (that is, classes of allied health practitioners who do not require supervision by a physician) to their medical staffs.[5] If the hospital admits a practitioner to its medical staff, it also must grant the practitioner delineated clinical privileges.[6] While "dependent" allied health practitioners (that is, those who must be supervised) are precluded from medical staff membership, the hospital *may* grant them delineated clinical privileges, thus permitting them to treat patients at the hospital.[7] The hospital is not required to grant them clinical privileges, however. Under JCAH standards, practitioners admitted to the medical staff must be eligible for membership on the medical executive committee.[8] Practitioners with clinical privileges must be accorded fair hearing and appellate review rights.[9]

Not surprisingly, the many different types of allied health practitioners have become more vocal in their demands for access to the hospital, which has led to an increasing number of antitrust cases challenging their exclusion.[10] Only one case, however, presently on appeal, has resulted in a final judgment for the plaintiff.[11] At least one was settled favorably to both the plaintiff nurse anesthetist and the state attorney general, who joined the litigation as parens patriae.[12] Another case, brought by forty-six chiropractors against nine hospitals, was dismissed and the plaintiffs ordered to pay the defendants' attorneys fees because the suit was frivolous.[13] As competition among different types of practitioners becomes more heated, the frequency of antitrust litigation by allieds against hospitals and their medical staffs will probably increase. The substantive antitrust analysis of staff privilege suits brought by allied practitioners is the same as that of suits involving physicians. The first article in this series discussed the relevant principles of law and how they apply,[14] and that analysis will not be repeated. Suffice it to say that the allied practitioner whose application for privileges is denied will allege that his or her exclusion resulted from a conspiracy between the hospital and its medical staff, or among members of the medical staff, which unreasonably restrained competition.

Although the antitrust legal analysis is the same, applications from allied practitioners can present some important practical problems that typically do not arise in connection with credentialing actions involving physicians. This article will focus on what these problems are and will provide some general guidance about how they can be handled. Often, for example, neither the hospital's corporate bylaws nor the medical staff bylaws even mention allied health practitioners. Neither set of bylaws may provide a hint as to whether particular types of practitioners may practice at the hospital, whether they may join the medical staff or another staff, whether they may obtain clinical privileges, whether they will have a special credentialing procedure, and other similar issues. In these circumstances, what should be done when an allied practitioner asks the hospital about staff membership or privileges?

If the hospital's response is simply that the medical staff bylaws preclude consideration of an application, then the allied practitioner could argue that this itself shows a conspiracy among the medical staff members to exclude their competitors. In such a view, the medical staff bylaws, themselves, could constitute the requisite conspiracy because they constitute an "agreement" among medical staff members and between the medical staff and the hospital.

A second major problem is that the medical staff might have substantial difficulty in assessing an allied practitioner's credentials rationally because, aside from possible preconceived biases against a particular class of allied practitioner, medical staff members may be unfamiliar with the profession involved, its schools, and the value of references that the applicant submits. Thus, when an allied practitioner inquires about privileges, the hospital and its staff might have to educate themselves about the particular profession of which the applicant is a member.

### Handling Inquiries From Allied Practitioners

The key to minimizing antitrust and other types of legal exposure resulting from the privilege applications of allied practitioners is careful planning before a potential problem has the chance to arise. Too many hospitals and medical staffs simply are unprepared to handle unexpected applications from different classes of allied practitioners.

A worst possible scenario occurs, for example, when a letter of inquiry is received from an allied practitioner, the letter is shunted off to the medical staff president because the hospital administration does not know what to do with it, and the president does not know what to do with it, and the president, on behalf of the medical staff, writes the potential applicant that "the medical staff has agreed, through its bylaws, not to grant clinical privileges to quacks." Another dangerous response is a letter from the med-has enough physicians who provide the type of services the allied practitioner would provide. These kinds of responses can occur when the hospital and its medical staff have not developed a thoughtful strategy for handling inquiries and applications from allied practitioners.

Early on, therefore, the hospital's governing body, with input from (but not control by) the medical staff, must decide several important questions. The answers to these questions will have significant effects upon competition among practitioners and can thus lead to antitrust litigation. Important questions that must be considered include:

1. What classes of allied practitioners will be permitted to practice at the hospital?
2. Should the hospital have an allied practitioner staff? If so, will certain types of "independent" allied practitioners be permitted to join the medical staff as opposed to the allied staff?
3. What types of allied practitioners will be required to work under physician supervision? How stringent will the supervision be, and what form it will take? For example, must the supervising physician only be available (that is, on call or in the hospital), or must he or she actually be present during treatment rendered by the allied practitioner? What happens if physicians refuse to supervise allied practitioners because they perceive that it would increase their malpractice exposure or reduce their income, or because they simply lack the necessary time?
4. How do the hospital and the medical staff obtain the requisite knowledge to credential the applicants? Who should bear the cost of obtaining this knowledge? Who should credential them? What type of procedure will be used?
5. What types of allied practitioners, if any, should be granted delineated clinical privileges? If the practitioner is not granted delineated clinical privileges, what procedure will be established to define the scope of the practitioner's activities in the hospital and to ensure that he or she does not exceed that scope?
6. Should the delineated clinical privileges granted the allied practitioner be commensurate with the practitioner's scope of practice under state law, or should they be narrower? If narrower, how will this be justified? Should written protocols be developed? If so, by whom?
7. What effect, if any, might granting privileges to different classes of allied practitioners have on the hospital's malpractice exposure or malpractice insurance?
8. How will quality assurance and peer review of the allied practitioner's work be handled? Who on the medical staff is qualified to do it?

9. Aside from antitrust considerations, are there state laws that restrict the ability of hospitals to deny medical staff membership or clinical privileges to particular classes of allied practitioners?[15]
10. Which, if any, allied practitioners will be granted admitting privileges? Should a co-admission procedure be developed? How will it work?
11. Should the governing body or one of its committees hold informal hearings at which allied practitioners and the staff appear to provide information that may help answer some of these questions? In particular, should this informal hearing format be used to determine whether a particular class of allied practitioner will be permitted to practice at the hospital?

There is no blanket requirement under the antitrust laws (or under JCAH standards or the Health Care Quality Improvement Act of 1986)[16] that hospitals grant any type of allied practitioner either membership on the medical staff or delineated clinical privileges. When an exclusion is likely to occur, however, especially the exclusion of an entire class of practitioners, thought, planning, and caution are essential.

Most important, at least from the standpoint of antitrust exposure, the decision about the classes of practitioners that may use the hospital should be made by the hospital's governing body—not by the medical staff. Indeed, it is wise to specify in the hospital's corporate bylaws the classes of practitioners that can render services at the hospital. Very little antitrust risk accrues when the hospital, as opposed to members of the medical staff, decides who may practice at the hospital. Related to this, inquiries about privileges from allied practitioners should be handled by the hospital administration after discussion with the hospital attorney. In sum, the hospital and its medical staff should have a well-conceived strategy in place before the issue arises, rather than handling it on an ad hoc basis.

## II. Exclusive Hospital-Physician Contracts

An exclusive hospital-physician contract is an arrangement by which a hospital and a physician (or single group of physicians) agree that only that particular physician (or group) will be permitted to render certain medical services at the hospital. Accordingly, applications from other practitioners to render these services are denied. Similarly, a hospital may determine that a previously "open" department should be operated on an exclusive or "closed" basis, and it will then attempt to prevent incumbent staff members from rendering the services in question.[17] The physician-beneficiary of the exclusive may be an employee of the hospital or, as is more frequently the case, an independent contractor.

Exclusive contracts are used most frequently in radiology, anesthesiology and pathology—the hospital-based medical specialties.[18] Exclusive contracts can achieve substantial efficiencies in the delivery of the medical services they cover, but, under certain economic conditions, they can result in significant anticompetitive effects. In particular, anticompetitive effects are most likely where the medical specialty in question is practiced only at the hospital, and there are very few hospitals in the geographic area.

## The Illegal Tying Arrangement

A physician challenging an exclusive contract under the antitrust laws typically alleges that the arrangement results in an illegal tying agreement and is an illegal exclusive dealing arrangement violative of Section 1 of the Sherman Antitrust Act.[19] A tying agreement results where there is an understanding between a seller and a buyer that the seller will sell one service to the buyer (called the "tying" product) only if the buyer purchases another service (called the "tied" product) from the seller or from someone designated by the seller.[20] In effect, the purchaser is coerced into purchasing a service from someone designated by the seller before the seller will sell another service to the purchaser. As a result, competitors of the seller's designee may effectively be precluded from competing in the market and, in the extreme, the designee can exercise monopoly power. In claiming that an exclusive contract with a radiologist (for example) results in a tying arrangement, the plaintiff physician might allege that the hospital agrees with its patients to sell them use of the *hospital's* radiology room, equipment, and personnel to perform radiological tests (the tying product) only if they agree to purchase interpretational services from the *radiologist chosen by the hospital* (the tied service).

As a practical matter, an illegal tying arrangement results only if: (1) the tying and tied services actually are *two* services instead of one,[21] (2) the seller of the tying services has significant market power in the market for the tying services and thus can coerce the purchaser into buying the tied product from the designated source,[22] and (3) the seller of the tying services has some economic interest in the sale of the tied service.[23] In finding that use of a hospital's operating room facilities and anesthesiology services provided by physicians were two separate services, the U.S. Supreme Court explained in a landmark 1984 case that a "package" contains separate services if consumers view the services as distinguishable and thus might choose a physician other than the one chosen by the hospital if given the opportunity.[24]

the seller's use of its economic power in one market to foreclose competition in another market. The only hospital in an area, for example, may use its market power over surgical facilities to force patients to use the anesthesiological services of the anesthesiologist with whom the hospital has an exclusive contract. As a rule of thumb, the hospital's share of the tying product market must be at least 30% before serious concern should arise.[25]

Finally, a number of cases have held that no illegal tying arrangement can exist unless the seller of the tying service receives some direct financial benefit from the sale of the tied service in the form of a profit, commission, rebate, or the like.[26] Otherwise, the seller of the tying service has not "invaded" the market for the tied service-the market in which the alleged anticompetitive effect results.[27] A hospital likely has the requisite economic interest in the sale of the tied service where the physician with the exclusive contract is a salaried hospital employee, because his or her services probably generate a profit for the hospital.[28] The same may be true where the physician with the exclusive contract, even if an independent contractor, splits his or her remuneration with the hospital. The requirement probably is not met where the physician is an independent contractor, the physician and the hospital bill separately for their services, and the physician does not share his or her revenues with the hospital.[29]

## Exclusive Dealing Arrangements

The potential anticompetitive effect of an exclusive dealing arrangement is that competitors of the physician with the exclusive contract may be foreclosed from serving a significant percentage of customers and thus be unable to compete. Exclusive dealing arrangements are tested under the rule of reason,[30] and the most important variable in analyzing their legality, after the relevant product and geographic markets are proved, is the percentage of foreclosure resulting from the contract.[31]

Judicial decisions provide little guidance as to what specific percentage of foreclosure should cause alarm but, as a rule of thumb, a percentage of 10% or less is safe while 30% or more is very troublesome.[32] Moreover, the duration of the contract is important in assessing its competitive effect—the shorter the contract, the less the anticompetitive effect. Another important variable is the procompetitive efficiency in delivering the service in question that results from an exclusive arrangement.[33]

If the hospital merely substitutes a new exclusive provider for an old one,[34] there likely is no antitrust problem. In this situation, competition usually is not decreased but rather stays at the same level. Finally, if the physician with the exclusive contract is a hospital employee, there will likely be no "agreement" between the physician and the hospital, in an antitrust sense, because they are treated as a single entity for purposes of the antitrust laws.[35] Accordingly, an exclusive dealing agreement claim under Section 1 of the Sherman Antitrust Act is not viable,[36] since one requirement for a Section 1 violation is an agreement. A tying claim, however, is possible because the "agreement" under that theory is between hospital and its patients rather than between the hospital and its exclusive physician.

## Minimizing Antitrust Exposure

It follows from this analysis that exclusive contracts of rural hospitals, everything else being equal, create greater antitrust exposure than those of metropolitan facilities. In confronting a tying claim, the rural hospital will likely be seen as having greater power in the market for the tying service. In an exclusive dealing contract claim, the percentage of foreclosure in a rural hospital setting will likely be higher than in a metropolitan hospital. In any even, hospitals and their medical staffs can take several steps to minimize whatever antitrust risk arises from the use of exclusive contracts:

1. The decision whether to use an exclusive contract should be made by the hospital's governing body—not by the medical staff, and especially not by the physician who would be given the exclusive.
2. The reasons for using an exclusive arrangement should be well documented by the governing body, with emphasis on the various types of efficiencies that the arrangement achieves.
3. If the hospital plans to move from an open departmental arrangement to an exclusive arrangement, it is helpful to retain a consultant and have the recommendation for change come from the consultant.
4. The decision not to grant an applicant's application for privileges because of an exclusive contract should be made by the governing body. The medical staff should base its recommendation about the applicant only on his or her professional competence and conduct and not on the hospital's needs. Indeed, from an antitrust standpoint (although state law or the medical staff bylaws might dictate otherwise), it probably is best that the administration handle the application itself and that the normal credentialing procedure not be used.
5. In determining which physician should be awarded an exclusive contract, a hospital should foster competition among physicians for the contract to the extent practicable.
6. The contract should be of short duration (one or two years, if possi-

ble), should not renew automatically, and, at the end of the period, the governing body should reconsider both whether to continue using an exclusive arrangement and, if so, to whom it should be awarded.

7. The hospital and physician should bill separately for their services, and the physician should not split his or her revenues with the hospital.

8. Although not required by the antitrust laws, the hospital should notify a physician with whom it contracts in writing, about the effect that termination of the contract will have on his or her medical staff membership and clinical privileges.[37] Indeed, the contract should cover this, and the medical staff bylaws should state clearly that the contract's termination does not trigger fair hearing and appellate review procedures unless the termination results in loss of medical staff appointment or clinical privileges *and* was based on the physician's lack of competence or inappropriate professional conduct.

## III. Conclusion

A common theme running through these discussions about allied practitioners and exclusive contracts is the importance of careful planning before a potential problem arises. Regarding allied practitioners, the hospital and its medical staff need to have answered each of the questions listed above. Regarding exclusive contracts, they need to have "eyeballed" the hospital's market power and the contract's foreclosure effects and have documented the efficiency reasons for using an exclusive arrangement.

A second theme is that, at least from the standpoint of antitrust exposure, the hospital rather than the medical staff should be the real decisionmaker about who obtains medical staff membership and clinical privileges. While this may not be to the medical staff's liking, it is crucial to minimize antitrust risk. The hospital can and should seek substantial input and advice from the medical staff, but its final decision must be based on what is in the best interests of the hospital and its patients. In the overwhelming majority of cases, the hospital's decision, based on this standard, will be precisely the same as the medical staff would have made had it been the decisionmaker.

## References


1. *See* Miles, *Antitrust and the Credentialing of Physicians*, MED STAFF COUNSELOR, Summer 1987, at 16.
2. 42 U.S.C.A. §§11101-52 (1986).

3. See Miles, The Health Care Quality Improvement Act of 1986: An Overview of Its Immunity Provisions, MED. STAFF COUNSELOR, Fall 1987, at 1.

4. The Act's lack of applicability to credentialing decisions affecting allied health practitioners is specific. *See* U.S.C.A. §11115(c) (1986). Regarding exclusive contracts, the Act's protection against damages applies only to peer review decisions based on a physician's "competence and professional conduct," 42 U.S.C.A. §11151(9) (1986); a denial of privileges because the hospital has an exclusive contract with another physician probably would not meet this requirement.

5. *See* JOINT COMM'N ON ACCREDITATION OF HOSPS., ACCREDITATION MANUAL FOR HOSPITALS 1987, MS. 1.1.1, at 109 (1986) (hereinafter "1987 AMH'); *see generally* AMERICAN HOSP. ASS'N, AN ANALYSIS OF THE REVISED MEDICAL STAFF STANDARD STANDARDS OF THE JOINT COMMISSION ON ACCREDITATION OF HOSPITALS (1984) (hereinafter "AHA ANALYSIS").

6. 1987 AMH, MS. 1.1.2, at 109. Indeed, all independent allied practitioners must have clinical privileges. *Id.*, MS. 4.1, at 117.

7. Although the 1987 AMH does not mention this issue, the AHA ANALYSIS states as follows:

> [I]t may be inferred from the fact that the revised standards are silent concerning the delineation of clinical privileges for dependent practitioners that the hospital may, if it chooses, extend limited clinical responsibilities and duties to nonphysician practitioners who are participating in the management of patients under the direction or supervision of a physician or other party with designated responsibility for that supervision.

AHA ANALYSIS at 33 (footnote omitted).

8. 1987 AMH, MS 3.5.1, at 115.

9. *Id.*, MS. 4.2.10, at 119.

10. *See, e.g.*, Cooper v. Forsyth County Hosp. Auth., 789 F.2d 278 (4th Cir.), *cert. denied*, 107 S. Ct. 474 (1986); Bhan v. NME Hosps., Inc., 772 F.2d 1467 (9th Cir. 1985); Kaczanaski v. Medical Center Hosp. of Vt., 612 F. Supp. 688 (D. Vt. 1985); Feldman v. Jackson Memorial Hosp., 571 F. Supp. 1000 (S.D. Fla. 1983).

11. Oltz v. St. Peter's Community Hosp., 1987-1 Trade Cas. (CCH) ¶ 67,477 (d. Mont. 1987).

12. Ables v. City of Parkersburg, No.84-A106 (S.D. W. Va., *filed*, Feb. 1, 1983).

13. Colorado Chiropractic Council v. Porter Memorial Hosp., 650 F. Supp. 231 (D. Colo. 1986).

15. *See, e.g.*, D.C. CODE ANN. § 32-1307(c) (1987 Cum. Supp.) (requiring hospitals to consider nurse anesthetists, nurse, midwives, nurse practitioners, podiatrists, and psychologists for clinical privileges and all categories of medical staff membership).

16. *See* 42 U.S.C. § 11115(b) (1986).

17. As a practical matter, the risk of litigation from using an exclusive contract is greater when its implementation adversely affects incumbents as opposed to when a potential new staff member's application is denied. Two examples include Drs. Steurs and Latham, P.A.v. National Medical Enters., Inc., No. 7:87-454-3 (D.S.C. Amended Complaint, *filed*, July 1, 1987) (pathology), and Ritter v. North Penn Hosp., No.85-6849 (E.D. Pa., *filed*, Nov. 27, 1985) (anesthesiology).

18. For a discussion about the frequency of exclusive contracts, *see* Morrisey & Brooks, *The Myth of the Closed Medical Staff*, HOSPITALS, July 1, 1985, at 75.

19. Section 1 of the Sherman Act, 15 U.S.C. § 1 (1982), prohibits agreements that unreasonably restrain competition.

20. *See generally* AMERICAN BAR ASS'N, ANTITRUST LAW DEVELOPMENTS 72 (2d ed. 1984).

21. *See, e.g.*, Collins v. Associated Pathologists, Ltd., 1987-1 Trade Cas. (CCH) ¶ 67,603 (C.D. Ill. 1987) (hospital services and pathological services *not* separate products).

22. *See, e.g.*, Ezpeleta v. Sisters of Mercy Health Corp., 621 F. Supp. 1262 (N.D. Ind. 1985), *aff'd on other grounds*, 800 F. 2d 118 (7th Cir. 1986).

23. *See, e.g.*, White v. Rockingham Radiologists, Ltd., 820 F. 2d 98 (4th Cir. 1987); Griffing v. Lucius O. Crosby Memorial Hosp., 1984-1 Trade Cas. (CCH) ¶ 65,854 (S.D. Miss. 1984).

24. Jefferson Parish Hosp. Dist. No. 2 v. Hyde, 466 U.S. 2 (1984).

25. *Id*; *see also* U.S. DEPT. OF JUSTICE, VERTICAL RESTRAINTS GUIDELINES § 5.3 (Jan. 23, 1985).

26. In addition to the cases cited in note 23 *supra*, *see* Robert's Waikiki U-Drive, Inc. v. Budget Rent-A-Car Sys., 732 F. 2d 1403 (7th Cir. 1984); General Motors Corp. v. Gibson Chem. & Oil Corp., 1987-1 Trade Cas. (CCH) ¶ 67,621 (E.D.N.Y. 1987).

27. *See* Carl Sandburg Village Condominium Ass'n No. 1 v. First Condominium Dev. Co., 758 F.2d 203 (7th Cir. 1985).

28. *See, e.g.*, McMorris v. Wiliamsport Hosp., 597 F. Supp. 899 (M.D. Pa. 1984).

29. For example, this was the situation in White v. Rockingham Radiologists, Ltd., 820 F. 2d 98 (4th Cir. 1987), and thus there was no illegal tying agreement.

29. For example, this was the situation in White v. Rockingham Radiologists, Ltd., 820 F. 2d 98 (4th Cir. 1987), and thus there was no illegal tying agreement.
30. *See, e.g.,* Tampa Electric Co. v. Nashville Coal Co., 365 U.S. 320 (1961); Dos Santos v. Columbus-Cuneo-Cabrini Medical Center, 684 F.2d 1346 (7th Cir. 1982).
31. *See generally* Ryko Mfg. Co. v. Eden Services, 1987-1 Trade Cas. (CCH) ¶ 67,614 (8th Cir. 1987). Roughly speaking, the percentage of foreclosure is the percentage of patients in a market which competitors of the physician with the exclusive cannot serve because of the exclusive contract. Typically, it will proximate the hospital's market share.

     The size of the percentage of foreclosure is quite sensitive to whether the hospital or the patient is perceived as the "purchaser" of services under the exclusive contract. If the former is, then the geographic market in which to assess the degree of foreclosure is probably nationwide because physicians across the country might compete for the contract. Any foreclosure percentage from the contract then would be insignificant. If the patient is viewed as the purchaser, the market likely is local because patients typically will not travel long distances for the service. The degree of foreclosure in this situation could be substantial. See generally Collins v. Associated Pathologists, Ltd., 1987-1 Trade Cas. (CCH) ¶ 67,603 (C.D. Ill. 1987) (nationwide market); *see also* Lynk, *Restraint of Trade Through Hospital Exclusive Contracts: An Economic Appraisal of the Legal Theory,* 9 J. HEALTH POL., POL'Y & LAW 269 (1984).
32. *See* U.S. Dept. of Justice, Vertical Restraints Guidelines (Jan. 23, 1985); see generally Miles, Hospital Exclusive Contracts and the Department of Justice Vertical Restraints Giudelines, AHA HEALTH L. VIGIL, Mar. 8, 1985.
33. *See* Jefferson Parish Hosp. Dist. No.2 v. Hyde, 466 U.S. 2, 32 (1984) (O'Connor, J., concurring); Roland Equip Co. v. Dresser Indus., 749 F.2d 380 (7th Cir. 1984).
34. *See, e.g.,* Fishman v. Wirtz, 807 F.2d 520, 565 (7th Cir. 1986) (Easterbrook, J., dissenting) ("a swap of one contractor for another cannot violate the antitrust laws"); Trepel v. Pontiac Osteopathic Hosp., 599 F. Supp. 1484 (E.D. Mich. 1984), *aff'd without opinion,* 780 F. 2d 1023 (6th Cir. 1985).
35. *See generally* Copperweld Corp. v. Independence Tube Corp., 467 U.S. 752 (1984); Weiss v. York Hosp., 745 F.2d 786 (3d Cir. 1984), *cert. denied,* 470 U.S. 1060 (1985).
36. *See* McMorris v. Williamsport Hosp., 597 F. Supp. 899 (M.D. Pa. 1984).
37. *See* 1987 AMH, MS. 1.2.3.1.14.1 & 4.2.12, at 111 & 119.

# The Board's Role in Medical Staff Credentialing

James E. Orlikoff and Mary K. Totten

## Introduction

Perhaps the board's most important quality assurance responsibility is the credentialing of the hospital's medical staff. For most hospital boards, this is the most difficult of all the governance functions to perform effectively.

For many hospital trustees, the issue of the board's role in medical staff credentialing causes much anxiety and doubt. "After all," many trustees have said, "how can a board composed of mostly *laymen* decide whether a physician is qualified or competent enough to be on the medical staff?" This issue of why and how a lay board decides which physicians can practice at the hospital and what procedures they can perform is very intimidating to most trustees. It is also an issue that can be very threatening to physicians. Hence the controversial nature of the board's role in medical staff credentialing.

*Medical Staff Credentialing* encompasses the policies, procedures, and all activities surrounding the initial appointment and reappointment of physicians (and other health care practitioners, such as dentists) to the hospital's medical staff. Medical staff credentialing also involves granting and renewing of clinical privileges to medical staff members. Basically, then, credentialing involves deciding which physicians may join the medical staff, which physicians may remain on the medical staff, which procedures each physician will be allowed to perform, and which diseases or categories of diseases the physician will be allowed to treat. Although the medical staff *recommends* these credentialing decisions, it is the hospital board that actually makes the final decision.

The primary purpose of your hospital's medical staff credentialing system is to ensure that only qualified physicians are granted practice privileges and that physicians practice within the scope of their capabilities and expertise. Because this evaluation is done *prior* to a physician's initial appointment or reappointment, credentialing, when properly conducted, is an excellent example of prospective quality assurance (discussed in chapter 4). Development and use of an appropriate credentialing system is essential if your hospital is to achieve and maintain a desired level of quality care and minimize the risks of medically related patient injury that can result in malpractice losses.

Physicians, as clinical decision-making authorities in the hospital, profoundly affect the hospital's overall level of quality of care. Yet despite physicians' impact on quality and the board's ultimate accountability for physician performance, many boards continue to discharge their credentialing oversight responsibility in an ineffective, outdated, and inappropriate mode. Unfortunately these governing boards merely "rubber stamp" the medical staff's recommendations about who should be a medical staff member and what privileges they should have.

A recent survey on disagreements among hospital governing boards, executives, and medical staffs (Joint Commission on Accreditation of Healthcare Organizations, 1987, p. 7) found that physician credentialing ranked among the top 10 points of conflict among these groups. This finding is not really surprising, given the long history of individual physician responsibility for patient care quality and the board's relatively recent involvement in and accountability for it.

Yet governing boards that choose the rubber stamp approach to credentialing to avoid conflict are exposing themselves and their hospitals to significant potential liability. At the same time, they are missing an important opportunity to strengthen their relationship with the medical staff by collaboratively discharging this critical leadership responsibility.

Hospital boards that are effectively operating in an active oversight mode have trustees who know the board's responsibility and accountability for medical staff credentialing and understand the credentialing process and their role in it. This chapter discusses the board's accountability for medical staff credentialing and describes the roles of the board, medical staff, and hospital executives in effectively conducting the credentialing process. This chapter also suggests a collaborative approach that can be used to help your hospital board make more consistent and objective credentialing decisions on medical staff candidates.

## The Board's Expanding Accountability

As mentioned in chapter 3, the landmark case of *Darling v. Charleston Memorial Hospital* was the beginning of a wave of legal cases that further delineated the governing board's ultimate accountability for patient care quality. As chapter 3 also demonstrated, many of these cases focused on the hospital's, and therefore the governing board's, responsibility for physician capability, competence, and performance. Legal cases such as those listed in chapter 3 (and others that your hospital CEO will be able to provide you) all expand and reinforce the hospital board's ultimate responsibility for patient care quality through the medical staff credentialing function.

In addition to its quality implications, credentialing also has *liability* implications for the hospital and its board. A hospital board that oversees a credentialing system that allows incompetent physicians to join or remain on the medical staff, or that allows physicians to practice procedures they are not qualified to practice, increases the risk of medically related patient injury and malpractice liability. On the other hand, a board that condones a credentialing system that unfairly denies medical staff membership or privileges to qualified physicians runs the risk of a physician suing the hospital and board for restraint of trade or antitrust violations. Thus credentialing can be a double-edged sword of liability, with either patients or physicians suing the hospital.

## Legal Mandates

Although many legal cases regarding physician credentialing have been decided in favor of the hospital (Orlikoff and Totten, 1988, p. 15), liability has been incurred when governing boards failed to ensure that an appropriate credentialing process exists and was in fact conducted. Hospitals have been found liable when patient injury resulted from lack of appropriate diligence in conducting physician credentialing. Liability also can occur when physicians successfully claim that inappropriate credentialing resulted in economic loss to them through the hospital's antitrust activities, which was the situation in *Patrick v. Burget* (1988).

In this case, Dr. Timothy Patrick, a general and vascular surgeon practicing in Astoria, Oregon, contended that his denial of privileges at Columbia Memorial Hospital, Astoria's only hospital, was motivated by a desire to restrict competition. He claimed that the hospital's peer review activities had been initiated and conducted by physicians who were staff members at the hospital and members of the Astoria Clinic. The clinic was a group practice in which Dr. Patrick had declined to accept partnership, preferring to set up his own practice in competition with it.

After Dr. Patrick established his own practice, the clinic physicians refused to have professional dealings with him, declining to provide consultations or back-up coverage for his patients. At the same time, they criticized him for failing to obtain consultations or coverage and complained about his medical practices to the State Board of Medical Examiners. Clinic physicians also requested review of Dr. Patrick's hospital privileges. After the hospital's medical staff executive committee voted to terminate Dr. Patrick's privileges, clinic physicians also participated in the hearing he requested to review the termination.

Dr. Patrick filed suit, claiming that the clinic physicians participated in the hospital's peer review activities to reduce competition rather than to improve the quality of patient care. The clinic physicians denied the assertion and the court turned the matter over to a jury, which supported Dr. Patrick's claim. Antitrust damages of approximately $2 million were awarded to Dr. Patrick.

Upon appeal, the circuit court ruled that despite the motivation of the clinic physicians to use peer review to restrict competition, the matter was exempt from federal antitrust scrutiny. The court reasoned that hospital peer review instead fell under the state action doctrine.

The case went to the U.S. Supreme Court, which reversed the appeals court. The Supreme Court found that whereas the state of Oregon had a policy favoring peer review, the state did not actively supervise hospital peer review decisions and, therefore, the state action exemption did not apply. Ultimately, the district court's $2 million judgment in favor of Dr. Patrick was upheld.

It is important that all trustees on your board understand that the hospital's accountability and liability for the credentialing function exist primarily to protect patients as well as to ensure fair, thorough, and consistent consideration of physician requests for privileges. Trustees must ensure that their credentialing process is thorough, fair, and free from conflicts of interest such as those that existed in the *Patrick* case.


### Legislative Mandates

In addition to a body of legal cases that clearly demonstrates board accountability for medical staff credentialing, the 1986 Health Care Quality

Improvement Act also focuses squarely on hospital requirements for participation in the credentialing process. The act provides limited immunity from liability for hospitals that participate in both contributing data to, as well as consulting, a National Practitioner Data Bank. The data bank contains information such as restrictions or revocations of medical staff membership and clinical privileges, malpractice payments, state licensure, and society membership actions.

Hospitals are required to submit information on reduction, suspension, denial, revocation, restriction, nonrenewal, or surrender of medical staff privileges lasting longer than 30 days. Hospitals also must report information related to malpractice payments made on behalf of licensed health practitioners. Hospitals must query the data bank every two years concerning reappointment of medical staff members and those holding clinical privileges. They also must access the bank when screening applicants for initial appointment and granting of privileges ("Data banking," 1989, p. 6). Hospitals that fail to comply with the reporting requirements of the act can face substantial penalties: fines of up to $10,000 per occurrence and loss of immunity protection for a three-year period (National Practitioner Data Bank [Title IV Regulations, Oct. 1989, pp. 5,7]).

Although implementation of the data bank and questions about its utility and effectiveness will take several years to resolve, hospital boards should be aware of hospital responsibilities related to the bank as well as potential problems it poses. For example, some experts are concerned that the data bank will have a chilling effect on medical staff participation in the credentialing process and may even worsen rather than improve the way credentialing is conducted ("Key problems," 1990, p. 1).

Hospital medical staff committees and hospital boards must now, more than ever before, make sure that medical staff applications and requests for privileges are handled carefully and completely. Governing boards must ensure that the hospital has in place and is using a thorough, consistent, and fair credentialing process and that trained personnel participate in both contributing information to the bank and querying and using the information appropriately for reviewing medical staff candidates.

In reaching final decisions on medical staff applicants, boards should remember that the data bank is only one source of information that should be used as part of a broader investigation into the candidate's capability and competency to practice. Even though the data bank may indicate a clean record, a more extensive investigation might uncover a different picture of the candidate. To help protect themselves and their hospitals from potential liability, boards must rely on sources other than the data bank, such as internal hospital quality and risk management information. Careful review and interpretation of data bank information is required by all participants in the credentialing process to ensure that final decisions on each applicant are made first in the best interests of the patients the hospital serves, and then the practitioner.

## Regulatory Mandates

In addition to legal and legislative imperatives, the Joint Commission on Accreditation of Healthcare Organizations also specifies the board's ultimate accountability for medical staff appointment and privileges delineation. As mentioned in chapter 3, the Joint Commission standards require the medical staff executive committee to make recommendations for approval by the governing body regarding mechanisms to review credentials and delineate individual clinical privileges. The standards also require board approval of medical staff recommendations regarding individual medical staff membership and specific clinical privileges for each eligible practitioner.

These legal, legislative, and regulatory mandates clearly indicate the board's accountability for medical staff appointment and privileges delineation. Yet many boards that continue to "rubber stamp" their medical staff's recommendations do so not only to avoid conflict but also because they simply do not understand how the credentialing process works and how the board can most effectively participate in it. Because they are not familiar with the process and are not aware of the information that typically is reviewed on each candidate, many trustees are uncomfortable asking questions or seeking additional information before making final decisions on medical staff recommendations.

The next section of this chapter discusses the key players and their roles in credentialing and reviews the steps in the process to help you gain a basic understanding of how to meaningfully participate in this critical quality assurance responsibility.

## The Basics of Credentialing

Credentialing consists of two separate processes: appointment to the medical staff and delineation of clinical privileges. Each process has its own objective.

The *appointment process*, which is composed of initial appointment to the medical staff and periodic reappointments thereafter, is designed to evaluate the individual practitioner's *capability* to practice at the hospital. The appointment process focuses on a review of a practitioner's eduction, training, licensure, certification, references, and other credentials that testify that the individual is eligible to be a member of the hospital's medical staff.

When candidates apply for medical staff membership, they generally also apply for specific privileges to practice at the hospital. The *delineation of clinical privileges process* focuses on assessing the practitioner's *competence* to treat various illnesses or perform various procedures. In granting privileges to individual physicians, the board is specifying the scope of that individual's competence to practice within his or her areas of skill and expertise (Orlikoff, 1990, p. 63).

Once physicians gain initial appointment and privileges, they enter a provisional period of medical staff membership, usually lasting six months to a year, during which their performance is monitored closely. If at the end of this time the physician and the hospital have found the experience mutually satisfactory, the physician gains full membership status and is subject to periodic reappraisal and reappointment, usually conducted at least every two years (Orlikoff and Totten, 1988, p. 15). This reappraisal may result in an alteration (restriction, expansion, or revocation) of delineated clinical privileges.

## Relative Roles of Participants in the Credentialing Process

Before learning the specifics of the credentialing process, it is helpful to understand who participates in it and the roles of each participant. Each member of the hospital leadership team—the governing board, the medical staff, and the hospital management group—has a role to play.

As you might suspect, the bulk of the review and analysis of a physician's capability and competency is conducted by the *medical staff* because a physician's peers are best able to assess and make recommendations regarding the practitioner's background and expertise. It is the medical staff that establishes the applicant evaluation process in its bylaws and works with candidates to obtain appropriate information for review. Once a completed application has been received, the medical staff credentialing committee (or its equivalent) reviews the information to assess the candidate's professional competence, performance, character, and fitness and then makes a recommendation regarding the candidate. Frequently this recommendation is reviewed by the medical staff executive committee, which then sends the recommendation to the governing board.

In discharging its responsibilities for credentialing, the medical staff often relies on support from the hospital's management group. *Hospital managers* have an important role to play in ensuring that adequate staff and other resources and support are available to the medical staff to gather and verify applicant information. Hospital executives also can facilitate the flow of information, such as hospital quality assurance and risk management data, that should be used in evaluating candidates. Finally, the hospital chief executive officer should help facilitate the flow of medical staff recommendations and supporting documentation to the governing board and help establish a collaborative process between the board and medical staff for reaching final decisions on medical staff candidates.

Ultimately it is up to the *governing board* to render final decisions on each medical staff applicant. Although the governing board does not actively participate in data collection and validation for each candidate, the board is responsible for ensuring that the medical staff bylaws provide for a credentialing procedure and that this procedure is in fact conducted thoroughly and consistently for each candidate. The board must ensure that appropriate information on each candidate has been received and reviewed (see the next section) and that all questions regarding the applicant have been satisfactorily answered. The board must make sure it understands the medical staff's recommendation and compares it against the criteria established in the medical staff's credentialing procedure. Finally, the board must make a determination on staff membership and privileges for each candidate (Orlikoff, 1990, pp. 63-64).

## The Appointment and Privileges Delineation Processes

Trustees who understand the information received and reviewed during the appointment and privileges delineation processes are best able to participate knowledgeably and meaningfully in reaching final decisions on applicants. This section reviews initial appointment and reappointment to the medical staff and discusses the granting of medical staff privileges in more detail.

## The Initial Appointment Process and Provisional Membership

The hospital often has its first opportunity to become familiar with a practitioner during the initial appointment process. Much of the information reviewed during this process is supplied from outside sources, so the medical staff and board must be especially thorough and diligent in obtaining and reviewing all relevant and appropriate information. The essential minimum information that should be received and reviewed on each candidate is:

- Validation of licensure in all states that apply

- Evidence of completed training, including undergraduate and medical school education, and residency, fellowship, or other training, if claimed
- Disciplinary actions by previous hospitals, professional societies, or specialty boards, if any
- Current good standing at other hospitals
- Current and adequate malpractice insurance
- Valid board certification, if claimed or required by the hospital
- Satisfactory recommendations regarding professional performance, clinical skills, ethical character, ability to work with others
- Statement of health history, including substance abuse or chronic illnesses, if any
- Malpractice claims history
- Privileges granted at other hospitals and evidence of special training and experience, especially in conducting high-risk or unusual procedures

The board should make sure that any questions regarding the practitioner's capabilities are answered satisfactorily prior to initial appointment. The burden of proof to obtain medical staff membership resides with the applicant and, therefore, this is the best time to catch any potential problems. It is usually much easier to prevent a physician with a questionable background from joining the medical staff than to remove a physician once he or she has become a medical staff member.

Once the initial appointment process has been successfully completed, the applicant undergoes a period of provisional membership on the medical staff. This period, though frequently underused, is the one opportunity that allows the hospital to monitor the physician in action and to gain firsthand experience with physicians prior to admitting them to the medical staff. Hospitals that use the provisional period well can acquire valuable information that will help the board make a more informed decision about whether to confer full membership status or grant the privileges requested by physician applicants. For these reasons, your board should ensure that the medical staff bylaws specify a monitoring process to be used during the provisional period be submitted to the board prior to making final decisions about admitting physicians to the medical staff.

## The Reappointment Process

Each medical staff member must reapply for medical staff membership and undergo a reappointment process at least every two years. This time the emphasis is on actual physician performance at the hospital during the past two years. In addition to the type of information reviewed during initial appointment, the hospital should now rely on several sources of internal information in assessing candidates.

For example, mortality statistics, infection rates, or malpractice claims can be provided by the hospital's quality assurance and risk management department. The board and medical staff also have access to a variety of performance-specific information. Compliance with hospital and medical staff bylaws, rules, and regulations; patterns of adverse clinical outcomes; and reduction or revocation of privileges are examples of some of the performance indicators that should be considered during reappointment. Such data should be carefully gathered and considered because the burden of proof lies with the hospital in the event reappointment is denied. Ultimately, a thorough, fair, and consistent approach to appointment and reappointment is in the best interest of the hospital, its practitioners, and its patients.

## The Privileges Delineation Process

Generally practitioners will submit a request for medical staff privileges along with their applications for appointment. The delineation of privileges is practitioner specific and defines the types of illnesses that can be treated or the procedures that can be performed. Privileges usually are developed by each clinical department in the hospital using one of several approaches. They can be specified by practitioner's specialty, patient risk category, lists or groups of procedures and diseases, or combinations of these. The specificity required for delineating privileges may vary for each hospital based on its size, complexity, and staffing.

The process for granting clinical privileges also requires review of the appointment information listed previously, with special emphasis on assessing the candidate's competency to treat the diseases or perform the procedures specified. In assessing the candidate's level of expertise, the medical staff may review the individual's initial and continuing education, overall use of privileges previously granted, volume of cases seen or procedures performed, and specific outcome indicators (unplanned returns to surgery or number of missed diagnoses). After the review is completed, the medical staff can make any of a number of recommendations, including to approve, deny, revoke, restrict, reduce, suspend, or expand the practitioner's privileges, as appropriate.

Boards that participate effectively in the appointment and privileges delineation processes balance their responsibility for ensuring quality care with the physician's interest in practicing at the hospital. If the board decides, for example, to deny, modify, or revoke a medical staff member's privileges, it must do so according to the hospital's bylaws and be consistent with constitutional or common law requirements of due process. These requirements usually call for fair and consistent application of criteria based on professional standards of care, the legitimate objectives of the hospital, and the character and ethical behavior of the applicant (Orlikoff and Totten, 1988, p. 15).

### Economic Credentialing

Although most credentialing processes largely focus on the *clinical* skills of the physician, some recent court cases have upheld denial of medical staff privileges based on *economic* results of the physician's practice, such as overutilization of hospital resources. This is called *economic credentialing*, and hospitals that set resource use standards must include them in the hospital bylaws, apply them fairly and consistently to all practitioners, and give those whose practice patterns deviate from the standards an opportunity to comply.

To understand the reason for economic credentialing, consider the following situation. A physician at your hospital is up for reappointment to the medical staff and meets all the clinical and administrative criteria for reappointment; in other words, the physician's quality of care is good. However, the physician consistently costs the hospital huge sums of money by requesting extra tests and treatments. The physician also has a history of extended patient stays, which results in frequent payment denials by Medicare, insurers, and other third-party payers. Now imagine that your hospital is in economic trouble and has a negative operating margin.

Clearly, in this situation the hospital must act to control the physician's inappropriate resource use, which is costing the hospital money it can ill afford to lose. If counseling and education—the first-line approaches—do not change the physician's expensive behavior, then the hospital might establish criteria to conduct economic credentialing in the future.

Bear in mind, however, that the issue of economic credentialing is a controversial one that is likely to cause concern among physicians. It is an issue that can generate litigation and, if improperly approached, liability for the hospital and the board. Yet it also is an issue that many hospitals and boards likely will find they must confront in the near future (Blum, 1990, p. 30).

### Common Problems in Credentialing

Now that you know the basic process of credentialing, you also should know about problems that commonly occur in credentialing. The first and foremost problem is confusion between the role of the medical staff and the role of the board. This role confusion frequently results in disagreement, conflict, and ineffective credentialing.

In a nutshell, here is the difference in roles: The medical staff does the actual work of credentialing; that is, it develops criteria, evaluates applicants, and makes recommendations. The board, on the other hand, makes certain that the medical staff has done it right and has used the same process consistently for each candidate; that is, the board reviews medical staff recommendations against credentialing criteria, verifies that the recommendations are appropriate, and makes final decisions.

The next problem is that even if relative roles are known and understood, the medical staff credentialing criteria are often so vague that it is impossible for the board to do its job meaningfully. Most medical staff criteria relate to administrative issues such as licensure, meeting attendance, and the like. A physician's clinical skill and performance, on the other hand, usually are determined by the particular medical staff department head.

In most hospitals, the critical judgment of the medical staff department head is a subjective one. If the credentialing process, and specifically the privileges delineation process, relies too heavily on the subjective judgment of medical staff department heads, then it is impossible for the board to verify the appropriateness of a particular recommendation *or* to ensure that the process is equally and consistently applied to all applicants.

How can the board know the appropriateness of a subjective judgment—in essence, what went on in the mind of a medical staff department head or credentials committee? How does the board know the department head or credentials committee would make the same recommendation for two different physician applicants if both had similar clinical skills and performance records but different social or economic relationships with these evaluators? How can the board know that certain department heads are *not* making the negative credentialing recommendations when they *should* be, because they fear being sued by the physician applicant? Unfortunately the answer to these and similar questions is that, under the vast majority of credentialing systems, *the board simply cannot know.*

Often there is no evidence that the *past practice* of renewal applicants is systematically evaluated and relied on by medical staff department heads and credentials committees to recommend privileges renewal, expansion, restriction, or revocation. This also is due to the subjectivity of the process.

A similar problem is that there rarely is evidence that the results of the hospital's quality assurance activities are meaningfully integrated into the reappointment and privileges renewal process. Each physician who reapplied for membership and privileges has had two years' worth of quality assurance monitoring and evaluation and peer review of the quality of his or her care. This is *precisely* the information that the reappointment process should rely on. Unfortunately it rarely does. What is the point of the hospital conducting these activities if the information they yield is not used?

To summarize, the most common credentialing problems are lack of definition of relative roles between the medical staff and the board; vagueness of medical staff criteria relating to clinical performance of applicants, or subjectivity of the process; failure to systematically evaluate past practice of the applicant; and failure to objectively integrate results of quality assurance and peer review activities into the process. These common problems usually will undermine a hospital's medical staff credentialing system, thus rendering it ineffective. Do any of these problems exist in your hospital's credentialing system? The next section will suggest a process to help overcome these common problems.

### Reaching a Final Decision

As mentioned, the board's role is to understand and evaluate the credentialing process used by the medical staff and to reach a final decision on appointment and privileges delineation for each candidate. To understand the process and recommendations made by the medical staff, the board needs to be aware of the criteria used by the medical staff to evaluate each candidate. These criteria then can be used by the board to evaluate the medical staff's decision-making process.

Decision-making criteria should be developed jointly by the medical staff and the board, incorporated into the medical staff bylaws, and consistently applied to each applicant. Using such criteria can help make the process of reaching a final decision more objective and can help establish a basis of fairness in consideration of all candidates.

When the board receives the medical staff's recommendation, it should be accompanied by the criteria used to evaluate the applicant and by a summary of the information received and verified by the medical staff, indicating which criteria were met. Then the board can use the decision criteria to evaluate the medical staff's review and recommendation process and to independently determine whether its final decision coincides with the medical staff's recommendation. If it does, the board can then approve the recommendation. However, if the board determines that the medical staff's decision is not consistent with the criteria, the board should reverse the recommendation in favor of a final decision that is in fact based on the criteria profile specific to each candidate. The board also should direct the medical staff to follow the criteria in considering all candidates. In this way the board both verifies whether the established credentialing process has been followed and also makes a final decision that is consistent with the process and the criteria that support it (Orlikoff, 1990, pp. 67-68).

This is an important point to stress. The board simply compares the medical staff recommendation for a particular applicant to that applicant's criteria profile. If the medical staff recommendation is consistent with the criteria, the board votes to approve the medical staff recommendation. If the recommendation and profile are inconsistent, *the board votes a decision that is mandated by the criteria.*

Obviously, for the credentialing process to work, there must be objective, measurable criteria for the medical staff to use in evaluating applicants and for the board to use in evaluating and voting on the recommendations of the medical staff. The next section discusses a method for developing such a criteria-based credentialing system.

### A Level 1 and Level 2 Criteria System

Hospital boards and medical staffs can take a variety of approaches to developing decision criteria. A simple two-level system is one approach.

Level 1 criteria would be an essential, minimum set; that is, if even one criterion is not met, the candidate would not be appointed or granted privileges to practice at the hospital. Examples of such "deal-breaker" criteria are:

- Valid medical license in all states that apply
- Verification of medical school, residency, or other required training
- Adequate and current malpractice insurance
- A completed application

For those physicians reapplying for medical staff membership, these additional level 1 criteria are usually added:

- Must have attended at least 50 percent of all medical staff meetings
- Must not have delinquent medical records for more than _________ (a specified period of time)

If your hospital is like the vast majority of hospitals, only level 1 criteria are used. That is, because every single criterion must be met for an applicant to join or remain on the medical staff, *every* criterion is a potential "deal-breaker."

The problem with the level 1 approach is its inflexibility. As a result, the medical staff resists the development and use of *criteria that measure the clinical skill and performance of a physician.* It is precisely these types of criteria that should be used in the credentialing process, but most medical staff would not like the idea of a negative credentialing decision being triggered by missing *one* clinical criterion (such as a high infection rate).

This is the reason why clinical criteria are nonexistent or vague in most hospitals' medical staff credentialing systems. This is also a fundamental reason why many trustees are uncomfortable with the credentialing process; they see objective, measurable criteria used for *administrative issues* but see no such criteria for *clinical issues*. The trustees get the sense that they must blindly trust the subjective judgment of the medical staff regarding clinical issues.

A way to correct this serious flaw in a credentialing system is to create level 2 criteria. Whereas failure to meet any single level 2 criterion would not result in denial of staff appointment or privileges, failure to meet a predefined threshold, perhaps 3 of 10, would trigger a negative credentialing decision.

This level 2 criteria system allows a great deal of flexibility and thus facilitates the use of objective *clinical* criteria. Bear in mind that the medical staff would develop both the level 2 criteria *and* the criteria threshold for a negative decision. Examples of possible level 2 criteria that are primarily clinically or quality related are shown in table 1.

Under this system, a board would get a criteria profile sheet for each physician applicant. It would show whether all level 1 criteria were met; what the level 2 criteria threshold was for negative action—missing 4 out of 8 or 3 out of 7 criteria, for example; which level 2 criteria were met; and the recommendation of the medical staff. The board then simply *compares* the recommendation for each candidate to that candidate's *criteria profile* and votes accordingly. If the recommendation is consistent with the criteria profile, the board votes to approve the recommendation. If inconsistent, the board votes *consistent with the criteria* and then communicates with the medical executive committee to determine why their recommendation was inconsistent with the established criteria.

A sample level 1 and level 2 evaluation form is shown in table 2. This form, initially developed and used by the medical staff, shows established criteria thresholds, which level 1 and level 2 criteria were met or not met, and the recommendation of the medical staff regarding Dr. Scalpel's reappointment. The board can easily review this form, make sure the medical staff's evaluation and recommendation are consistent with the criteria thresholds, and then vote. As the medical staff and the board gain experience in developing and using this evaluation method, new criteria may be added or existing criteria tightened or revised.

The level 1 and level 2 criteria system, developing various levels of criteria and then assigning different decision outcomes to each level, has several

**Table 1. Examples of Level 2 Medical Staff Quality-Related Credentialing Criteria**

1. Nosocomial (hospital-acquired) infection rates. (Note: Infection rate criteria and other quality-related criteria are usually rated in comparison to the arithmetic mean of the medical department in question. For example, a nosocomial infection rate that is *1 standard deviation* above the mean of the infection rate for the entire Internal Medicine Department can be used as a level 2 criterion.)

2. Inpatient mortality rates.

3. Surgical wound infection rates.

4. Unplanned returns to operating room; this can be expressed as a set percentage of a surgeon's cases or can be compared to the mean of the department.

5. Maximum cesarean section rates (as a percentage of an individual's cases).

6. Perioperative mortality rates.

7. Neonatal mortality rates.

8. Rates of unplanned readmissions to hospital.

9. Rates of unplanned transfers or returns to special care units.

10. Patient complaint rates.

11. Number of malpratice claims or filed lawsuits; either as an absolute number per year or as a statistical comparison to other physicians in the same department or on the entire medical staff.

12. Adequate use of privileges previously granted; frequency criteria for procedure-specific privileges delineation.

13. Abusive or disruptive behavior. (Note: This must be more specifically defined, such as arguments with patients, arguments with staff, sexual harassment of patients or staff, assaults on either patients or staff, inebriation or intoxication, or drug use. Also, this criterion is expressed as a defined maximum number of occurrences and *not* as a comparative percentage—for example: two instances of abusive or disruptive behavior during a 12-month period.

14. Department-specific requirements for continuing medical education *in addition to* those requirements for medical staff membership.

### Table 2. Sample Level 1 and Level 2 Evaluation Form

| Reappointment: Dr. Sam Scalpel<br>General Surgeon | Level 1: Must meet all<br>Level 2: Must meet 4 or more | |
|---|---|---|
| **Level 1 Criteria** | Evaluation<br>Meets | Evaluation<br>Does Not Meet |
| 1. Has a valid medical license (expiration date: 1992) | × | |
| 2. Has current and valid medical malpractice insurance ($1 million/$3 million coverage; expiration date: 1992) | × | |
| 3. Attended a minimum of 50% of all medical staff and medical staff department meetings | × | |
| 4. Had no medical records delinquent for more than 30 days | × | |
| Total | 4 | |
| **Level 2 Criteria** | | |
| 1. Surgical wound infection rate less than or equal to 10% of all cases | × | |
| 2. Unplanned returns to operating room less than or equal to 1 standard deviation above the mean for all surgeons in the department | | × |
| 3. Mortality rate less than or equal to 2 standard deviations above the mean for all surgeons in the department | × | |
| 4. Abusive/disruptive behavior (documented arguments with or assaults on patients and/or staff) occurred 4 or fewer times in the past 2 years | × | |
| 5. Patient complaints occurred in 7% or less of all cases treated | | × |
| 6. Four or fewer malpractice suits or claims occurred in the past 2 years | | × |
| 7. Obtained at least 30 hours of category 1 continuing medical education (CME) in the past 2 years | × | |
| 8. During the past 2 years has performed at least 1 of all procedures for which privileges are currently held | × | |
| Total | 5 | 3 |

Recommended for reappointment:     Yes __×__     No ______

______________ Chief, Department of Surgery

______________ Chair, Medical Staff Credentialing Committee

______________ Chair, Medical Executive Committee

advantages. Such criteria make the decision-making process more objective, consistent, and verifiable by the board; furthermore, they help ensure that several important criteria, which alone may not be actionable, nevertheless are considered during the evaluation process. The level 1 and level 2 criteria system also allows the integration of critically important clinical and quality criteria into the credentialing process. Joint development and use of the level 1 and level 2 criteria system also can lead to more informed, productive, and improved relationships throughout the hospital leadership team.

## Conclusion

Hospital governing boards, executives, and medical staffs that understand and adhere to the credentialing process and their respective roles in it can most effectively ensure a medical staff that is capable and competent to provide high-quality patient care. You and members of your board must remember that your primary responsibility in the credentialing process is to ensure that a criteria-based evaluation process exists and is being applied fairly and consistently to each medical staff candidate. Once you are assured that such a process is being used in the hospital, then the board can review the medical staff's recommendation against the established criteria, verify that the recommendation is appropriate, and make a final decision for each applicant.

Although the medical staff initiates establishment of the evaluation criteria and thresholds for decision making, your board should ensure that the criteria developed address administrative as well as clinical or quality-related issues as indicated in the level 1 and level 2 system described in this chapter. Such a system is the only way you can ensure thorough, objective, consistent, and fair evaluation of each candidate. And it is this approach to the credentialing process that leads to successful fulfillment of this critical board quality assurance responsibility.

## References

Blum, J. Study examines role of hospital boards in physician evaluation: economic credentialing may raise legal, political issues. *Modern Healthcare* 20(3); 30-31, Jan. 22, 1990.

Data banking. *QRC Advisor* 5(12):1, 6-8, Oct. 1989.

Joint Commission on Accreditation of Healthcare Organizations. *Report on the Joint Commission's Survey of Relationships among Governing Bodies, Management, and Medical Staffs in the United States Hospitals.* Chicago: JCAHO, 1987.

Key problems of the National Practitioner Data Bank. *Staff Privileges Report* 2(12):1-2, Jan. 1990.

National Practitioner Data Bank for Adverse Information on Physicians and Other Health Care Practitioners. 45 CFR Part 60 of §§401-432 of the Health Care Quality Improvement Act of 1986. Pub. L. 99-660, 100 Stat. 3784-3794, as amended by §402 of Pub. L. 100-177 Stat. 1007-1008 (42 U.S.C. 11101-11152).

Orlikoff, J. *Quality from the Top: Working with Hospital Governing Boards to Assure Quality Care—A Guide for Quality Assurance Professionals.* Chicago: Pluribus Press, 1990.

Orlikoff, J., and Totten, M. Medical staff appointments and privileges: key role of the governing board. *Trustee* 41(4):14-15, Apr. 1988.

Patrick v. Burget, 108 S.Ct. 1658 (1988).

# Credentialing: A Current Perspective and Legal Background

Arthur L. Pelberg, MD

This article reviews the development of physician credentialing for hospital privileges over the last 30 yr. Important developments are discussed in the admitting and clinical privilege areas. The second part of the article considers the legal aspects to credentialing and the avenues for challenging credentialing denials. Finally, a generic credentialing form for physicians is presented for use by health care organizations.

The first step in controlling the quality and utilization of any health care program is to obtain the appropriate physicians to provide the services. This is done through the organization's credentialing process. This paper gives a current perspective of credentialing including a discussion of some of the legal issues. The final section of the paper is a generic credentialing form that health care organizations can use.

A physician may have either admitting privileges, clinical privileges, or both. As recently as 20 years ago, a physician received his privileges very informally. The privileges were for life, were not re-evaluated, and were only revoked if the physician committed a major crime.[1] The criteria for privileging were very loose, and formal checking of credentials was rare.

Reprinted by permission of REVIEW PHYSICIAN'S NEWSLETTER, Volume 4, Page 8, 1989. Copyright American College of Utilization Review Physicians.

## Formalizing the Credentialing Process

Over the last 20 yr, several factors arose causing the credentialing process to become structured. These factors mainly impacted the hospitals and caused them to re-evaluate their processes for granting privileges to physicians. The first factor was the demand from third party payors, government, and other agencies to control utilization, quality, and appropriateness of services; the second, the high cost of medical technology limiting the hospital's ability to provide desired equipment for an unregulated medical staff; and the third, the recognition that financial resources for health care are limited.[2] These factors made credentialing a way for the hospital to ration limited hospital resources among physicians. This becomes even more important when looking to the future with a 30% surplus of physicians projected for the yr 2000.[2] A decrease in acute care hospital beds is also expected at the same time, creating more competition for hospital privileges among physicians and other health care providers.

## The Darling Case

The major cause for formalizing the credentialing process came from the *Darling v. Charleston Community Hospital* lawsuit, which formally established the principles of corporate negligence and corporate liability for hospitals.[1] Corporate negligence is the failure of those responsible for providing accommodations and facilities necessary to carry out the purposes of the hospital corporation to follow the established standards of conduct.[2] These include establishing the competence of the physicians on staff at the hospital. The Darling case went further in stating that the hospital will be considered a "health care provider" in supervising the competence of its visiting or attending staff.[2] The various committees and department heads act on behalf of the hospital. The hospital owes the patient a duty of care. Many cases have supported the Darling decision over the last 20 yr. The courts have stated that hospital liability is not limited to cases of actual knowledge of carelessness, but also includes cases where the hospital should have known which practitioners' conduct and practice of medicine were substandard.[1] This means the hospital was now responsible for formally checking the applicants for privileges to protect itself from liability in malpractice. The hospital could find itself responsible for a malpractice settlement if the physician on the staff committed malpractice while attending patients in the hospital. Over the past 20 yr, the hospital has become firmly established as a source of monetary gain in the litigious atmosphere of health care. Formalizing the credentialing process is one way hospitals can decrease their overall liability, both financially and operationally.

Since 1983 there has been an average increase of 50-60% in the number of applications for hospital privileges by physicians.[3] The total physician population grew by 40% from 1975-1985.[4] All this leads to greater competition for hospital privileges, at a time when the actual number of acute care hospitals is decreasing, for the first time this century. It also increases the potential for more litigation involving denial by hospitals for physician privileges, a subject to be covered later in this paper.

## The Purposes of Credentialing

There are many reasons why staff and clinical privileges are important for the physician and the hospital. From the physician's viewpoint, privileges potentially allow him or her to provide a higher standard of practice. Hospital practice has become an integral part of most physicians' professional activities and allows for increased medical care for the patient and increased income production for the physician. The hospital gives the physician access to technology and interaction with medical specialists, sub-specialists, and other staff members. Hospitals can provide ancillary services and continuing education. Finally, social and other informal benefits (e.g., practice management) can be obtained by being on staff.

The hospital needs credentialing of its physician staff to ensure the standards of quality and efficiency of patient care. Credentialing allows the hospital to control costs as well as capture market share in its geographic area. Corporate liability and negligence become more controlled through credentialing physicians. Hospital malpractice cases increased 53% from 1983 to 1985. Hospitals paid an average of $40,300 per claim in 1985 and insurance premiums for hospital liability rose to $1.3 billion in 1985.[5] Credentialing can allow the hospital to project needs for new programs, to change programs, or to delete programs. It also can help the hospital budget for successive years by knowing who is on staff and how those physicians utilize their clinical privileges.

## The Credentialing Process

The institutional criteria for credentialing are established by the board of directors of the hospital. These criteria relate to effective resource allocation, financial efficiency, quality of care, and institutional objectives.[3] The board must also make sure that the hospital has the facilities to care for the patients of applicant physicians. The medical staff is required to set

the professional criteria, including professional competence, eduction, training, performance, professional character, and fitness of the applying physician. Further requirements are set up by the Joint Commission on Accreditation of Healthcare Organizations in their *Accreditation Manual for
Hospitals.*[6] The medical staff recommends physicians for staff privileges
and the governing board has the final authority to approve or deny privileges.

The medical staff by-laws must have an objective set of criteria for granting, postponing, and denying staff privileges. The by-laws must be applied
uniformly to all physicians seeking staff privileges. This is an area where
litigation may arise in the credentialing process. If privileges are to be
denied, that denial must be based on quality of care issues or operational
efficiency of the hospital; some courts have approved denial of privileges
for economic reasons.[5] Physicians with personality problems have been
denied privileges legally as well.

State law determines the types of health professionals eligible for staff
privileges. In California, dentists, podiatrists, psychologists, and physicians can obtain staff privileges. In Pennsylvania, only physicians and dentists can be on staff. The District of Columbia allows nurse practitioners,
nurse midwives, and nurse anesthetists to be on staff.[2]

Initially, it can take up to four months before all the information is
processed and a decision on granting privileges can be made. If the privileges are approved, the physician serves in a provisional category for a
designated period of time (usually 6 months) to permit evaluation of his
or her quality and performance. Upon successful completion of the provisional period, he or she will be granted privileges in one of that hospital's
staff categories, which typically include courtesy, consulting, active, temporary, honorary, provisional, or other designations.


## Clinical Privileges

Clinical privileges are those privileges that permit the physician to provide medical or other patient care services in the granting institution. These
privileges must be within well defined limits, based on the individual's
professional license, experience, competence, ability, and judgment.[6] Clinical privileges are the "job description" for each physician practicing in the
hospital. The Joint Commission on Accreditation of Healthcare Organizations mandates that all providers who give patient care services in the
hospital must have clinical privileges.[7] These privileges must be based on
evidence of expertise as supplied by the physician and as personally checked
by the granting hospital. Clinical privilege determinations are mandated
because the Joint Commission on Accreditation of Healthcare Organiza-

tions states that "within the medical staff department, across department or services, and between members and nonmembers of the staff who have delineated clinical privileges the same level of quality must be assured."[7]

The criteria for granting clinical privileges in a certain clinical department (e.g., Internal Medicine, Pediatrics, Surgery) are established by the medical staff of that department. The medical staff will recommend to the hospital board of directors to grant or deny the clinical privileges. It is the board of directors who have final approval or denial of each physician's clinical privileges. The process and requirements for granting the clinical privileges must be clearly documented in the medical staff by-laws and uniformly applied to all applicants, as is done for staff privileges. Criteria for clinical privileges should be as detailed and specific as possible.[17] The physician usually requests the clinical privileges he or she plans to use.

## Categories of Clinical Privileges

There are several ways of categorizing clinical privileges. Four of the most commonly used categories are:

1. Practitioner Specialty—A physician who is board-eligible or -certified in the specialty is presumed to be qualified to perform all the diagnostic and therapeutic activities within that specialty.[7]
2. Patient Risk—Each patient admitted to the hospital is classified according to their severity of illness and risk. The practitioner's degree of training or experience determines the category of patient for which he or she can have privileges.[7]
3. Procedure List—This is a comprehensive list of procedures each division of clinical practice supplies for the physician to check off. This can also be a list of illnesses, injuries, treatments, or conditions.[7]
4. Combined—This is a combination of the above categories.[7] Usually, it includes a procedure list and a patient risk category. Currently, the combined category is becoming popular for hospital use.

There are drawbacks to each of the above categories. Under the practitioner's specialty, the extent of training for each specialist in the same category may be different. This could lead to one specialist having certain skills and another not having those skills, yet both having the same clinical privileges. It is often very difficult to assign each patient to a risk category on admission to the hospital. Also, the patient's risk could change while in the hospital and the physician caring for the patient may not have privileges to care for the patient in the new category. The physician would have to call in a consultant who had the proper clinical privileges. The procedure list is often very cumbersome and incomplete. It is also very difficult to apply to physicians in the more cognitive fields of medicine. Combining the categories seems to decrease the individual drawbacks.

Clinical privileges are not static. A physician can apply for new privileges at any time. The Joint Commission on Accreditation of Healthcare Organizations requires that clinical privileges be renewed at least every 2 yr. Through this review, the hospital is obligated to assure that the physician has maintained his or her expertise and that new deficiencies have not developed. The hospital is required to check the national clearinghouse for physicians, AMA files, state medical boards, personal references, as well as other sources for information about the physician. This process protects the patient, the hospital, and the physician.

## Denial of Privileges

The granting of privileges is a two-step process. The physician needs to have staff privileges to admit the patient to the hospital and then the physician needs clinical privileges to provide medical services to the patient in the hospital. Either of these privileges can be denied to the physician. There has been increasing litigation between physicians and hospitals over the denial of or decrease in hospital privileges—either staff or clinical. Before litigation occurs, the physician usually has gone through a grievance process outlined in the medical staff by-laws.

The hospital must be sure that it is very familiar with its by-laws, it observes the time requirements, the committee is impartial, and it documents the reasons (usually patient care or hospital operation issues) for denial of privileges.[8] Privileges may also be denied if the hospital is unable to care for the type of patients the physician will be admitting. Other reasons include a closed medical staff and exclusive physician contracts. In a closed medical staff, the physician is denied privileges not because of his or her qualifications but because of a problem in the utilization of hospital facilities, equipment, personnel, or beds.[2]

Denial of privileges has been approved by the courts under the arrangements of exclusive contracts between a hospital and a physician or physician group. The courts have stated that if the contracts promote better control and standardization of the specialized department, assurance of full-time coverage and continuity of care for patients, or higher quality of patient care and teaching, then consultative services or privileges to other physicians of the same specialty may be denied.[8] In 1984, hospitals in the United States had exclusive contracts with physicians in the following percentages: Pathology services, 62.3%; Radiology, 59.9%; Emergency Services, 48.7%; Anesthesia, 30.2%; Cardiology, 12.7%; and Internal Medicine, 11.8%.[4] Under exclusive contracts, the hospital becomes specifically responsible for the action of the physicians under the doctrine of agency — vicarious liability and respondent superior.[1] If privileges are denied, the hospital must furnish a written notice to the physician in a defined period of time, which may vary.

## Legal Challenges to the Denial of Privileges

The physician has several avenues to challenge the hospital's denial of his or her staff or clinical privileges. Under due process, the physician whose staff privileges have been denied is entitled to a reasonable opportunity to prepare for a hearing and be heard by an unbiased tribunal. Adequate and appropriate notice must be provided to the physician.[9] Notice must include the charges and nature of the hearing and all evidence and witnesses to be used in the hearing against the physician. If any of the notices or hearings is not conducted properly, the physician's due process has been violated and legally he or she may be able to have privileges reinstated. Included in due process is the physician's right not to have his or her reputation slandered or libeled before, during, or after a meeting held to determine staff privileges. In California the question of substantive due process was raised by the court in Anton v. San Antonio Community Hospital: did the facts of the case support the conclusion of denial of privileges to the physician?[1] The American Medical Association (AMA) and the Joint Commission on Accreditation of Healthcare Organizations in their official policy uphold strict observance of a physician's right to due process in the credentialing procedures. Presently, the law requires that the governing board of a hospital adhere to a minimum of due process in its appointment of physicians to its medical staff and not to engage in arbitrary and capricious or malicious exercise of its discretion.[9] Most medical staff bylaws substantially exceed the minimal requirements for due process and the number of legal cases supported by the lack of due process in credentialing denials has decreased.

The physician can challenge a denial of credentials under the Civil Rights Act of 1871, section 1963. The physician must allege that the committee acted under "color of state law" (color of state law include any hospital receiving funds under Hill-Burton, Medicare, or Medicaid) and that the committee violated the denied physician's rights on the basis of race, sex, color, or national origin.[1]

In the case of *Wills v. Santa Ana Community Hospital Association*, the question of civil conspiracy was raised in the denial of a physician's privileges.[1] Civil conspiracy is a combination of two or more persons, joined together to accomplish an unlawful purpose by concerted action or some purpose, not in itself unlawful, by unlawful means.

The questions of violation of the Sherman Antitrust Law have been increasing in the denial of clinical privileges for physicians. To sustain a case action under the Sherman Act, the plaintiff must establish by evidence: 1) a connection with interstate commerce sufficient to involve federal jurisdiction; 2) a contract, combination, or conspiracy among the defendants that results in; 3) an unreasonable restraint of trade; and 4) resultant injury to the plaintiff's business or property.[11] Physicians can allege that one or more channels of interstate commerce have been affected by the denial of privileges through treatment of patients who traveled across state lines; the hospital's delivery of services to out-of-state patients; purchase by the hospital or physician of drugs, supplies or equipment marketed in interstate commerce; and interstate flow of insurance payments including those of Medicare, Medicaid, and private carriers.

In *Zambi v. William Beaumont Hospital*, the Supreme Court held that the local nonprofit hospital business sufficiently affected interstate commerce to place hospitals within the jurisdictional reach of the antitrust laws.[1] Generally, courts have been making it easier to challenge denial of staff privileges under the antitrust laws.

Due process, civil rights, and antitrust provisions are presently the major litigation tools physicians are using in challenging the denial or restriction of their clinical or staff privileges by a hospital. It can take from 3-5 yr before a case actually gets to court.


## Future Questions

The future of hospital credentialing holds many unanswered questions. Who will be eligible for credentials? What mechanisms will be used for credentialing by hospitals and other health care organizations? How will litigation over credentials change the relation between hospitals and physicians? Are we moving to a national credentialing center with the formation of a national clearinghouse for lawsuits involving physicians under PL99-660, the Health Care Quality Improvement Act of 1986? The future will be interesting.


## Acknowledgements

I would like to thank Joseph Trautlein, M.D. for his review and comments on the manuscript and Bonnie Brandt for her accurate and efficient processing of this article.

## References


1. Hirsh H. The Physician and Hospital Privileges. Transactions and Studies of the College of Physicians of Philadelphia 1983;5:285-308.
2. Affeldt J. Clinical privileges—what ahead. Connecticut Medicine 1983;47:779-783.
3. Brook D, Morrisey M. Credentialing: Say goodbye to the rubber stamp. Hospitals 1985;59:50-52.
4. Guinklein D. Impact of exclusive contracts on medical staff bylaws. Quality Review Bulletin 1987:215-218.
5. Burda D. Liability reshapes hospital physician relationships. Hospitals 1987:56-60.
6. Joint Commission on Accreditation of Hospitals. *Accreditation Manual for Hospitals/88*. Chicago 1987, p. 101.
7. Jessee W. "Delineating Clinical Privileges," Quality Review Bulletin, June 1987, pp. 209-214.
8. Lombardo Trostorff, D. "Medical Staff Privileging: How to Avoid Pitfalls in the Administrative Process," Quality Review Bulletin, June 1987 pp. 198-204.
9. Winters, A. and R. Toth, "Texas Physicians Entitled to Due Process in Privileges Dispute," Texas Medicine, November 1986, 82, pp. 50-51.
10. Cowan, R., and C. Montgomery. "Hospital Credentialing" Journal of the Mississippi State Medical Association 28(1), January 1987, pp. 9-12.
11. Tabor, W. "The Battle for Hospital Privileges III The Antitrust Frontier," Journal of the American Medical Association 251 (12), March 23-30, 1984 pp. 1602-1605.


## Appendix

The final portion of this paper is a generic credentialing form to be used by hospitals as well as other health care organizations for staff privileges. The form covers the requirements of the Joint Commission on Accreditation of Health Care Organizations. The form can be placed on a word processor and have the various fields changed to the needs of the health care organization. The first page lists the essential data to be collected on the physician. Under the miscellaneous section, item two asks for letters from training directors, other hospitals, or chairmen of departments, stating the physician has competence to perform any procedures he or she may list on the clinical privileges form. The physician will often have a list of actual chart numbers, or the names of patients on whom they have performed procedures. Item eight asks for any activities the physician has carried out to help support or enhance the health care organization's image. This may include speaking engagements, articles in a local paper, or television or radio shows.

The third page is a listing of procedures and clinical activities including severity of illness with a comparison to hospital norms. The outpatient section may be used as it becomes appropriate for the health care institution.

The fourth page covers the inpatient aspect of the physician's practice covering morbidity and mortality. The areas with an asterisk indicate that a file with further written documentation should be kept to explain the variations in the physician's practice. Item eighteen includes patients hospitalized for research and special study purposes which could affect the utilization review issues under item seventeen. Many times research patients may be denied days or reimbursement but should not be considered in the normal pool of patients. The last three items under general questions should be completed by the department chairman, dean, or chief of staff.

### Generic Credential File

### General Information
  1. Name
  2. Office and Home addresses and phone numbers
  3. Spouse and Dependents
  4. Previous Employer
  5. Social Security Number
  6. Present Health Status/Chronic or Communicable Disease
  7. Malpractice Insurance
  8. Privileges at other hospitals

### Special Medical Information
  1. Department
  2. Specialty
  3. Subspecialty
  4. Other
  5. Current Staff Category
  6. Past Staff Categories
  7. Years Since Initial Appointment
  8. Academic Position

### Medical Background
  1. Medical Education
  2. Internship and Residency

3. Fellowship
4. Other Training/Education
5. Board Certifications and Dates (Number of Specialty Board Certificates)
6. Medical License state/states (License Numbers)
7. Privileges at other hospitals (Name of Hospital, Type of Privilege)

**Miscellaneous**
1. Letters of Recommendation. List the names and addresses of three physicians who will be writing letters on your behalf
2. Letters/lists of proven competence for procedures
3. Statement of investigation or loss of license, loss of privileges or membership on medical staffs, loss of professional society or specialty board status, loss of privileges with an HMO, PPO, or other managed health care system
4. Statement of any and all malpractice activity including being named in a lawsuit, settlement of a lawsuit, or loss of a lawsuit
5. Letters for reappointment from the Department Chairman or others
6. Documentation of Continuing Education
7. Publications/Lectures
8. Public Relations
9. Research Activities

# Credentialing of Emergency Physicians: Support for Delineation of Privileges in Invasive Procedures

Edward A. Ramoska, MD, Alfred D. Sacchetti, MD, Todd M. Warden, MD

The American College of Emergency Physicians states in its "Guidelines for Delineation of Clinical Privileges in Emergency Medicine" that a qualified emergency physician "performs such definitive treatment as falls within the physician's competence."[1] The exact definition as to what treatments or procedures an emergency physician is competent to perform, though, remains nebulous.

The resuscitation and stabilization of critical patients is one of the hallmarks of the emergency physician; yet in many institutions emergency physicians are granted very restricted clinical privileges. New emergency physicians or even entire groups of physicians may meet severe resistance from the hospital staff when requesting privileges for invasive procedures. Personal experience has shown this problem of credentialing to be most evident in institutions in which the style of emergency medicine changes abruptly from passive to active with the introduction of newer career emergency physicians.

Why emergency physicians should undergo a different credentialing process from the remainder of the medical staff is unclear. Other generalists or specialists need only cite their completion of a residency or special course to be granted specific privileges, whereas emergency physicians may have to petition specific department chairmen for permission to perform inva-



**373**

sive procedures. In other situations emergency physicians have to establish credibility with existing hospital staff who may have traditionally performed the same procedures. In fact, the first time an invasive procedure is performed by an emergency physician, that same physician may find himself or herself defending those actions before the chairman of another department.

The source of this restriction of clinical privileges is multifactorial and probably varies from institution to institution. Past experiences with less competent or less aggressive emergency physicians certainly prejudice many physicians' perceptions of emergency personnel. Ignorance of the specialty of emergency medicine, our training programs, or the commitment of practice-track physicians is a very real problem.[2] Ego infringement, protection of turf, and financial considerations may also play a role in restriction of clinical procedures.

Most discussions concerning the credentialing of emergency physicians are based strictly on personal opinions. In an effort to provide more objective evidence to support emergency physicians, we studied the competence of emergency physicians to perform specific invasive procedures.

## Materials and Methods

Methodist Hospital is an acute care university-affiliated community hospital having a 280-bed capacity located in Philadelphia, Pennsylvania. The emergency department has an annual census of 26,000 visits with a mix of medical, surgical, trauma, pediatric, and gynecologic patients.

All patients undergoing an invasive procedure by a board-certified emergency physician during a 1-year period were included in the study. The characteristics of the study physicians are presented in Table 1. Procedures performed by emergency medicine, internal medicine, surgery, or gynecology residents under the direct supervision of an emergency physician were not included. Procedures attempted by residents but not successfully performed and subsequently completed by the attending emergency physician were included. Invasive procedures are defined as the following: central venous catheterization, endotracheal intubation, tube thoracostomy, transvenous pacemaker insertion, lumbar puncture, peritoneal lavage, indwelling arterial catheterization, cricothyroidotomy, and thoracotomy. Procedures such as peripheral intravenous access, Foley catheter placement, and nasogastric intubation, although technically invasive, were not included in the study because these procedures rarely present credentialing problems.

On patients meeting the inclusion criteria, a data sheet including the following information was completed: patient name, hospital number, procedure(s) performed, exact technique employed, immediate patient outcome and complications, patient follow-up and delayed complications, and results at surgery or autopsy. Immediately available information was collected at the completion of the procedure, and information on delayed complications was obtained through monitoring the patient's hospital course. In cases of death in the emergency department, complications were identified clinically if no diagnostic studies were obtained.

Information concerning the difficulty of any particular procedure was recorded under a Comments section on the data sheet. Procedures requiring multiple attempts or alternate approaches were recorded along with the complications of any of the attempts.

## Results

A total of 408 procedures were performed on 267 patients. Table 2 lists these procedures along with the number of times each was performed and their complications. The average number of procedures per patient was 1.53, with 157 patients undergoing one procedure, 91 undergoing two, 11 undergoing three, 4 undergoing four, and 4 undergoing five. In all patients in whom a procedure was attempted, it was successfully completed, although some patients required multiple attempts or alternate approaches. For example, a patient unable to be intubated nasally may have been orally intubated, or a failed supraclavicular central venous catheter may have subsequently been placed infraclavicularly.

**Table 1. Characteristics of Board-certified Emergency Physicians Studied**

| Physician | Age | Residency Training (length of Training [yrs]) | Years in Practice* |
|---|---|---|---|
| 1 | 33 | Emergency medicine (3) | 4.5 |
| 2† | 33 | Emergency medicine (3) | 4.5 |
| 3† | 32 | Emergency medicine (3) | 3.5 |
| 4 | 32 | Emergency medicine (3) | 2.5 |

*Number of years after residency that physician has been practicing emergency medicine at the time of study.

†Full-time emergency physicians but devote 50% of practice at study emergency department and 50% at a different emergency department.

Endotracheal tube placement was correctly assessed at the time of the procedure in all intubated patients. Supportive ventilation through the endotracheal tube was not attempted in any patient prior to proper tube placement.

A total of 13 complications were encountered during the study, all of which occurred with either the central venous catheterizations or the intubations. With the exception of hoarseness, all of the complications occurred in the immediate postprocedure period.

Twenty-two (11%) of the intubated patients were extubated in the emergency department, and of these, 20 were discharged to home after a short observation period. All of the discharged patients had had drug overdoses. Thirteen of the intubated patients were in infants, 8 of whom were premature. The intubations on these premature infants were performed in the obstetrics/nursery suite, when emergency physicians were called to help with unusually difficult situations.

---

**Table 2. Invasive Procedures Performed by Emergency Physicians**

| Procedure | No. Performed | Complications |
|---|---|---|
| Intubations | | |
| Oral | 100 | 2* |
| Nasal | 98 | 7‡ |
| Total | 198 | 9 |
| Central Venous Catheterization | 143 | 4‡ |
| Tube thoracostomy | 22 | — |
| Lumbar puncture | 19 | — |
| Peritoneal lavage | 9 | — |
| Tranvenous pacemaker insertion | 8 | — |
| Arterial catheterization | 4 | — |
| Thoracotomy | 3 | — |
| Cricothyroidotomy | 2 | — |
| TOTAL | 408 | 13 |

*Laryngitis
†One laryngitis, one arrhythmia, five moderate epistaxis (defined as bleeding controlled with pressure but not requiring packing).
‡Three arterial punctures, one pneumothorax. (The 143 cannulations required a total of 160 puncture attempts.)

## Discussion

That emergency physicians can successfully perform complex and invasive procedures has been one of the intuitive cornerstones of the field of emergency medicine. One need only look at Roberts and Hedges' *Clinical Procedures in Emergency Medicine* to appreciate the array of technical skills employed by emergency physicians.[3] Within the specialty and at institutions familiar with emergency medicine, proficiency in invasive techniques is axiomatic. In hospitals unaccustomed to aggressive emergency management, the ability of the emergency physician to perform these tasks successfully must be proved. The proof of this competency may be obtained through multiple meetings with the chairmen of more traditional departments, letters of reference, or even trial periods of limited privileges.

Little objective data exist documenting the competency of emergency physicians in performing procedures. One previous study has shown emergency physicians competent in the stabilization of pediatric patients.[4] The data presented in this study demonstrate objective evidence that emergency physicians can successfully complete specific invasive procedures in the emergency department.

The overall success rate and complication rate of central venous catheterizations and intubations compare well with results reported in previous studies.[4-14] Tables 3 and 4 present a comparison of our data with those of other groups. These comparisons, although supportive, are not entirely

| Table 3. Comparison of Complication Rates for Intubation | |
|---|---|
| Complication Rate | Reference |
| Epistaxis (moderate) | |
| 5/98 = 5.1% | |
| 5/71 = 7.0% | 5 |
| Laryngitis | |
| 3/198 = 1.5% | |
| 14/317 = 4.4% | 6 |
| = 3.0% | 7 (review) |
| = 33–50% | 8 (review) |
| Total complication rates | |
| 9/198 = 4.5% | |
| 9/300 = 10.0% | 9 |
| 7/71 = 10.0% | 5 |
| 38/43 = 88.4% | 10 |

valid, because the previous studies examined primarily the competence of house officers rather than attending physicians. All of the complications encountered have been reported previously and have occurred even with meticulous attention to technique.

The lack of complications with the other procedures studied may only be a function of the small number performed during the study period. It is inevitable that should a sufficient number of procedures be collected, complications would occur. Again, however, the fact remains that the procedures performed were technically correct and the physicians demonstrated an ability to do them properly.

The purpose of these data, however, is not to prove that emergency physicians are better than other medical groups at performing invasive proce-

| Table 4. Comparison of Complications of Central Venous Catheterizations* | |
|---|---|
| Complication Rate | Reference |
| Arterial puncture | |
| 3/160 = 1.9% | |
| 6/554 = 1.1% | 11 |
| 8/500 = 1.6% | 12 |
| 6/210 = 2.9% | 13 |
| 2/61 = 3.3% | 14 |
| Pneumothorax | |
| 1/160 = 0.6% | |
| 3/554 = 0.5% | 11 |
| 5/500 = 1.0% | 12 |
| 5/210 = 2.4% | 13 |
| 3/61 = 4.9% | 14 |
| Total | |
| 4/160 = 2.5% | |
| 18/500 = 3.6% | 12 |
| 22/554 = 4.0% | 11 |
| 20/210 = 9.5% | 13 |
| 8/61 = 13.1% | 14 |

*Because each attempt may cause a problem, complication rates are based on puncture attempts rather than number of catheters placed. This same calculation technique is used in all the comparison studies.

dures, but only to document their competency in doing them. The fact that all these procedures were done emergently provides further support for this argument.

That emergency physicians should be performing invasive procedures cannot be disputed. It is totally unrealistic to expect a physician completely capable of performing a life-saving intervention to withhold care pending the arrival of a consultant. This situation becomes even more absurd when it is the less-experienced resident of the consultant who arrives to actually perform the procedure. Despite the logic of this argument, it may be difficult to convince a department chairman who has never seen a career emergency physician perform the given procedure. Personal experience has shown that discussions about training programs and past accomplishments often do little to overcome preconceived opinions. It is only through direct exposure to good emergency medicine, usually under a very attentive eye, that many skeptics are converted.

The heterogeneity of many emergency department staffs also presents difficulties in the delineation of privileges. Critics will often cite the performances of noncareer emergency physicians as evidence for limiting the privileges of an entire emergency staff.

Despite these differences, emergency physicians must insist that credentialing of their staff be performed in the same manner as other physician members of the hospital. Credentialing must be on an individual basis and through the chairman or director of the emergency department. It must not be generic for an entire department. In internal medicine and surgery departments, privileges are granted on an individual basis. Specifically trained internists are permitted to place Swan-Ganz catheters or perform endoscopy, whereas only certain surgeons are granted thoracic or vascular privileges. Variability in training of emergency physicians must be approached in a like manner.

The data presented in this study demonstrate that emergency physicians can perform invasive procedures. Whether a particularly obstructive member of a credentialing committee is willing to accept this information when he or she will not accept arguments about prior residency training is unknown. However, emergency physicians can present the argument, "Here are data showing that physicians with training similar to mine are competent with these invasive procedures. The credentials committee must now provide evidence to the contrary."

It is also valuable to collect this type of information in an ongoing fashion. Such cumulative data serve as an excellent referral source during any discussions concerning a recent complication. One additional benefit to this manner of prospective data collection is that it complies well with the recently revised Joint Commission on Accreditation of Hospitals Standards for Quality Assurance.

## References


1. American College of Emergency Physicians: Guidelines for Delineation of Clinical Privileges. Ann Emerg Med 1985;14:1218-1220
2. Lowe RA, Knopp RK: Respect and commitment in emergency medicine. Am J Emerg Med 1987;5:174-176
3. Roberts JR, Hedges JR: Clinical Procedures in Emergency Medicine. Philadelphia, Saunders, 1985
4. Sacchetti A, Carraccio C, Warden T, et al: Community hospital management of pediatric emergencies: implications for pediatric emergency medical services. Am J Emerg Med 1986;4:10-13
5. Tintinalli JE, Claffey J: Complications of nasotracheal intubations. Ann Emerg Med 1981;10:142-144
6. Jones G, Hale DE, Wasmuth CE, et al: A survey of acute complications associated with endotracheal intubation. Cleve Clin Q 1968;35:23-31
7. Lewis RN, Swerdlow M: Hazards of endotracheal anaesthesia. 1964;36:504-515
8. Blanc VF, Tremblay NG: The complications of tracheal intubation: a new classification with a review of the literature. Anesth Analg 1974;53:202-213
9. Danzl DF, Thomas DM: Nasotracheal intubations in the emergency department. Crit Care Med 1980;8:677-682
10. Taryle DA, Chandler JE, Good JT, et al: Emergency room intubations—complications and survival. Chest 1979;75:541-543
11. Eisenhauer ED, Derveloy RJ, Hastings PR: Prospective evaluation of central venous pressure catheters in a large city-county hospital. Ann Surg 1982;196:560-564
12. Sterner S, Plummer DW, Clinton J, et al: A comparison of the supraclavicular approach and the infraclavicular approach for subclavian vein catheterization. Ann Emerg Med 1986;15:421-424
13. Schug CB, Culhane DE, Knopp RK: Subclavian vein catheterization in the emergency department: a comparison of guidewire and non-guidewire techniques. Ann Emerg Med 1986;15:769-773
14. Abraham E, Shapiro M, Podolsky S: Central venous catheterization in the emergency setting. Crit Care Med 1983;11:515-517

# Denying Hospital Privileges to Non-Physicians: Does Quality of Care Justify a Potential Restraint of Trade?

Gayle Reindl

## I. Introduction

Much of the recent increase in antitrust litigation in the health care field is due to suits by health care professionals alleging antitrust violations when hospitals have denied them staff privileges.[1] In addition to individual physicians, non-physician health care providers such as podiatrists, clinical psychologists, nurse-midwives, nurse-anesthetists, and chiropractors seek hospital privileges and have legally challenged privilege denials.[2] The large number of cases indicates the strength of the competing interests involved.[3] For a health professional, access to a hospital is vital to fully practice his profession. For a hospital, the ability to be selective in choosing its staff is vital to the quality of its service.

A plaintiff's allegation that the denial of privileges is an illegal group boycott and the hospital's assertion in defense that it must maintain its quality of care present special problems to an antitrust court. The variety and inconsistency of judicial approaches to analyzing quality of care as a justification for exclusion[4] suggest the difficulty of reconciling these competing interests under the antitrust laws in a way that prevents anticompetitive abuses without interfering with the legitimate functioning of hospitals. In struggling with these cases, courts have not adequately distinguished between denial of privileges to an individual physician and exclusion of an entire group of non-physicians.[5] However, there are clear differences between quality of care as a rationale for excluding an individual physician and as a justification for barring a group of non-physicians. Because of these differences, exclusion of a group merits heightened antitrust scrutiny.

Beginning with an overview of group boycott law, this Note discusses the issue of hospital privileges, focusing on specific non-physician groups seeking privileges. After examining a denial of privileges as a group boycott and quality of care as a defense, this Note surveys judicial approaches to such a defense. As this Note will show, there are significant differences between a quality of care rationale asserted against individuals and asserted against groups. Because of these differences, primarily the greater potential anticompetitive effects of excluding an entire group of competitors, this Note concludes with a recommendation that judicial scrutiny of quality of care as a defense be based on a substantial relation and least restrictive alternative test when quality is asserted as a justification for excluding a group. A court should demand that a quality standard invoked to deny privileges to non-physicians be substantially related to the procompetitive justification asserted for the standard and that the standard be the least restrictive alternative for achieving that procompetitive justification.

## II. Overview of Antitrust Law

Section one of the Sherman Act states that "[e]very contract, combination in the form of trust or otherwise, or conspiracy, in restraint of trade or commerce among the several States, or with foreign nations, is declared to be illegal."[6] Relatively early in the history of litigation under this provision, the United States Supreme Court decided that Congress could not have intended such a potentially broad proscription of trade.[7] The Court, therefore, formulated the "rule of reason," declaring that only conduct that unreasonably restrains trade violates the Sherman Act.[8] Under the rule of reason, a court analyzes in detail the challenged conduct in a specific market and weights the procompetitive and anticompetitive effects. Where anticompetitive effects predominate, the conduct will be declared unreasonably restrictive of trade, thus illegal.[9]

Because applying the rule of reason consumed much judicial time and because certain practices were repeatedly found to be anticompetitive in various contexts, the Court has, over the years, declared certain trade restrictions per se illegal.[10] Having specific, clearly defined per se offenses conserves judicial time and enhances predictability in the conduct of business.[11] Because a per se offense includes a presumption of anticompetitive effect,[12] a plaintiff need not show the challenged conduct has an anticompetitive effect in a specific market, but only that a defendant did the act alleged.

One type of conduct that has been accorded per se status is a group boycott or concerted refusal to deal,[13] recently defined by the Court as "joint efforts . . . to disadvantage competitors by 'either directly denying or persuading or coercing suppliers or customers to deny relationships the competitors need in the competitive struggle.'"[14] A group boycott is a somewhat amorphous offense because almost any joint conduct that results in denial of a business relationship to a competitor may be characterized as a group boycott.[15] Therefore, the courts have not found that anything a plaintiff labels a group boycott is per se illegal, but have instead applied the rule of reason in certain contexts, so that only conduct with clearly anticompetitive effects would be found illegal.[16] Group boycotts thus became a quasi per se offense. In *Northwest Wholesale Stationers, Inc v. Pacific Stationery and Printing Co.*,[17] the Supreme Court attempted to clarify the confusion in group boycott law by declaring that only where a plaintiff can show that a defendant "possesses market power or exclusive access to an element essential to effective competition,"[18] may a court find an alleged group boycott per se illegal.[19] Where a plaintiff cannot make this showing, the alleged group boycott should be evaluated under the rule of reason.[20]


## III. Hospital Staff Privileges


### A. Overview of Staff Privileges

A health care provider must have staff privileges in order to admit his patients to a hospital and to care for them there.[21] A hospital's decision whether to grant these privileges is typically made by a committee of the medical staff, physicians who have privileges at the institution, by applying criteria in the hospital's by-laws.[22] This decision may be reviewed by the entire medical staff and is subject to approval by the hospital's board of directors or trustees.[23]

The Joint Commission on Accreditation of Hospitals (JCAH), a body formed and run by physicians and hospitals, is responsible for accrediting most of the hospitals in the country.[24] The JCAH has established several categories of hospital privileges. These categories include "clinical privileges," whereby a provider may not admit patients to a hospital but he may provide treatment there, as well as privileges providing for varying levels of participation on the medical staff itself.[25] The most advantageous category for a practitioner is full membership on the medical staff, with its attendant admission privileges and voting rights in setting medical policy.

Whether an applicant is granted privileges is critical to him, both professionally and economically.[26] If certain tasks of his profession, such as surgical procedures, must be done in a hospital, the lack of privileges means that his range of practice is significantly curtailed. If he has no privileges and one of his patients needs treatment that can only be provided in a hospital, he must refer the patient to a provider with privileges and he may never get the patient back. Furthermore, if patients know the applicant cannot use a hospital, they may elect not to go to him at all.[27]

There has historically been some degree of conflict between physicians on the medical staff, concerned primarily that the hospital provides the facilities, support staff, and equipment the doctors need, and the hospital administration, concerned primarily with budgetary and efficiency matters.[28] Recent economic changes in the market for health and hospital services are likely to intensify this conflict with regard to admission privileges. There is currently a surplus of some types of physicians, which is expected to increase in the future.[29] The resulting increased competition for patients may lead physicians on staff to deny privileges to unwanted competitors.[30] In addition, the recent change to a prospective payment method for Medicare payments to hospitals has led to empty beds because hospitals are discharging patients earlier.[31] While hospitals may have an incentive to increase their medical staff to provide patients to fill the empty beds, hospitals must also appease the doctors already on staff to encourage them to admit more patients.[32] Finally, the development of preferred provider organizations (PPO's) promises to increase price competition among hospitals. One commentator predicts this will only increase tension between the medical staff and hospital administration as physicians respond to the increased competition by trying to close the staff while administrators want a larger staff to increase business.[33]

## B. Non-Physicians and Hospital Privileges

Until 1985, the Joint Commission on Accreditation of Hospitals required that medical staff membership be restricted to physicians and dentists.[34] However, partially because of antitrust suits against the JCAH by non-physician groups categorically denied staff privileges,[35] the JCAH relaxed its criteria and now permits each hospital to decide for itself whether to grant staff privileges to independent non-physician health care providers.[36] This change may encourage non-physicians to apply for privileges and to sue under the antitrust laws if privileges are denied.

Several specific non-physician groups desire hospital privileges and have legally challenged privilege denials in the past. One such group is podiatrists. Podiatrists receive four years of graduate level education in the diagnosis and medical and surgical treatment of diseases of the foot and are licensed in all states.[37] Podiatrists seek hospital privileges because some complex podiatric surgical procedures can best be performed in a hospital or because surgical patients have chronic medical diseases and require close monitoring and observation available only in a hospital setting.[38] Podiatrists compete with orthopedic surgeons in the market for foot surgery.[39]

A major antitrust suit by a podiatrist who lost his hospital admitting and surgical privileges due to the previous JCAH restriction was *Levin v. Doctors Hospital*.[40] After Levin successfully joined the JCAH as a defendant,[41] the suit was settled out of court. As part of the settlement, the JCAH established a separate category of clinical privileges for podiatrists whereby, at the discretion of the individual hospital, a podiatrist and a physician could collaborate on admitting and treating a podiatric patient.[42] In the twenty years since *Levin*, podiatrists have succeeded in gaining some type of privileges at over fifty percent of the hospitals in this country.[43] However, two recent cases in which podiatrists lost antitrust challenges to the categorical denial of staff privileges attest to the continuing vitality of physicians' resistance to podiatrists obtaining hospital privileges.[44]

Clinical psychologists, who compete with physician psychiatrists in the market for psychotherapy and treatment of mental illness, seek hospital privileges to admit and treat patients experiencing acute emotional crises or patients requiring constant protection against self-harm.[45] Psychologists have been less successful than podiatrists in getting a foot in the door regarding hospital privileges.[46] The major psychologists' privileges case was instituted by the Attorney General of Ohio, who alleged that the categorical denial of staff privileges to psychologists foreclosed consumer choice in the market for mental health care and stabilized prices at non-competitive levels.[47] The case became moot, however, when the Ohio legislature enacted a statute that restricted hospital admission privileges to physicians.[48]

Another non-physician group interested in obtaining staff privileges is nurse-midwives.[49] Nurse-midwives are registered nurses who have completed six to twenty-four months of additional specialized training and who are certified to provide health care for women during all phases of the reproductive cycle and to deliver babies of women with low-risk pregnancies.[50] By statute, nurse-midwives must be supervised by physicians for some aspects of their practice.[51] In 1982, nurse-midwives delivered only

1.8 percent of the babies born in the United States, but this proportion was an eighty percent increase from 1976.[52] Nurse-midwives directly compete with obstetricians in the market for childbirth services. Legal battles involving hospital privileges for nurse-midwives have been reported in several states and the District of Columbia, although no antitrust case has yet been decided on the merits.[53]

The most recent group to challenge denial of privileges under the antitrust laws is nurse-anesthetists. Nurse-anesthetists are registered nurses who receive a minimum of two years of additional training in administering anesthesia.[54] Like nurse-midwives, they must work under physician supervision.[55] Historically, nurses were the primary group responsible for administering anesthesia in this country, and nurse-anesthetists are still responsible for more than fifty percent of anesthetic procedures.[56] Today, nurse-anesthetists' primary competitors are physician anesthesiologists, and in a market with an increasing supply of anesthesia providers, the competition is intense.[57]

Neither nurse-anesthetists nor physician anesthesiologists actually admit patients to a hospital. They generally work under a contractual arrangement to provide anesthesia to surgical patients.[58] Consequently, the conflict has not been over staff privileges per se, but over potential anticompetitive abuses where contractual arrangements have been changed to replace nurse-anesthetists with physician anesthesiologists.[59] In Maine, the state attorney general accused anesthesiologists who attempted to close a nurse-anesthetist training program of violating antitrust law.[60] The physicians entered into a consent decree enjoining them from raising prices, negotiating exclusive contracts, and interfering with the employment or training of nurse-anesthetists.[61] In West Virginia, the state attorney general also alleged antitrust violations where two hospitals changed their staff by-laws to block nurse-anesthetists from obtaining staff privileges, and also reached a settlement in which the anesthesiologists involved would not raise prices, enter into exclusive contracts, or jointly participate in any privileges decision regarding nurse-anesthetists.[62] Finally, in a case from California, the Ninth Circuit declared that nurse-anesthetists compete with physician anesthesiologists despite a state statutory requirement that nurse-anesthetists be supervised by physicians, thus permitting a nurse-anesthetist barred from hospital practice to proceed with his antitrust suit.[63]

Chiropractors are another group seeking access to hospitals, although chiropractors may not actually compete with physicians. At least one study suggests consumers do not view chiropractors' services as a substitute for physicians'.[64] Nevertheless, chiropractors have been challenging exclusionary behavior by the medical establishment for years.[65] Regarding hospital access, chiropractors do not necessarily want admitting privileges, but merely the ability to refer patients to a hospital's laboratory or x-ray facilities as an aid in diagnosis.[66] In the past, the JCAH has warned hospitals that cooperating with chiropractors even to this extent might threaten the hospital's accreditation.[67] In light of the recent relaxation of JCAH standards for privileges,[68] however, each individual hospital may now apparently decide whether to accommodate chiropractors. In general, chiropractors have not fared well in their legal efforts to gain access to hospitals,[69] although suits by chiropractors against medical associations may be partially responsible for the change in JCAH standards.

## IV. Hospital Privilege Denials as a Group Boycott

As a result of United States Supreme Court decisions in the 1970's and early 1980's, health care providers can challenge the denial of hospital privileges under the antitrust laws. In *Hospital Building Co. v. Trustees of Rex Hospital*[70] and *McLain v. Real Estate Board of New Orleans*,[71] the Court relaxed its definition of interstate commerce, so that a plaintiff's showing that the challenged restraint affects the purchase of supplies out-of-state or the billing of out-of-state insurers is enough to satisfy the Sherman Act's interstate commerce requirement.[72] More significantly, in *Goldfarb v. Virginia State Bar*[73] and in *Arizona v. Maricopa County Medical Society*,[74] the Court made it clear that professionals, including physicians, are not exempt from the antitrust laws.[75] These changes cleared the way for a deluge of antitrust suits challenging privilege denials, many of which were brought by individual physicians.[76] Because an excluded privileges applicant competes with physicians on the hospital's medical staff, the denial of hospital privileges can be characterized as a group boycott. The staff's recommendations to deny or terminate privileges is a joint decision by competitors that deprives the applicant of access to the hospital, a resource essential to his ability to compete.[77]

Because a group boycott is a violation of section one of the Sherman Act, a critical issue in a hospital privileges suit brought on a group boycott theory is the existence of a conspiracy or concerted action by competitors. Some defendants have asserted that the denial of privileges resulted from merely unilateral action by the hospital; thus, there was not the combination or conspiracy required for a section one violation.[78] However, although the hospital board makes the final decision on whether to grant privileges, hospital boards almost always defer to the medical expertise of physicians and agree with the medical staff's or staff committee's recommendation.[79] According to one federal district court, the individual physicians on the staff or on the reviewing committee are more than the mere agents of the hospital in making this recommendation because the doctors have a personal economic interest in the outcome of the privileges decision.[80] Therefore, the board's approval of this recommendation does not immunize the staff's action from antitrust scrutiny. In *Weiss v. York Hospital*,[81] the Third Circuit held that as a matter of law, a medical staff is a combination of competitors.[82] This court also noted the individual economic interest of staff members in the outcome of a privileges decision.[83] According to this view, the potentially illegal conspiracy is not between the staff and the hospital, but within the staff itself.

The absence on the reviewing committee of a direct competitor of an applicant should not mislead a court to conclude that there was no anticompetitive conduct.[84] Commentators have noted the immense power of the referral network among physicians.[85] Because physician specialists depend on their physician colleagues for patient referrals and for coverage on days off, there is great incentive for physicians to conform to their colleagues' wishes.[86] Peer pressure subtly exerted on the members of a reviewing committee could easily induce them to deny privileges to their colleagues' unwanted competitors.

Although a group boycott can be a per se antitrust offense,[87] most courts faced with hospital privileges cases have applied the rule of reason, on several bases. One basis is that hospital privileges decisions are a form of industry self-regulation.[88] Because industry self-regulation can have significant procompetitive benefits, whether a particular restraint is unreasonable can only be determined after detailed analysis under the rule of reason.[89] Also, although the Supreme Court in *Maricopa* made it clear that per se rules may apply to learned professions,[90] dicta in this and other Supreme Court decisions suggest that the rule of reason is the proper approach when restraints of trade by a profession are premised on public service or ethical norms.[91] A denial of privileges because the applicant fails to meet a quality standard has such a premise.[92] Some courts have used the rule of reason because the judiciary lacks experience applying antitrust laws to the health care industry.[93] These courts are wary of per se condemnation of a particular industry practice until they can be more confident that the practice will almost always be anticompetitive.

Finally, despite the Supreme Court's recent statement in *Northwest Wholesale Stationers, Inc v. Pacific Stationery and Printing Co.*[94] that the per se rule may apply to a group boycott if the defendant has market power,[95] where the defendant hospital in a privileges case has market power, a trial court might use the rule of reason. Dicta in *Northwest Stationers* suggesting that "plausible arguments that [the restraints] were intended to enhance overall efficiency and make markets more competitive"[96] may weaken the per se rule's presumption of anticompetitive effect and make the rule of reason the appropriate judicial approach. Particularly in rural areas, a hospital may have market power simply because it is the only hospital in a county. Applying the per se rule when rural hospitals deny staff privileges while applying the rule of reason to the same practice by urban hospitals would be illogical and could deny rural hospitals necessary discretion to qualitatively screen individual applicants, for fear of per se antitrust liability.[97] Supreme Court dicta in an earlier hospital privileges case emphasizing "the hospital's unquestioned right to exercise some control over the identity and the number of doctors to whom it accords staff privileges"[98] further support application of the rule of reason to a hospital privileges case, even where the defendant hospital has market power.


## V. Quality of Care as a Defense

### A. Overview

Under the rule of reason, a defendant may not justify a privileges denial merely by asserting that restricting hospital privileges to the most highly-qualified practitioners promotes the public health or welfare.[99] In *National Society of Professional Engineers v. United States*,[100] the Supreme Court emphasized that the rule of reason permits only justifications based on the procompetitive effects of an alleged restraint.[101] The Court stated that to permit an antitrust defense based on protecting the public welfare would be "tantamount to a repeal"[102] of the Sherman Act and suggested that such an argument is more properly directed to the legislature.[103]

The Court recently repeated this position in *Federal Trade Commission v. Indiana Federation of Dentists*.[104] The Federal Trade Commission had found that a collective refusal by a group of dentists to submit dental x-rays to insurers to enable the insurers to assess the appropriateness of care was an unreasonable restraint of trade.[105] The dentists attempted to justify their boycott by asserting that they were protecting the quality of dental care.[106] The Supreme Court rejected this argument and reaffirmed its position in *Professional Engineers* that quality of service considerations unrelated to enhancing competition are not available as a justification under the rule of reason.[107]

In *Wilk v. American Medical Association*,[108] a case in which chiropractors alleged antitrust violations in various exclusionary acts by organized medicine, the Seventh Circuit also emphasized that under the rule of reason, the effect of the challenged restraint on competition is the "critical and sole factor"[109] in determining whether a practice is illegal. Nevertheless, the Seventh Circuit, citing Supreme Court dicta regarding the application of the antitrust laws to professions, fashioned a new rule of reason defense for physicians where their exclusionary conduct is motivated by an ethical concern for their patients' well-being.[110] Commentators have been critical of this judicial creation of a special rule, pointing out that the Supreme Court's suggestions that the antitrust laws might operate differently for the service and ethical aspects of a profession can be satisfied by a special sensitivity to the unusual features of competition in professional markets.[111] Such a unique rule for physicians threatens to undermine the basic premise of the rule of reason, that effect on competition is the sole yardstick for legality, and threatens to legitimize professional usurpation of the legislative function of deciding what is in the public interest.[112]

Under the rule of reason, an exclusion based on quality of care is defensible, however, because quality is a major competitive variable in the health care industry. Because third-party insurers pay such a large proportion of health care bills, patients are relatively unconcerned about price when they purchase health services, leading to minimal price competition among physicians or hospitals.[113] Quality, instead of price, is a major factor patients and physicians use to select a hospital.[114] Therefore, where an exclusion improves the overall quality of a hospital, the restriction is procompetitive and quality of care may be asserted as a defense.[115]

Where non-physicians have been excluded, quality of care as a justification has arisen primarily in cases involving podiatrists and chiropractors,[116] although a similar rationale could apply to barring psychologists, nurse-midwives and nurse-anesthetists. The essence of this defense in a group context is that because physicians are the only group trained and licensed to independently diagnose and treat the whole person, only physicians should have hospital privileges.[117] Granting privileges to less qualified providers would threaten the overall quality of care in the institution; thus, the exclusion is procompetitive.


## B. Judicial Approaches to Quality of Care as a Defense

Courts have taken a variety of approaches in evaluating quality of care as a procompetitive justification for denying hospital privileges to individual physicians or to groups of non-physicians. Some courts have almost totally deferred to medical authority, labeling the privileges decision professional rather than commercial. For example, in *Hackett v. Metropolitan General Hospital*,[118] a case brought by an individual physician under state antitrust law, the court, using federal antitrust concepts, stated, "[E]ven when serious anticompetitive effects exist[,] . . . professional decision-making relative to the quality or efficiency of health care should not be subject to antitrust constraints and, therefore, impeded."[119] Similarly, in a suit by podiatrists challenging a categorical denial of hospital privileges, a federal district court granted a summary judgment for defendant hospitals, finding in the record "nothing by way of the Sherman Act to call upon the courts to intrude upon a responsibility reserved to medical decision-makers."[120] In addition to deviating from the rule of reason's mandate that the proper judicial focus is on the impact on competition, this approach ignores the fact that privileges decisions have both professional and commercial aspects and, in some cases, could be economic decisions disguised as professional.[121]

Other courts have looked to whether the exclusionary decision was made in good faith or was not arbitrary or capricious. For example, the federal district court in *Williams v. Kleaveland*,[122] a case involving an individual physician, invoked the professional-commercial distinction noted above and recognized a good faith defense, based on a bona fide concern for the public welfare.[123] A similar standard was used in a podiatrist's case in which the court granted a summary judgment for the defendant based on a "good faith judgment that high quality care requires that surgery . . . only be performed by physicians educated and trained to treat the whole person."[124] The court failed to consider the denial's impact on competition, although the court said it was applying the rule of reason.[125]

A third judicial approach has been to require a mere rational relation between the decision to exclude and quality of care. The court in *Kaczanowski v. Medical Center Hospital of Vermont*,[126] a podiatrists' case, thought that "common sense dictates that the use of sensitive medical instruments, which may engage highly technical diagnostic equipment . . . should not be entrusted to applicants who fail to meet a high level of advanced medical training."[127] The court did not address the facts that the plaintiff podiatrists had spent several years in professional school learning how to use the sensitive instruments and that the state legislature had decided it was proper for podiatrists to perform the surgical procedures at issue.[128]

Some courts have applied a higher level of scrutiny and required that a quality rationale for denial of privileges or other exclusionary conduct in a health care context be objectively reasonable. In *Feminist Women's Health Center v. Mohammad*,[129] the defendants were charged with a group boycott and other antitrust violations in persuading physicians not to work at an abortion clinic. Reversing (on other grounds) a summary judgment for the defendants, the Fifth Circuit stated that under the rule of reason, the tests for evaluating a defense based on maintenance of professional standards are "the genuineness of the defendants' justification, the reasonableness of the standards themselves, and the manner of their enforcement."[130] In *Virginia Academy of Clinical Psychologists v. Blue Shield of Virginia*,[131] the Fourth Circuit found that a requirement that third-party payment for psychologists' services be billed through a physician was patently unreasonable as a quality assurance measure because it permitted supervision by any physician, not just those knowledgeable about mental illness.[132] The court noted that "we are not inclined to condone anticompetitive conduct upon an incantation of 'good medical practice.' "[133]

In *Pontius v. Children's Hospital*,[134] a federal district court established the test under the rule of reason for evaluating termination of an individual physician's hospital privileges as "valid reasons supported by substantial evidence."[135] Because evaluating individual competence is largely subjective, the court stated it would not attempt to decide whether the privileges committee was correct, but would make sure there was substantial evidence to support the decision.[136] Perceptively noting a difference between exclusion of an individual and exclusion of a group of physicians, the court suggested that the validity of excluding a group on a quality basis is more capable of objective evaluation.[137] Although the court used the example of a categorical exclusion of a group of physicians from a specific medical school, exclusion of a group of non-physicians on a quality basis should be amenable to the same objective evaluation.

Finally, commentators and at least one court have advocated a "purpose-based rule of reason," requiring a dominant anticompetitive purpose for a denial of privileges to violate the Sherman Act.[138] One difficulty with purpose as the determinative criterion is that a hospital staff might have mixed purposes for a particular privileges denial or might assert a purpose to maintain the quality of care while the covert purpose is to suppress competition. Uncovering the true or dominant purpose will necessarily require a lengthy trial.[139] A second problem with this approach is that it is inconsistent with the rule of reason's primary focus on anticompetitive effect. According to Justice Brandeis' classic statement of the rule of reason in *Chicago Board of Trade v. United States*,[140] "[t]he true test of legality is whether the restraint imposed is such as merely regulates and perhaps thereby promotes competition or whether it is such as may suppress or even destroy competition."[141] Justice Brandeis explained that a court may consider the purpose of the restraint, "not because a good intention will save an otherwise objectionable regulation or the reverse; but because knowledge of intent may help the court to interpret facts and to predict consequences."[142] Thus, while purpose is relevant, it is not determinative.[143]

## VI. Differences Between Denial of Privileges to an Individual and to a Group

In general, the lower courts have attempted to find a way to "guard against . . . anticompetitive abuses without disrupting the legitimate interests of hospitals and medical staffs in providing efficient and high quality medical care."[144] Except for the court in *Pontius v. Children's Hospital*, however, these courts have not clearly distinguished between denial of hospital privileges to individual physicians and denial to groups of non-physicians and have, therefore, applied the same variety of levels of scrutiny to both types of cases. There are at least four fundamental differences between denial of privileges to an individual and to a group: differences in the substantive validity of the quality rationale for exclusion, in the operation of due process, in procompetitive justifications, and in anticompetitive effects. Because of these distinctions, denial of privileges to a group merits antitrust scrutiny beyond a mere rational relation or good faith standard.

### A. Differences in the Substantive Validity of the Quality Justification

In contrast to a quality of care justification for denying privileges to an individual physician, there are inherent weaknesses in a quality rationale when applied to exclude a group of non-physicians. Although physicians are probably best qualified to assess a fellow physician's skill, training, and experience, they are not necessarily experts about the capabilities of allied health practitioners. Members of the medical staff may have little experience with or knowledge about the group being excluded. For example, only twenty-seven percent of physicians questioned in one study knew that podiatrists receive four years of graduate level podiatry education in addition to undergraduate studies.[145] Most physicians underestimated the extent of podiatry training.[146] There may be reason to question the validity of physicians' opinions of podiatric care if physicians lack even basic knowledge about podiatrists' education. Furthermore, physicians' evaluations of the quality of care rendered by non-physicians may be baised by the physicians' professional ego.[147] Because the training and experience of doctors may lead them to believe in their own superiority, their ability to judge objectively the competence of a group with different or less training may be distorted.[148]

There are also inherent weaknesses in the argument that allied groups should not obtain privileges because they are not qualified to treat the whole person.[149] Non-physicians do not necessarily want to treat the whole person; they want only to provide professional care within the scope of their licenses, whether it be care of the feet or the psyche.[150] As long as physicians are readily available to treat health problems beyond the scope of the non-physician's expertise, there is no reason to exclude the non-physician. Also, many physician specialists might fail to measure up to this "whole person" criterion. For example, a physician who has specialized in psychiatry for many years may no longer be competent to regulate insulin dosages in a newly diagnosed diabetic and would, as a matter of course, seek consultation from a more qualified physician. In an era of increasing specialization, there may be few health care providers who are truly qualified to treat the whole person.[151] Finally, this "whole person" argument is weakened by the fact that hospital privileges were available to dentists even under the pre-1985 JCAH standards.[152] Dentists clearly are not trained to treat the whole person, but neither do they compete with physicians as directly as the excluded non-physician groups do.

Additionally, denying an entire professional group the opportunity to provide services for which it was trained and licensed has the effect of partially negating the licensure law. The courts have clearly declared that a license does not automatically give an individual the right to practice in any hospital.[153] A state licensure law is, however, a legislative determination that in general, people with the requisite training and knowledge can safely provide whatever service they are licensed to provide.[154] A hospital's denial of privileges to an entire licensed group on a quality basis is, in effect, a declaration that despite the legislature's judgment, no one with that particular license is competent to provide that service. The courts have been hostile to industry self-regulation that is so extensive that the industry acts as a private government and threatens to usurp the legislature's prerogative of determining what is in the public interest.[155]

A quality rationale for excluding a group may be further flawed if research demonstrates the safety or effectiveness of treatment by non-physicians. Although there are few such studies of patient-outcomes, an assertion that an allied health group given inferior care is inherently suspect if scientific investigations document the quality of care given by non-physicians.[156] Nurse-midwives are one group for which such outcome studies exist. These studies consistently show no difference in patient outcomes or even better outcomes when childbirth care is provided by nurse-midwives as compared with physicians.[157] Thus, any exclusion of nurse-midwives as a group on the basis that they give lower quality care would be highly questionable.

## B. Differences in the Effects of Due Process

Courts deciding privileges cases should also be sensitive to the differences in the operation of due process when a group of non-physicians has been excluded as opposed to an individual physician. Notice of the reason for denial and an opportunity to be heard can serve as effective safeguards for an individual physician against competitive abuses. A hearing and an internal appeal procedure provide an individual physician threatened with denial or termination of privileges an opportunity to show how his personal qualifications meet a presumably valid standard.[158] In contrast, when privileges are limited to physicians, a non-physician applicant, no matter how expert in his own field, is automatically barred. He is faced with trying to persuade the medical staff not only that he is highly qualified, but that the standard should be changed. Thus, a hearing and an appeal procedure may be of little help to the non-physician when the barrier is the standard itself.[159]

## C. Examination of Procompetitive and Anticompetitive Effects

In applying the rule of reason to privilege denials and weighing the procompetitive and anticompetitive effects, courts must first recognize that there are three distinct markets involved: hospitals compete for patients, hospitals compete for providers, and providers compete for patients.[160] What is procompetitive in one market may be anticompetitive in another.[161]

Courts should also recognize that the structure of the market for inpatient hospital services creates a conflict of interest for physicians. Although the hospital sells its services to patients, the physician acts as the patient's agent in the decision to purchase hospital services.[162] The physician decides whether the patient needs hospital care, what kind of care, and for how long. Aware that physicians thus control hospital utilization, hospitals compete for patients indirectly by competing for physicians.[163] Hospital decisions regarding what services to offer and who should offer them are aimed at making the hospital attractive to physicians.[164] On the other side of the hospital-patient transaction, physicians on the medical staff advise the hospital what services to offer. The power of physicians on both sides of this transaction creates a conflict of interest.[165] When a group of non-physicians is denied hospital privileges based on the advice of physicians on the medical staff, antitrust courts should be sensitive to this conflict of interest and scrutinize the extent to which the exclusion may serve the physicians' self-interest as well as or instead of the patient's interest.

*1. Differences in Procompetitive Justifications for Privilege Denials.—* One procompetitive justification for the denial of privileges to non-physicians that is no longer available to hospitals is that the denial is necessary to maintain the hospital's accreditation, which, in turn, is critical in qualifying for federal and private insurance payments.[166] The JCAH has recently changed its accreditation standards and no longer requires a hospital to restrict its staff to physicians and dentists to be accredited.[167]

From the perspective of the hospital-provider market, there is no price competition among hospitals for physicians because hospitals do not pay physicians. The main competitive variables here are quality and amenities; physicians want to be on staff at a hospital with a reputation for quality and at a hospital offering the services and equipment that facilitate the physician's work.[168] Thus, an exclusion that maintains or enhances a hospital's quality is procompetitive in the hospital-provider market.[169] In addition, a hospital's decision to deny staff privileges to non-physicians may be procompetitive in this market because the exclusion makes the hospital more attractive to physicians by insulating them from whole groups of competitors in the provider-consumer market for in-patient services.[170] The purpose of the antitrust laws, however, is to promote competition to benefit consumers.[171] A court faced with a privileges case should therefore focus on whether the denial is procompetitive from the consumer's viewpoint as well as from the physician's.

Other procompetitive justifications a hospital might assert for qualitatively screening individuals do not necessarily apply to the exclusion of entire groups of non-physicians. For example, because a hospital may be liable in tort for negligently screening or supervising members of its medical staff,[172] any exclusion that decreases the hospital's potential liability for malpractice is procompetitive in that it decreases the hospital's costs of doing business.[173] This rationale would justify excluding any individual who the hospital has reason to believe is likely to practice negligently, such as a physician with a history of several malpractice suits against him or a physician who attempts to practice beyond the scope of his expertise. This rationale would not justify excluding an entire group of non-physicians where there is no evidence that the group is prone to malpractice. For example, the rate of malpractice suits against nurse-midwives is one-tenth of the rate of suits against obstetricians.[174] The low rate for nurse-midwives is no doubt partially because nurse-midwives deliver primarily low-risk patients and because some nurse-midwives do no deliveries at all.[175] Nevertheless, a hospital should not be permitted to assert potential tort liability as a justification for excluding nurse-midwives.

This rationale may justify excluding chiropractors due to the hospital's potential liability for a chiropractor's misdiagnosis.[176] Orthodox health care providers do not agree with chiropractors that the cause of all disease is misalignment of the spine.[177] If, for example, a hospital x-ray for a chiropractor's patient revealed an operable tumor as the probable cause of the patient's symptoms, but the chiropractor proceeded to treat the patient by spinal manipulation, the hospital and its radiologist might be placed in a vulnerable position.[178]

Several statutes as well as accreditation bodies require members of a medical staff to conduct peer review.[179] Staff members might be discouraged from participating in peer review or being candid in evaluating their colleagues if an expelled provider institutes an antitrust suit against the members of a review committee that recommended termination of privileges.[180] This potential chilling of peer review by antitrust litigation is a proper judicial concern and a valid procompetitive justification in privileges cases involving individuals.[181] Although this rationale might justify a differential judicial approach where individual physicians lost hospital privileges as a result of peer review, the rationale does not support excluding an entire group of non-physician providers. If the group were granted privileges, evaluation by physicians or peers could still be done on an individual basis.

Another procompetitive effect of denying privileges to less qualified practitioners is that a hospital would incur high costs in monitoring these people if it could not initially qualitatively screen privileges applicants.[182] This rationale is another argument that does not, however, readily transfer from an individual to a group context because the rationale does not justify excluding an entire group unless there is some evidence that, in general, its members give inferior care.

If a specific non-physician group seeking privileges must have physician supervision of some aspects of its practice, the costs to the hospital of providing such supervision are a procompetitive justification for excluding the group.[183] Even the new, flexible JCAH standard restricts full medical staff membership to providers licensed to practice independently.[184] This justification would not apply, however, if the non-physician applicant has arranged for his own supervision by a doctor already on the staff. For example, although nurse-midwives legally require medical supervision for some types of services,[185] nurse-midwives challenging exclusion in *Nurse Midwifery Associates v. Hibbett*[186] had already arranged for the necessary supervision and did not ask the hospital to supply it.

Furthermore, even physicians require consultation with other physicians when they encounter an illness or clinical situation beyond their own fields of expertise. For example, a family physician may be required to call in an obstetrician when a maternity patient needs a caesarean section.[187] Although there is a distinction between medical supervision required by statute and consultation or back-up required by the hospital, hospitals and medical staffs have not found such cooperative arrangements unduly costly when only physicians were involved.

A hospital could assert, as a procompetitive justification for exclusion, that accommodating new types of staff members would create high costs in developing standards and review mechanisms for the new group.[188] The key legal question, however, is whether these initial costs are outweighed by the benefit to the consumer of the increased competition from the new group. This argument might be a valid justification for excluding chiropractors because chiropractic is based on an entirely different theory of disease then orthodox medicine.[189] It is difficult to imagine how an institution, the hospital, based on a scientific-medical model of diagnosis and treatment could even begin to articulate standards for an alien ideology.

Consumers may have problems making informed choices in purchasing health or hospital care because information about the skill of a provider or the quality of a hospital is difficult for a lay person to obtain and evaluate.[190] Thus, in the hospital-patient market, the hospital's selectivity in staff membership is procompetitive because it reduces consumers' information search costs. The uninformed consumer can rely on the hospital's screening to provide at least some assurance that the hospital itself and the providers on its staff meet a professionally determined level of quality.[191] As applied to groups of non-physicians, however, the hospital's screening serves this function only if the group excluded in fact gives low quality care.[192] It is, therefore, reasonable to demand of a hospital that asserts this justification for excluding a group some qualitative evidence beyond the fact that the members of the group are not physicians.

Most of these procompetitive benefits are achievable by screening individuals and do not require excluding an entire group. Because the major factor on which hospitals compete with each other is quality, an antitrust ruling that decreases a hospital's ability to select among individuals on a quality basis would greatly diminish competition among hospitals. However, the consequences of prohibiting a hospital from excluding an entire group without substantive evidence of a quality deficiency would not be as destructive of competition. The hospital could still be selective as to individuals within the group.

*2. Differences in Anticompetitive Effects.*—From the consumer's perspective, there are clear differences between excluding an individual and excluding a group in terms of anticompetitive effects. Denial of hospital privileges to an entire group of non-physicians has a much greater effect in foreclosing consumer choice than denial of privileges to an individual physician. According to the Seventh Circuit, "[A] consumer has no interest in the preservation of a fixed number of competitors greater than the number required to assure his being able to buy at the competitive price."[193] In the consumer-health care provider market, such factors as personalization of care, convenience, and variations in treatment modalities may be added to price as the salient competitive variables. Where the excluded individual offers essentially the same array of services at a similar price as other physicians in the geographic market, the loss of one physician has a minimal anticompetitive effect.[194] However, where the excluded individual offers a different, but still reasonably substitutable package of services, and the exclusion means that consumers will be unable to select that package at all, the anticompetitive effect is much greater. For example, in a market where six obstetricians and one nurse-midwife compete to sell health care to pregnant women, the loss of the midwife, who may have been offering more personalized care, greater flexibility in choices for delivery, and more health education,[195] forecloses consumer choice much more drastically than the loss of one of the obstetricians. In a recent antitrust case involving dentists, the Supreme Court emphasized that it does not look favorably upon agreements among competitors that limit consumer choice, "absent some countervailing procompetitive virtue."[196]

Also, the non-physicians who are barred from offering in-patient services generally charge less than the physicians with whom they compete. Podiatrists charge less than orthopedic surgeons,[197] psychologists charge less than psychiatrists,[198] nurse-midwives charge less than obstetricians,[199] and nurse-anesthetists charge less than physician anesthesiologists.[200] Therefore, denying privileges to allied health groups has the anticompetitive effect of maintaining higher prices in the provider-consumer market. The same is not true of the exclusion of an individual physician whose prices may be similar to those of other physicians in the market.

Another anticompetitive effect of excluding a group of non-physicians that does not apply to the exclusion of an individual physician is that restricting hospital privileges to physicians stifles innovation in health care delivery. From the consumer's perspective, where services offered by non-physicians are reasonably substitutable for services by physicians, the two groups compete.[201] However, where non-physicians also offer treatments not generally used by physicians, denying privileges to non-physicians retards the development of alternative approaches, even where such treatments have been proven safe and effective.[202] For example, nurse-midwives are inclined to use natural childbirth techniques rather than anesthesia,[203] and psychologists may offer biofeedback training rather than drugs as a treatment for chronic pain.[204] In addition to limiting consumers' options, barring these groups from hospital practice slows the acceptance of these safe and effective alternatives.

Finally, although excluding a single physician from hospital practice has a minimal anticompetitive effect in the provider-consumer market, excluding an entire group of non-physicians protects the dominant group (physicians) from all competition from an alternative group offering reasonably substitutable services at lower prices. Defending such an exclusion under the rule of reason on a quality basis is, in effect, an assertion that non-physicians should not be allowed to compete in hospitals. This assertion comes close to arguing that competition itself is unreasonable, an argument the Supreme Court flatly rejected in *National Society of Professional Engineers v. United States.*[205]

## VII. Suggested Judicial Approach

A relatively deferential judicial approach might be appropriate in privileges cases involving exclusions of individual physicians.[206] Physicians are better qualified than judges to evaluate other physicians. The content of the quality standard on which the exclusion is based, as the standard relates to training, experience, and expertise, is not suspect. Due process can effectively curb anticompetitive abuses. Most significantly for antitrust purposes, there is a minimal anticompetitive effect in any market.

However, because of the greater anticompetitive effect of precluding competition from an entire group, as well as other differences noted above, a quality of care standard invoked to exclude a group should be substantially related to the procompetitive justifications the hospital asserts.[207] A court should not merely defer to physicians' subjective opinions or allow a good faith defense. It is not unreasonable to demand some evidence that in general, the group excluded in fact provides inferior care.[208] Such a demand is consistent with the Supreme Court's recent decision in *Federal Trade Commission v. Indiana Federation of Dentists.*[209] "[E]ven if concern for the quality of patient care could under some circumstances serve as a justification for a restraint of [trade],"[210] defendants must produce sufficient evidence that the restraint in fact improves the quality of care. Mere expert opinion testimony may not be enough.[211]

A court should also require that the exclusionary standard be the least restrictive way to achieve the particular procompetitive benefit used to justify the standard. The least restrictive alternative concept appears in several antitrust cases involving industry self-regulation. Evaluating the antitrust liability of stock exchange self-regulation in *Silver v. New York Stock Exchange,*[212] the Supreme Court articulated "the principle that exchange self-regulation is. . . justified in response to antitrust charges only to the extent necessary to. . . [achieve]. . . the aims of the Securities Exchange Act[.]"[213] In a concurring opinion in *Professional Engineers,*[214] Justice Blackmun found that even if one accepted a quality argument for the engineers' policy against competitive bidding, the "rule is still grossly overbroad."[215]

The Court of Appeals for the District of Columbia Circuit cited these aspects of *Silver* and *Professional Engineers* in a case involving the exclusion of an individual from a health professional association and held that "even if evidence existed in the record to support the asserted justification that the [limitation] improved the quality of patient care, *it must be shown that the means chosen to achieve that end are the least restrictive available.*"[216] Similarly, the Seventh Circuit, also citing *Silver* and *Professional Engineers,* has declared that where a patient care motive is used to justify exclusionary behavior by a health professional association, the defendant's conduct must meet a least restrictive alternative test.[217] Scholarly commentary also recommends a least restrictive alternative standard for potentially anticompetitive acts that result from industry self-regulation.[218]

As applied to individual practitioners, denial of hospital privileges is the least restrictive alternative for achieving various procompetitive benefits. When a hospital has reason to believe that an individual will provide low quality care because of deficient training, poor references, or a history of malpractice suits, forcing the hospital to nevertheless grant privileges, but closely monitor the individual's practice, would generate costs and potential liabilities for the hospital.

However, there are methods other than categorical exclusion of a non-physician group that can safeguard the quality of hospital care without limiting competition. A hospital could be selective as to individual non-physician applicants just as it is with physicians. Instead of barring all non-physicians, the hospital could provide for non-physicians' privileges, but admit only the most highly qualified podiatrists or psychologists, for example. With regard to standards of training, the appropriate focus is not on whether the training is less than that of physicians, because non-physician applicants are not seeking to practice medicine. Rather, a court should consider whether the training is deficient in relation to what the applicant intends to do in the institution. For example, where podiatrists seek to perform more elaborate surgical procedures, a hospital could reasonably require advanced residency training or Board certification.[219]

Another less restrictive alternative is for a hospital to grant staff membership to non-physician groups, but limit specific clinical privileges, a practice analogous to the current policy of some hospitals which permit family physicians to deliver babies but require that an obstetrician perform caesarean births.[220] A court should be careful, however, that such limits are not so narrow as to be a sham. In *Davidson v. Youngstown Hospital Association*,[221] a podiatrist's privileges case brought on public policy grounds, podiatrists were permitted to cut toenails and trim callouses on a physician's order.[222] It is hard to believe that seven or eight years of professional education qualify podiatrists to do no more than cut toenails.[223] Finally, to avoid institutional costs of providing medical supervision for legally dependent providers, a hospital could require that an applicant needing physician back-up arrange for his own medical supervision by a staff member.[224]

## VIII. Conclusion

Hospital privileges cases have presented courts with the thorny problem of protecting against anticompetitive abuses while guarding the legitimate interest of hospitals in maintaining high quality care.[225] A first step in resolving this problem is recognizing the clear differences between denial of staff privileges to an individual physician and denial to a group of non-physicians, differences in the substantive validity of the quality rationale for exclusion, differences in the application of due process, differences in procompetitive justifications and differences in anticompetitive effects. A relatively deferential judicial approach to the exclusion of an individual physician might be appropriate. Because of these differences, however, when quality of care is invoked to justify excluding a non-physician group, judicial scrutiny should be based on a substantial relation and least restrictive alternative test. This approach would ensure that the rule of reason is not applied so deferentially as to insulate one powerful group of competitors from competition. In addition, this heightened scrutiny would uphold the fundamental principle that the purpose of the antitrust laws is to protect competition, not competitors.[226]

## References

1. Nearly half of health care antitrust cases involve staff privileges. *Attempts to Gain Access to Hospitals Are Prevalent in Health Care Actions*, [Jan.-June] Antitrust & Trade Reg. Rep. (BNA) No. 1150, at 187 (Feb. 2, 1984).
2. *See, e.g.*, Bhan v. NME Hosp., Inc., 772 F.2d 1467 (9th Cir. 1985) (nurse-anesthetist); Wilk v. American Med Ass'n, 719 F.2d 207 (7th Cir. 1983), *cert. denied*, 467 U.S. 1210 (1984) (chiropractors); Kaczanowski v. Medical Center Hosp. of Vt., 612 F. Supp. 688 (D. Vt. 1985) (podiatrists); Nurse Midwifery Assocs. v. Hibbett, 54 F. Supp. 1185 (M.D. Tenn. 1982) (nurse-midwives); *Ohio Charges Accreditation Association with Preventing Competition in Provision of Psychological Care*, [Jan.-June] Antitrust & Trade Reg. Rep. (BNA) No. 948, at D-2 (Jan. 24, 1980) [hereinafter *Ohio Charges Accreditation Association*] (clinical psychologists).
3. Enders, *Antitrust and Health Care: Reconciling Competing Values—Medical Staff Issues*, 6 Whittier L. Rev. 737, 737 (1984).
4. *See infra* notes 118-38 and accompanying text.
5. *See infra* notes 118-44 and accompanying text.
6. 15 U.S.C. § 1 (1982).
7. Standard Oil Co. v. United States, 221 U.S. 1, 60 (1911). Because a contract to sell a product to one buyer effectively precludes others from buying that particular product, a literal reading of section one could conceivably bar all contracts to sell. *Id.*
8. *Id.*
9. National Soc'y of Professional Eng'rs v. United States, 435 U.S. 679, 690-92 (1978).
10. Northern Pac. Ry. Co. v. United States, 356 U.S. 1, 5 (1958) (listing price fixing, division of markets, group boycotts, and tying arrangements as per se offenses).
11. Arizona v. Maricopa County Medical Soc'y, 457 U.S. 332, 343-44 (1982).
12. *Id.*
13. Silver v. New York Stock Exch., 373 U.S. 341, 347-48 (1963); Klor's v. Broadway-Hale Stores, 359 U.S. 207, 212 (1959).
14. Northwest Wholesale Stationers, Inc. v. Pacific Stationery & Printing Co., 105 S. Ct. 2613, 2619 (1985) (quoting L. SULLIVAN, LAW OF ANTITRUST 261-62 (1977)).
15. P. AREEDA, ANTITRUST ANALYSIS ¶ 370 (3d ed. 1981) ("boycotts are not a unitary phenomenon").

16. *See, e.g.*, Kreuzer v. American Academy of Periodontology, 735 F.2d 1479, 1491-93 (D.C. Cir. 1984); United States Trotting Ass'n v. Chicago Downs Ass'n, 665 F.2d 781, 788-90 (7th Cir. 1981); Virginia Academy of Clinical Psychologists v. Blue Shield of Va., 624 F.2d 476, 484-85 (4th Cir. 1980), *cert. denied*, 450 U.S. 916 (1981); Hatley v. American Quarter Horse Ass'n, 552 F.2d 646, 652-53 (5th Cir. 1977).

17. 105 S. Ct. 2613 (1985).

18. *Id.* at 2621. "Market power" is "the capacity to act other than as a perfectly competitive firm would;" it often results from having a large market share. P. AREEDA, *supra* note 15, at ¶ 201.

19. 105 S. Ct. at 2621.

20. *Id.*

21. JOINT COMM'N ON ACCREDITATION OF HOSPS., ACCREDITATION MANUAL FOR HOSPITALS, 1986 111 (1985).

22. *Id.* at 101-02, 107. *See generally* M. ROEMER & J. FRIEDMAN, DOCTORS IN HOSPITALS 43-46, 225 (1971).

23. JOINT COMM'N ON ACCREDITATION OF HOSPS., *supra note 21, at 101-02, 114; see also* M. ROEMER & J. FRIEDMAN, *supra* note 22.

24. Jost, *The Joint Commission on Accreditation of Hospitals: Private Regulation of Health Care and the Public Interest*, 24 B.C.L. REV. 835, 839 (1983).

25. For example, in addition to the "active medical staff," a hospital may establish an "associate medical staff," consisting of "physicians and dentists who are being considered for advancement to the active medical staff;" a "courtesy medical staff," with "privileges to admit and treat only an occasional patient;" and a "consulting medical staff" of physicians who are not in another category, but who come to the hospital to consult. JOINT COMM'N ON ACCREDITATION OF HOSPS., ACCREDITATION MANUAL FOR HOSPITALS 89-96 (1984); *see also* Quinn v. Kent Gen. Hosp., 617 F. Supp. 1226, 1231 (D. Del. 1985) (physician appointed to consulting staff challenged exclusion from active medical staff where only active medical staff could admit patients); Jost, *supra* note 24, at 873.

26. Enders, *supra* note 3, at 737.

27. *See* Wolf v. Jane Phillips Episcopal-Memorial Medical Center, 513 F.2d 684, 686 (10th Cir. 1975).

28. M. ROEMER & J. FRIEDMAN, *supra* note 22, at 283.

29. Tarlov, *Shattuck Lecture—The Increasing Supply of Physicians, the Changing Structure of the Health Services System, and the Future Practice of Medicine*, 308 NEW ENG. J. MED. 1235, 1237-38 (1983).

30. Spivey, *The Relation Between Hospital Management and Medical Staff Under a Prospective-Payment System*, 310 NEW ENG. J. MED. 984, 984 (1984).
31. *Patients are Leaving Hospitals Sooner and Sicker, Study Says*, 85 AM. J. NURSING 828 (1985). Under the new prospective payment method, Medicare pays a hospital for a specified number of days of care based on a patient's diagnostic category. If the patient's hospitalization lasts longer than predicted based on his diagnosis, the hospital is not paid for the extra days. Conversely, if the patient is sent home in fewer than the established number of days, the hospital still receives the predetermined amount. Therefore, there is an incentive for hospitals to discharge patients quickly. Havighurst, *Doctors and Hospitals: An Antitrust Perspective on Traditional Relationships*, 84 DUKE L.J. 1071, 1077 n.14 (1984).
32. *See* Mechanic, *Some Dilemmas in Health Care Policy*, 59 MILBANK MEMORIAL FUND Q. 1, 4-5 (1981); Spivey *supra* note 30.
33. Spivey, *supra* note 30. *But see* Enders, *supra* note 3, at 738-39. A preferred provider organization is an arrangement whereby a group of doctors or hospitals contracts with an insurer or other purchaser of health care to provide services to insureds at set (usually discounted) fees. The disadvantage to the provider of the lower fees is offset by increased business from participating in the PPO. Built-in financial disincentives discourage patients from seeking care from other than a "preferred provider." *See* AMERICAN HOSP. ASS'N, LEGAL DEVELOPMENTS REPORT NO. 4, STATE REGULATION OF PREFERRED PROVIDER ORGANIZATIONS: A SURVEY OF STATE STATUTES iv (1984).
34. JOINT COMM'N ON ACCREDITATION OF HOSPS., *supra* note 25, at 89.
35. *See, e.g.*, Wilk v. American Medical Ass'n, 719 F.2d 207 (7th Cir. 1983), *cert. denied*, 467 U.S. 1210 (1984); Levin v. Joint Comm'n on Accreditation of Hosps., 354 F.2d 515 (D.C. Cir. 1965); Health Care Equalization Comm. of the Iowa Chiropractic Soc'y v. Iowa Medical Soc'y, 501 F. Supp. 970 (S.D. Iowa 1980); New York v. American Medical Ass'n, 1980-2 Trade Cas. (CCH) ¶ 63,456 (E.D.N.Y. 1980); Ohio Charges Accreditation Association, *supra* note 2. *See generally* AMERICAN HOSP. ASS'N, AN ANALYSIS OF THE REVISED MEDICAL STAFF STANDARDS OF THE JOINT COMMISSION ON ACCREDITATION OF HOSPITALS 1-2 (1984); Beardon, *JCAH Adopts Revised Medical Staff Standards*, 2 THE HEALTH LAWYER 4, 4 (1984); Jost, *supra* note 24, at 912. One report estimated the potential antitrust liability of the JCAH and other medical organizations named as defendants in four pending antitrust actions at over

$300 million. *JCAH Is Weighing Wider Access to Staff Privileges in Hospitals,* 83 AM. J. NURSING 1260 (1983).

36  *See* JOINT COMM'N ON ACCREDITATION OF HOSPS., *supra* note 21, at 101. *See generally* AMERICAN HOSP. ASS'N. *supra* note 35, at 2-13.

37.  Hollowell, *The Growing Legal Contest—Hospital Privileges for Podiatrists,* 23 ST. LOUIS U.L.J. 491, 492 & n.8 (1979).

38.  *See* Podell, *Issues in the Organization of Medical Care: An Illustrative Case Study—Podiatry in the United States,* 284 NEW ENG. J. MED. 586, 587 (1971).

39.  Skipper & Hughes, *Podiatry: Critical Issues in the 1980's,* 74 AM. J. PUB. HEALTH, 507, 507 (1984).

40.  233 F. Supp. 953 (D.D.C. 1964), *rev'd per curiam sub nom.* Levin v. Joint Comm'n on Accreditation of Hosps. 354 F.2d 515 (D.C. Cir. 1965).

41.  Levin v. Joint Comm'n on Accreditation of Hosps. 354 F.2d 515 (D.C. Cir. 1965).

42.  Hollowell, *supra* note 37, at 500-01 n.55.

43.  AMERICAN PODIATRIC MEDICAL ASS'N, FOOT CARE: A MAJOR PRODUCT LINE FOR TODAY'S COMPETITIVE HOSPITAL MARKETPLACE 1 (1985).

44.  Kaczanowski v. Medical Center Hosp. of Vt. 612 F. Supp. 688 (D. Vt. 1985); Cooper v. Forsyth County Hosp. Auth., 604 F. Supp. 685 (M.D.N.C. 1985), *aff'd,* 789 F.2d 278 (4th Cir. 1986). For earlier cases in which podiatrists challenged exclusion from hospitals on antitrust or constitutional grounds, *see* Shaw v. Hospital Auth. of Cobb County, 614 F.2d 946 (5th Cir.), *cert. denied,* 449 U.S. 955 (1980); Feldman v. Jackson Memorial Hosp., 571 F. Supp. 1000 (S.D. Fla. 1983), *aff'd mem.,* 752 F.2d 647 (11th Cir.), *cert. denied,* 105 S. Ct. 3504 (1985); Todd v. Physicians & Surgeons Community Hosp., 165 Ga. App. 656, 302 S.E.2d 378 (1983); Settler v. Hopedale Medical Found., 80 Ill. App. 3d 850, 400 N.E. 2d 577 (1980); Davidson v. Youngstown Hosp. Ass'n, 19 Ohio App. 2d 246, 250 N.E.2d 892 (1969). *See also Hospital Must Consider Podiatrists for Privileges,* [July-Dec.] Antitrust & Trade Reg. Rep. (BNA) No. 1238, at 742 (Oct. 31, 1985) (podiatrists successfully challenged denial of privileges by invoking state anti-discrimination statute); 50 Fed. Reg. 41,693 (1985) (consent agreement proposed Oct. 11, 1985, to settle complaint by Federal Trade Commission that a hospital's and medical staff's restrictions of podiatrists' surgical privileges restrained competition in violation of section 5 of Federal Trade Commission Act).

45.  Tanney, *Hospital Privileges for Psychologists—A Legislative Model,* 38 AM. PSYCHOLOGIST 1232, 1233 (1983).

46. *See* McGuire & Moore, *Private Regulation in Mental Health: The JCAH and Psychologists in Hospitals*, 7 L. & HUM. BEHAV. 235 (1983); Zaro, Batchelor, Ginsberg & Pallak, *Psychology and the JCAH: Reflections on a Decade of Struggle*, 37 AM. PSYCHOLOGIST 1342 (1982).

47. *Ohio Charges Accreditation Association*, *supra* note 2.

48. OHIO REV. CODE ANN. ¶ 3727.06 (Page Supp. 1985).

49. *See generally* COMMENT, *Hospital Privileges for Nurse-Midwives: An Examination Under Antitrust Law*, 33 AM. U.L. REV. 959 (1984).

50. Adams, *Nurse-Midwifery Practice in the United States, 1982*, 74 AM. J. PUB. HEALTH 1267, 1267 (1984); Levy, Wilkinson & Marine, *Reducing Neonatal Mortality Rate with Nurse Midwives*, 109 AM. J. OBSTETRICS & GYNECOLOGY 50, 51 (1971).

51. Levy, Wilkinson & Marine, *supra* note 50, at 51; *see, e.g.*, CONN. GEN. STAT. ANN. § 20-86(b) (West Supp. 1986); N.J. STAT. ANN. § 45:10-8 (West 1978); OHIO REV. CODE ANN. § 4731.33 (Page 1977).

52. Adams, *supra* note 50, at 1267, 1270.

53. *See* Nurse Midwifery Assocs. v. Hibbett, 549 F. Supp. 1185 (M.D. Tenn. 1982); *CNM's Seek Test of Right to Compete with MD's*, 85 AM. J. NURSING 599 (1985); *CNM's Pursue Admitting Privileges*, 83 AM. J. NURSING 1261 (1983).

54. Adams, *Nurse Anesthetist Clarifies Group's Responsibilities*, Am. Med. News, May 10, 1985, at 6, col. 1.

55. *Id.; see, e.g.*, OHIO REV. CODE ANN. § 4731.35 (Page 1977).

56. Adams, *supra* note 54; *CRNA's Battle a Trend to Phase Out Hospital Jobs*, 84 AM. J. NURSING 376, 386 (1984) [hereinafter CRNA's Battle].

57. *CRNA's Battle, supra* note 56, at 386, 390.

58. *See* Adams, *supra* note 54.

59. *See CRNA's Battle, supra* note 56, at 376-90.

60. State v. Anesthesia Prof. Ass'n, 1984-2 Trade Cas. (CCH) ¶ 66,081 (Me. Super. Ct. 1984).

61. *Id. See generally Maine Aims AT Blow at MD's and Saves the Day for CRNA's*, 84 AM. J. NURSING 600 (1985) (reports background of the litigation).

62. *Anesthesiologists Will Hold Down Prices Under Settlement with Attorney General*, [Jan.-June] Antitrust & Trade Reg. Rep. (BNA) No. 1258, at 551 (March 27, 1986).

63. Bhan v. NME Hosp., Inc. 772 F.2d 1467 (9th Cir. 1985).

64. Yesalis, Wallace, Fisher & Tokheim, *Does Chiropractic Utilization Substitute for Less Available Medical Services?*, 70 AM. J. PUB. HEALTH 415 (1980).

65. *See,* Wilk v. American Medical Ass'n, 719 F.2d 207 (7th Cir. 1983), *cert. denied,* 467 U.S. 1210 (1984); Ballard v. Blue Shield of S.W. Va., 543 F.2d 1075 (4th Cir. 1976), *cert. denied,* 430 U.S. 922 (1977); Aasum v. Good Samaritan Hosp., 542 F.2d 792 (9th Cir. 1976); Spears Free Clinic & Hosp. for Poor Children v. Cleere, 197 F.2d 125 (10th Cir. 1952); Chiropractic Coop. Ass'n of Mich. v. American Medical Ass'n, 617 F. Supp. 264 (E.D. Mich. 1985); Slavek v. American Medical Ass'n, 1982-1 Trade Cas. (CCH) ¶ 64,509 (E.D. Pa. 1982); Ballard v. Blue Shield of S.W. Va., 529 F. Supp. 71 (S.D. W. Va. 1981); Health Care Equalization Comm. of the Iowa Chiropractic Soc'y v. Iowa Medical Soc'y, 501 F. Supp. 970 (S.D. Iowa 1980); New York v. American Medical Ass'n, 1980-2 Trade Cas. (CCH) ¶ 63,456 (E.D.N.Y. 1980); Kentucky Ass'n of Chiropractors v. Jefferson County Medical Soc'y, 549 S.W.2d 817 (Ky. 1977); New Jersey Chiropractic Soc'y v. Radiological Soc'y of N.J., 156 N.J. Super. 365, 383 A.2d 1182 (1978); Boos v. Donnell, 421 P.2d 644 (Okla. 1966).

66. *See* Kissam, Webber, Bigus & Holzgraefe, *Antitrust and Hospital Privileges: Testing the Conventional Wisdom,* 70 CALIF. L. REV. 595, 675 (1982) [hereinafter Kissam & Webber]; Note, *Health Professionals' Access to Hospitals: A Retrospective and Prospective Analysis,* 34 VAND. L. REV. 1161, 1194 (1981).

67. Wilk v. American Medical Ass'n, 719 F.2d 207, 214 (7th Cir. 1983), *cert. denied,* 467 U.S. 1210 (1984); *see also* Aasum v. Good Samaritan Hosp., 395 F. Supp. 363, 370-71 (D. Ore. 1975), *aff'd,* 542 F.2d 792 (9th Cir. 1976).

68. *See supra* notes 35-36 and accompanying text.

69. *See, e.g.,* Aasum v. Good Samaritan Hosp., 395 F. Supp. 363 (D. Ore. 1975), *aff'd,* 542 F.2d 792 (9th Cir. 1976); Boos v. Donnell, 421 P.2d 644 (Okla. 1966); *cf.* Kentucky Ass'n of Chiropractors v. Jefferson County Medical Soc'y, 549 S.W.2d 817 (Ky. 1977) (chiropractors not permitted to use services of medical laboratories).

70. 425 U.S. 738 (1976).

71. 444 U.S. 232 (1980).

72. *Hospital Bldg. Co.,* 425 U.S. at 744; *McLain,* 444 U.S. at 242, 245. There is conflict among the federal circuit courts of appeal as to just how much *McLain* relaxed the definition, i.e., as to whether a plaintiff may show merely that a defendant's business activities in general affect interstate commerce or whether a plaintiff must show a nexus between the challenged restraint and interstate commerce. *See* Shahawy v. Harrison, 788 F.2d 636 (11th Cir. 1985); Seglin v. Esau, 769 F.2d 1274 (7th Cir. 1985); Hayden v. Bracy, 744 F.2d 1338 (8th Cir. 1984); Cardio-

Medical Assoc. v. Crozer-Chester Medical Center, 721 F.2d 68 (3rd Cir. 1983); Furlong v. Long Island College Hosp., 710 F.2d 922 (2d Cir. 1983); Mishler v. St. Anthony's Hosp. Sys., 694 F.2d 1225 (10th Cir. 1981); Crane v. Intermountain Health Care, Inc., 637 F.2d 715 (10th Cir. 1981) (on reh'g en banc); Capili v. Shott, 620 F.2d 439 (4th Cir. 1980).
73. 421 U.S. 773 (1975).
74. 457 U.S. 332 (1982).
75. *Goldfarb*, 421 U.S. at 787-88; Maricopa, 457 U.S. at 348-49.
76. *Attempts to Gain Access to Hospitals Are Prevalent in Health Care Actions*, [Jan.-June] Antitrust & Trade Reg. Rep. (BNA) No. 1150, at 187 (Feb. 2, 1984). In October 1986, Congress effectively elimi- nated antitrust suits by individual physicians by providing immu- nity from damages liability for peer review committees, their mem- bers, and the hospital where restrictions in clinical privileges are based on review of a physician's competence or professional conduct. Health Care Quality Improvement Act of 1986, Pub. L. No. 99-660, tit. IV. The statutory definition of immunized conduct refers only to "indi- vidual physician[s]," *id.* § 431(9), so presumably the statute does not cover applications for hospital privileges by non-physicians, nor does it preclude a physician seeking injunctive relief.
77. *See supra* notes 13-15 and accompanying text.
78. *See* Weiss v. York Hosp. 745 F.2d 786, 814-17 (3rd Cir. 1984), *cert. denied*, 105 S. Ct. 1777 (1985); Quinn v. Kent Gen. Hosp., 617 F. Supp. 1226, 1242 (D. Del. 1985); Feldman v. Jackson Memorial Hosp., 571 F. Supp. 1000, 1009 (S.D. Fla. 1983), *aff'd mem.*, 752 F.2d 647 (11th Cir. 1985), *cert. denied*, 105 S. Ct. 3504 (1985); Williams v. Kleaveland, 534 F. Supp. 912, 920 (W.D. Mich. 1981).
79. Redisch, *Physician Involvement in Hospital Decision Making*, in HOSPITAL COST CONTAINMENT 217, 220-21 (M. Zubkoff, I. Raskin & R. Hanft eds. 1978).
80. Robinson v. Magovern, 521 F. Supp. 842, 907 (W.D. Pa. 1981), *aff'd mem.*, 688 F.2d 824 (3rd Cir.), *cert. denied*, 459 U.S. 971 (1982).
81. 745 F.2d 786 (3rd Cir. 1984), *cert. denied*, 105 S. Ct. 1777 (1985).
82. *Id.* at 814.
83. *Id.* at 815-16.
84. Havighurst, *supra* note 31, at 1116-17.
85. *See, e.g.*, E. FREIDSON, PROFESSIONAL DOMINANCE—THE SOCIAL STRUCTURE OF MEDICAL CARE 72, 99, 190 (1970).
86. A clear example of how physicians can influence their colleagues' behavior without overt coercion appears in Feminist Women's Health Center v. Mohammad, where an obstetrician described how peer pres-

sure induced him to sever his relations with an abortion clinic. 586 F.2d 530, 536-37 (5th Cir. 1978), *cert. denied,* 444 U.S. 924 (1979).

87. Silver v. New York Stock Exch., 373 U.S. 341, 347-48 (1963); Klor's v. Broadway-Hale Stores, 359 U.S. 207, 212 (1959); *see also* Weiss v. York Hosp., 745 F.2d 786 (3d Cir. 1984), *cert. denied,* 105 S. Ct. 1777 (1985) (denial of privileges to osteopaths held to be per se illegal group boycott).

88. *See, e.g.,* Vuciecevic v. MacNeal Memorial Hosp., 572 F. Supp. 1424, 1428 (N.D. Ill. 1983); *cf.* Kreuzer v. American Academy of Periodontology, 735 F.2d 1479, 1491 (D.C. Cir. 1984) (rule of reason appropriate for evaluating professional association's exclusion of dentist based on application of standards).

89. *See, e.g.,* Silver v. New York Stock Exch., 373 U.S. 341, 348-49 (1963) (rule of reason may be appropriate approach where proper procedures have been followed in stock exchange self-regulation under Securities Exchange Act); Hatley v. American Quarter Horse Ass'n, 552 F.2d 646, 652 (5th Cir. 1977) (rule of reason appropriate where group boycott alleged in context of sports industry self-regulation); *see also* Ponsoldt, *The Application of Sherman Act Antiboycott Law to Industry Self-Regulation: An Analysis Integrating Nonboycott Sherman Act Principles,* 55 S. CAL. L. REV. 1, 33-34 (1981).

90. 457 U.S. at 348-49.

91. *Id.* (per se rule applicable where doctors' conduct "not premised on public service or ethical norms"); National Soc'y of Professional Eng'rs v. United States, 435 U.S. 679, 696 (1978) ("professional services may differ significantly from other business services, and, accordingly, the nature of the competition in such services may vary. Ethical norms may serve to regulate and promote this competition, and thus fall within the Rule of Reason."); Goldfarb v. Virginia State Bar, 421 U.S. 773, 788-89 n.17 (1975) ("The public service aspect, and other features of the professions, may require that a particular practice, which could properly be viewed as a violation of the Sherman Act in another context, be treated differently."); *see also* Federal Trade Comm'n v. Indiana Fed'n of Dentists, 106 S. Ct. 2009, 2018 (1986) ("we have been slow to condemn rules adopted by professional associations as unreasonable per se").

92. *See, e.g.,* Weiss v. York Hosp. 745 F.2d 786, 820 (3rd Cir. 1984), *cert. denied,* 105 S. Ct. 1777 (1985) (per se rule applied because "defendants have offered no 'public service or ethical norm' rationale"); Pontius v. Children's Hosp., 522 F. Supp. 1352, 1369-70 (W.D. Pa. 1982); *see also* Chiropractic Coop. Ass'n of Mich. v. American Medical Ass'n, 617

F. Supp. 264, 269 (E.D. Mich. 1985) (defendant physicians' assertion that exclusion of chiropractors was motivated by quality of care invokes rule of reason).

93. Vuciecevic v. MacNeal Memorial Hosp., 572 F. Supp. 1424, 1427 (N.D. Ill. 1983); Pontius v. Children's Hosp., 552 F. Supp. 1352, 1368 (W.D. Pa. 1982); Everhart v. Jane C. Stormont Hosp., 1982-1 Trade Cas. (CCH) ¶ 64,703, 73,897 (D. Kans. 1982).

94. 105 S. Ct. 2613 (1985).

95. *Id.* at 2621.

96. *Id.* at 2620.

97. *See* Pontius v. Children's Hosp., 552 F. Supp. 1352, 1370, 1377 (W.D. Pa. 1982).

98. Jefferson Parish Hosp. Dist. No. 2 v. Hyde, 466, U.S. 2, 30 (1984) (dictum).

99 Havighurst, *supra* note 31, at 1095; Kissam & Webber, *supra* note 66, at 646.

100. 435 U.S. 679 (1978).

101. *Id.* at 688-92, 694.

102. *Id.* at 695.

103. *Id.* at 689-90.

104. 106 S. Ct. 2009 (1986).

105. *Id.* at 2014-15.

106. *Id.* at 2015, 2020.

107. *Id.* at 2020-21. The Court hinted that there might be circumstances where quality of patient care could justify a restraint of trade. *Id.* at 2021. However, its focus here seems to be on situations where quality relates to ethical grounds or is otherwise "noncompetitive." In a hospital privileges context, because hospitals compete with each other largely on the basis of quality, such a "loophole" in the rule of reason is unnecessary. *See* infra notes 113-15 and accompanying text.

108. 719 F.2d 207 (7th Cir. 1983), *cert. denied,* 467 U.S. 1210 (1984).

109. *Id.* at 225.

110. *Id.* at 226-27 (citing *Professional Engineers,* 435 U.S. at 696; Goldfarb v. Virginia State Bar, 421 U.S. 773, 787 n.17 (1975)).

111. Kissam, *Antitrust Boycott Doctrine,* 69 Iowa L. Rev. 1165, 1214-15 (1984).

112. *Id.; see also* Havighurst, *supra* note 31, at 1103-04 n.101.

113. Salkever, *Competition Among Hospitals,* in COMPETITION IN THE HEALTH CARE SECTOR: PAST, PRESENT AND FUTURE 191, 201 (1978).

114. *Id.*

115. *See, e.g.,* Dos Santos v. Columbus-Cuneo-Cabrini Medical Center, 684 F.2d 1346, 1355 (7th Cir. 1982); Pontius v. Children's Hosp. 521 F. Supp. 1352, 1365 (W.D. Pa. 1982).

116. *See* Wilk v. American Medical Ass'n, 719 F.2d 207 (7th Cir. 1983), *cert. denied*, 467 U.S. 1210 (1984); Chiropractic Coop. Ass'n of Mich. v. American Medical Ass'n, 617 F. Supp. 264 (E.D. Mich. 1985); Kaczanowski v. Medical Center Hosp. of Vt., 612 F. Supp. 688 (D. Vt. 1985); Cooper v. Forsyth County Hosp. Auth., 604 F. Supp. 685 (M.D.N.C. 1985), *aff'd*, 789 F.2d 278 (4th Cir. 1986).

117. *See, e.g.*, Cooper v. Forsyth County Hosp. Auth., 604 F. Supp. 685, 687 (M.D.N.C. 1985), *aff'd*, 789 F.2d 278 (4th Cir. 1986).

118. 465 So. 2d 1246 (Fla. Dist. Ct. App. 1985).

119. *Id.* at 1252 n.3. This case defies easy categorization. The opinion approvingly cites a variety of approaches which, when blended, become very deferential.

120. Kaczanowski v. Medical Center Hosp. of Vt., 612 F. Supp. 688, 697 (D. Vt. 1985); *see also* Levin v. Doctors Hosp., 233 F. Supp. 953, 954-55 (D.D.C. 1964), *rev'd per curiam sub nom.* Levin v. Joint Comm'n on Accreditation of Hosps., 354 F.2d 515 (D.C. Cir. 1965).

121 Although not a hospital privileges case, Federal Trade Commission v. Indiana Federation of Dentists, 106 S. Ct. 2009 (1986), illustrates this possibility. In this case, dentists' assertions that their boycott of insurers was aimed at protecting the quality of dental care were substantially undermined by statements of a boycott leader that "We are fighting an economic war. . . . The name of the game is money." *Id.* at 2013 n.1.

122. 534 F. Supp. 912 (W.D. Mich. 1981).

123. *Id.* at 920.

124. Cooper v. Forsyth County Hosp. Auth., 604 F. Supp. 685, 687 (M.D.N.C. 1985), *aff'd*, 789 F.2d 278 (4th Cir. 1986).

125. *Id.*

126. 612 F. Supp. 688 (D. Vt. 1985).

127. *Id.* at 697. *See generally* Havighurst, *supra* note 31, at 1133-36, recommending a rational basis test for privileges denials based on quality maintenance, absent market power or a violation of section two of the Sherman Act. This recommendation is premised on the hospital's ultimate accountability to consumers for its business decisions. Such a premise may be questionable in light of the hospital's greater responsiveness to physicians than to consumers. *See infra* notes 162-65 and accompanying text.

128. *See* VT. STAT. ANN. tit. 7, § 321 (1975); *see also supra* note 37 and accompanying text.

129. 586 F.2d 530 (5th Cir. 1978), *cert. denied*, 444 U.S. 924 (1979).

130. *Id.* at 547.

131. 624 F.2d 476 (4th Cir. 1980), *cert. denied*, 450 U.S. 916 (1981).

132. *Id.* at 485.

133. *Id.* On remand, however, the federal district court found that determining a remedy for the boycotted psychologists had become a moot issue because of a Virginia Supreme Court decision that the state statute under which the plaintiff psychologists were demanding insurance reimbursement was unconstitutional. 501 F. Supp. 1232 (E.D. Va. 1980) (citing Blue Cross of Va. v. Commonwealth, 221 Va. 349, 269 S.E.2d 827 (1980)).

134. 552 F. Supp. 1352 (W.D. Pa. 1982).

135. *Id.* at 1372.

136. *Id.* at 1372-73.

137. *Id.* at 1370-71.

138. Hackett v. Metropolitan Gen. Hosp., 465 So. 2d 1246, 1255-57 (Fla. Dist. Ct. App. 1985); Kissam & Webber, *supra* note 66, at 660-62.

139. Havighurst, *supra* note 31, at 1109-10.

140. 246 U.S. 231 (1918).

141. *Id.* at 238.

142. *Id.*

143. *See also* NCAA v. Board of Regents of the Univ. of Okla., 468 U.S. 85, 101 n.23 (1984) ("It is. . .well-settled that good motives will not validate an otherwise anticompetitive practice."); Kreuzer v. American Academy of Periodontology, 735 F.2d 1479, 1492-93 (D.C. Cir. 1984) (effect, and not intent, is controlling factor in a rule of reason inquiry); Ponsoldt, *supra* note 89, at 63 (lower courts often give great weight to defendants' intent despite Supreme Court declarations that intent is not controlling.)

144. Kissam & Webber, *supra* note 66, at 597.

145. Dixon, *Hospital Privileges for Podiatrists*, 24 Hosp. & Health Services Ad. 63, 74 (1979).

146. *Id.*

147. *Cf.* Kissam & Webber, *supra* note 66, at 608 ("the professional pride of physicians often will be at stake. . .particularly when nonphysicians apply for privileges.").

148. E. Freidson, *supra* note 85, at 146-58.

149. *See* Cooper v. Forsyth County Hosp. Auth., 604 F. Supp. 685, 687 (M.D.N.C. 1985), *aff'd*, 789 F.2d 278 (4th Cir. 1986) (court accepted this argument and upheld denial of privileges to podiatrists).

150. *Cf.* Dolan, *Antitrust Law and Physician Dominance of Other Health Practitioners*, 4 J. Health Pol'y & L. 675, 679 (1980).

151. Tanney, *supra* note 45, at 1235.

152. JOINT COMM'N ON ACCREDITATION OF HOSPS., *supra* note 25, at 89.

153. Hayman v. City of Galveston, 273 U.S. 414, 416-17 (1927); Don v. Okmulgee Memorial Hosp., 443 F.2d 234, 239 (10th Cir. 1971); Stern v. Tarrant County Hosp. Dist., 565 F. Supp. 1440, 1447 (N.D. Tex. 1983); *rev'd on other grounds*, 778 F.2d 1052 (5th Cir. 1985), *cert. denied*, 106 S. Ct. 1957 (1986); Aasum v. Good Samaritan Hosp., 395 F. Supp. 363, 371 (D. Ore. 1975), *aff'd*, 542 F.2d 792 (9th Cir. 1976); Levin v. Doctors Hosp., 233 F. Supp. 953, 955 (D.D.C. 1964), *rev'd per curiam on other grounds sub nom.* Levin v. Joint Comm'n on Accreditation of Hosps., 354 F.2d 515 (D.C. Cir. 1965); Settler v. Hopedale Medical Found., 80 Ill. App. 3d 1074, 1075-76, 400 N.E.2d 577, 578 (1980).

154. *See* Gellhorn, *The Abuse of Occupational Licensing*, 44 U. CHI. I., REV. 6, 6 & 25 (1976); Moore, *The Purpose of Licensing*, 4 J. LAW & ECON. 93, 104 (1961). These articles argue that even licensing, although ostensibly to protect the public from incompetence, is too restrictive and results in protecting the licensees from competition.

155. Fashion Originators' Guild of Am. v. Federal Trade Comm'n, 312 U.S. 457, 465 (1941); American Medical Ass'n v. United States, 130 F.2d 233, 245-49 (D.C. Cir. 1942), *aff'd*, 317 U.S. 519 (1943). *See generally* 1 P. AREEDA & D. TURNER, ANTITRUST LAW ¶ 216b (1978).

156. Dolan, *supra* note 150, at 686.

157. Levy, Wilkinson & Marine, *supra* note 50; Mann, *San Francisco General Hospital Nurse-Midwifery Practice: The First Thousand Births*, 140 AM. J. OBSTETRICS & GYNECOLOGY 676 (1981); Slome, Wetherbee, Daly, Christensen, Meglen & Thiede, *Effectiveness of Certified Nurse-Midwives*, 124 AM. J. OBSTETRICS & GYNECOLOGY 177 (1976).

158. *See* Drexel, *The Antitrust Implications of the Denial of Hospital Staff Privileges*, 36 U. MIAMI L. REV. 207, 227 (1982).

159. *See, e.g.*, Cooper v. Forsyth County Hosp. Auth., 604 F. Supp. 685, 687 (M.D.N.C. 1985), *aff'd*, 789 F.2d 278 (4th Cir. 1986) (granting staff privileges to plaintiff podiatrist would have required change in hospital by-laws); *cf.* Jost, *supra* note 24, at 907 (exclusion of a class of providers subject to criticism as denying procedural fairness).

160. *See generally* Rafferty, *Comment*, in COMPETITION IN THE HEALTH CARE SECTOR: PAST, PRESENT AND FUTURE 207, 208 (1978).

161. *See infra* notes 168-71 and accompanying text.

162. Reinhardt, *Comment*, in COMPETITION IN THE HEALTH CARE SECTOR: PAST, PRESENT, AND FUTURE 156, 157 (1978); Somers, Comment, in COMPETITION IN THE HEALTH CARE SECTOR: PAST, PRESENT, AND FUTURE 469, 469-70 (1978).

163. Redisch, *supra* note 79, at 231.

164. Havighurst, *supra* note 31, at 1081; Salkever, *supra* note 113, at 197-98.

165. E. Freidson, *supra* note 85, at 146-69; Havighurst, *supra* note 31, at 1104.

166. Jost, *supra* note 24, at 843; *see also* Havighurst, *supra* note 31, at 1087-88. For cases in which accreditation is discussed in this manner, *see, e.g.,* Wilk v. American Medical Ass'n, 719 F.2d 207, 214 (7th Cir. 1983), *cert. denied,* 467 U.S. 1210 (1984); Williams v. Kleaveland, 1983-2 Trade Cas. (CCH) ¶ 65,486, 68,358 (W.D. Mich. 1983); Levin v. Doctors Hosp., 233 F. Supp. 953 (D.D.C. 1964), *rev'd per curiam on other grounds sub. nom.* Levin v. Joint Comm'n on Accreditation of Hosps., 354 F.2d 515 (D.C. Cir. 1965).

167. *See supra* notes 34-36 and accompanying text.

168. Salkever, *supra* note 113, at 198.

169. Enders, *supra* note 3, at 742.

170. *Cf.* Kissam & Webber, *supra* note 66, at 610 (even with respect to fellow physicians, there is an incentive for physicians to want staff membership restricted to inefficient levels to increase excess capacity and physicians' own prestige and income.)

171. NCAA v. Board of Regents of the Univ. of Okla., 468 U.S. 85, 107 (1984); Marrese v. American Academy of Orthopaedic Surgeons, 706 F.2d 1488, 1495 (7th Cir. 1983), *rev'd on other grounds,* 105 S. Ct. 1327 (1985).

172. Crumley v. Memorial Hosp., Inc., 509 F. Supp. 531 (E.D. Tenn. 1978), *aff'd mem.,* 647 F.2d 164 (6th Cir. 1981); Elam v. College Park Hosp., 132 Cal. App. 3d 332, 183 Cal. Rptr. 156 (1982); Joiner v. Mitchell County Hosp. Auth., 125 Ga. App. 1, 186 S.E.2d 307 (1971), *aff'd,* 229 Ga. 140, 189 S.E.2d 412 (1972); Darling v. Charleston Community Memorial Hosp., 33 Ill. 2d 326, 211 N.E.2d 253 (1965), *cert. denied,* 383 U.S. 946 (1966); Ferguson v. Gonyaw, 236 N.W.2d 543 (Mich. Ct. App. 1975); Johnson v. Misericordia Community Hosp., 99 Wis. 2d 708, 301 N.W.2d 156 (1981).

173. Kaczanowski v. Medical Center Hosp. of Vt., 612 F. Supp. 688, 696 (D. Vt. 1985); Williams v. Kleaveland, 1983-2 Trade Cas. (CCH) ¶ 65,486, 68,358 (W.D. Mich. 1983); Drexel, *supra* note 158, at 231.

174. *Malpractice Crisis Leaves Nurse-Midwives Without Coverage,* 4 PROF. REG. NEWS, July 1985, at 6.

175. Levy, Wilkinson & Marine, *supra* note 50, at 51; Adams, *supra* note 50, at 1267. *But see id.* at 1270, noting increased involvement of nurse-midwives with complicated births.

176. Note, *supra* note 66, at 1194. Although there are no large scale studies of the quality of chiropractic care, there are assertions that chiropractic education is inadequate and that chiropractors tend to exceed the scope of their competence. *See generally* Ballantine, *Will the Delivery of Health Care Be Improved By the Use of Chiropractic Services?*, 286 New Eng. J. Med. 237 (1972); Firman & Goldstein, *The Future of Chiropractic: A Psychosocial View*, 293 New Eng. J. Med. 639 (1975); Silver, *Chiropractic: Professional Controversy and Public Policy*, 70 Am. J. Pub. Health 348 (1980). There are also anecdotal reports of injuries caused by chiropractic treatment. *See, e.g.*, Braun, Pinto, DeFilipp, Lieberman, Pasternack & Zimmerman, *Brain Stem Infarction Due to Chiropractic Manipulation of the Cervical Spine*, 76 S. Med. J. 1507 (1983); Schmidley & Kock, *The Noncerebrovascular Complications of Chiropractic Manipulation*, 34 Neurology 684 (1984).

177. Silver, *supra* note 176, at 348.

178. *But cf.* Kissam & Webber, *supra* note 66, at 608-09 (suggesting hospital may not be liable for chiropractor's treatment error as long as hospital has exercised proper care in selecting chiropractor). Regarding the difficulty a hospital might have in screening chiropractors, *see infra* notes 188-89 and accompanying text.

179. *See, e.g.*, Ind. Code § 16-10-1-6.5 (a) & (c) (Supp. 1985); Me. Rev. Stat. Ann. tit. 24, § 2503 (1984-85); Mich. Comp. Laws Ann. § 333.21513 (West Supp. 1985); 63 Pa. Cons. Stat. Ann. § 425.1 (Purdon Supp. 1985); Joint Comm'n on Accreditation of Hosps., *supra* note 21, at 107-09, 113.

180. Where peer review is mandated by a state statute, staff members may have state action immunity to antitrust liability. Marrese v. Interqual, Inc., 748 F.2d 373 (7th Cir. 1984), *cert. denied*, 105 S. Ct. 3501 (1985); Lombardo v. Sisters of Mercy Health Corp., 1985-2 Trade Cas. (CCH) ¶ 66,749 (N.D. Ind. 1985). *But see* Jiriko v. Coffeyville Memorial Hosp. Medical Center, 628 F. Supp. 329, 333 (D. Kan. 1985) (no state action immunity where publicly-owned hospital did not provide due process to demoted physician); Quinn v. Kent Gen. Hosp., 617 F. Supp. 1226, 1236-40 (D. Del. 1985) (peer review not immune as state action because peer review statute does not reflect a legislative intent to displace competition with regulation).

181. *See* Pontius v. Children's Hosp., 552 F. Supp. 1352, 1376 (W.D. Pa. 1982); Williams v. Kleaveland, 534 F. Supp. 912, 920 (W.D. Mich. 1981). Indeed, concern with this chilling effect largely prompted Congress to enact, in late 1986, a statutory provision for antitrust dam-

ages immunity for peer review of individual physicians. *See* Health Care Quality Improvement Act of 1986, Pub. L. No. 99-660, tit. IV; *see also supra* note 76.

182. Drexel, *supra* note 158, at 232; Enders, *supra* note 3, at 743.

183. See Kissam & Webber, *supra* note 97, at 655.

184. JOINT COMM'N ON ACCREDITATION OF HOSPS., *supra* note 21, at 101.

185. *See supra* note 51 and accompanying text.

186. 549 F. Supp. 1185 (M.D. Tenn. 1982).

187. *See* M. ROEMER & J. FRIEDMAN, *supra* note 22, at 284.

188. Kissam & Webber, *supra* note 66, at 655. Although not basing its decision on antitrust analysis, a New Jersey state court found that a hospital's inability to establish standards and supervise the care given by a new type of staff member was a reasonable basis for denying adjunct staff privileges to a certified psychiatric nursing specialist. Wrable v. Community Memorial Hosp., 205 N.J. Super. 438, 501 A.2d 187 (1985). Broad application of this court's reasoning could make it impossible for any new category of provider to obtain privileges.

189. *See supra* note 177.

190. Pauly, *Is Medical Care Different?*, in COMPETITION IN THE HEALTH CARE SECTOR: PAST, PRESENT, AND FUTURE 19, 28-34 (1978).

191. *See* Quinn v. Kent Gen. Hosp., 617 F. Supp. 1226, 1239 (D. Del. 1985) (medical staff peer review "arguably procompetitive" by compensating for consumers' "relative lack of information about these matters"). *See generally* Jost, *supra* note 24, at 866-75 (while standards may thus reduce costs, they may also promote inefficiency if the standards are merely symbolic or force consumers to pay for something they don't need).

192. Jost, *supra* note 24, at 906.

193. Marrese v. American Academy of Orthopaedic Surgeons, 706 F.2d 1488, 1497 (7th Cir. 1983), *rev'd on other grounds*, 105 S. Ct. 1327 (1985).

194. *See* Williams v. Kleaveland, 534 F. Supp. 912, 920 (W.D. Mich. 1981); Hackett v. Metropolitan Gen. Hosp., 465 So. 2d 1246, 1257 (Fla. Dist. Ct. App. 1985). *See generally* R. POSNER, ANTITRUST LAW—AN ECONOMIC PERSPECTIVE 123 (1976) ("the elimination of an individual potential competitor can be expected to have no competitive significance at all"). *But see* Havighurst, *supra* note 31, at 1143 (elimination of a single physician may have anticompetitive ramifications justifying judicial oversight).

195. *See* Comment, *supra* note 49, at 963 (describing physicians' childbirth services as technological and surgical in contrast with nurse-midwives' as natural and personalized).

196. Federal Trade Comm'n v. Indiana Fed'n of Dentists, 106 S. Ct. 2009, 2018-19 (1986).

197. AMERICAN PODIATRIC MEDICAL ASS'N, *supra* note 43, at 4 (podiatrists' charges are ten to fifty percent less than orthopedists').

198. Tanney, *supra* note 45, at 1233.

199. *See* Nurse Midwifery Assoc. v. Hibbett, 549 F. Supp. 1185, 1188 (M.D. Tenn. 1982) (excluded nurse-midwives alleged higher costs for maternity care in a market with only obstetricians).

200. *FTC, Attorney General Come to Rescue of California CRNA*, 85 AM. J. NURSING 601, 601, 608 (1985).

201. *See* Bhan v. NME Hosps., Inc. 772 F.2d 1467, 1471 (9th Cir. 1985); *FTC Addresses Key Question: Can Nurses and Doctors Compete?*, 4 PROF. REG. NEWS, Jan. 1985, at 2, 3.

202. *See* Tanney, *supra* note 45, at 1235. *See generally* Ponsoldt, *supra* note 89, at 37-38 (analysis of how product standards created and enforced by dominant group of competitors result in eliminating competition from innovation).

203. Comment, *supra* note 49, at 963.

204. Tanney, *supra* note 45, at 1235.

205. 435 U.S. at 696; *see also* NCAA v. Board of Regents of the Univ. of Okla., 468 U.S. 85, 117 (1984) (rejecting rule of reason defense based on premise that competition itself is unreasonable).

206. *See* Havighurst, *supra* note 31, at 1133-35; Kissam & Webber, *supra* note 66, at 613, 638-39; *see also supra* notes 76 & 181.

207. *Cf.* Kreuzer v. American Academy of Periodontology. 735 F.2d 1479, 1494 (D.C. Cir. 1984) (test for application of the rule of reason to exclusionary conduct by health professionals when a quality defense is asserted is whether there is a close rational nexus between the standard and quality of care).

208. *See* Pontius v. Children's Hosp., 552 F. Supp. 1352, 1370-72 (W.D. Pa. 1982) (demanding substantial evidence to support exclusion of individual physician).

209. 106 S. Ct. 2009 (1986).

210. *Id.* at 2021.

211. *Id.* at 2020-21.

212. 373 U.S. 341 (1963).

213. *Id.* at 361 (emphasis added).

214. 435 U.S. 679 (1978).

215. *Id.* at 699 (Blackmun, J., concurring).

216. Kreuzer v. American Academy of Periodontology. 735 F.2d 1479, 1491 (D.C. Cir. 1984) (emphasis added).

217. Wilk v. American Medical Ass'n, 719 F.2d 207, 227 (7th Cir. 1983), *cert. denied,* 467 U.S. 1210 (1984).

218. Ponsoldt, *supra* note 89, at 40-43, 59. A least restrictive alternative test is also recommended for scrutinizing exclusionary acts of joint ventures. Brodley, *Joint Ventures and Antitrust Policy,* 95 HARV. L. REV. 1521, 1536, 1568 (1982). A hospital and its medical staff may be characterized as a joint venture. *See* Kissam & Webber, *supra* note 66, at 656-59; *see also* Havighurst, *supra* note 31, at 1128-29 (recommending least restrictive alternative scrutiny of the hospital-medical staff joint venture, but focusing only on the structure, rather than the substance, of a privileges decision).

219. Although podiatrists need only meet state licensure requirements in order to practice, podiatrists may obtain additional clinical training during a residency and demonstrate advanced knowledge by passing a Board examination. Of the 9,200 podiatrists in the United States, 2,400 are Board certified or Board eligible. AMERICAN PODIATRIC MEDICAL ASS'N, *supra* note 43, at 5. *But see* 50 Fed. Reg. 41,693, 41,695 (1985) (Federal Trade Commission charged that a hospital, in demanding that all podiatrists have a three-year residency without relating the residency requirement to specific surgical procedures, restrained competition in violation of the Federal Trade Commission Act).

220. M. ROEMER & J. FRIEDMAN, *supra* note 22, at 284.

221. 19 Ohio App. 2d 246, 250 N.E.2d 892 (1969).

222. *Id.* at 252-54, 250 N.E.2d at 897.

223. *See supra* note 37 and accompanying text.

224. *Cf.* Reynolds v. Medical and Dental Staff of St. John's Riverside Hosp., 86 Misc. 2d 418, 382 N.Y.S.2d 618 (Westchester County Sup. Ct. 1976), *aff'd* 55 A.D.2d 948, 391 N.Y.S.2d 382 (1977) (although hospital not obligated to directly employ a physician's assistant, it is obligated to provide appropriate privileges when assistant is employed by a physician staff member).

225. Kissam & Webber, *supra* note 66, at 597.

226. Brown Shoe Co. v. United States, 370 U.S. 294, 320 (1962).

# Privilege Delineation in a Demanding New Environment


James S. Roberts, MD;
Margaret Higgins Radany, MPP;
and David B. Nash, MD, MBA


The delineation of clinical privileges is one of the most important means for hospitals to ensure high-quality care. Competition, cost control, and public accountability have created the need for hospitals to assure effective privilege delineation processes. Hospitals should focus on issues of practice variation, continuity of care, volume of services provided and planned, and the integration of ethical consideration into clinical decisions. How information is obtained, verified, and acted upon is reviewed within the organizational framework of the hospital. Several leaders within the hospital, such as the clinical department chairs and members of the medical staff executive committee, have important functions in the clinical privilege delineation process. Granting clinical privileges is a critical hospital function that requires a commitment by the governing body, management, and medical staff leaders.

The delineation of clinical privileges, long a cornerstone of hospital quality assurance activities, has been a central means for hospitals to ensure high-quality care. In today's environment of new and powerful legal, health policy, economic, and statutory forces, privilege delineation is increasingly important and requires sound information and strong leadership. We will briefly describe the rationale for privilege delineation, a framework that determines the need for involvement of all key hospital leaders in privi-


Reprinted by permission of ANNALS OF INTERNAL MEDICINE, Volume 108, Page 880, 1988. Copyright American College of Physicians.

lege delineation and defines the nature and flow of the information needed to judge clinical competence.

## The Need for Privilege Delineation

Hospitals need to delineate the clinical privileges of independent practitioners because of laws requiring hospitals and practitioners to define their relationship. Hospital care in the United States is governed by two types of licensure laws. The first type concerns the licensure of physicians and other independent practitioners. These laws authorize the person to practice and, implicitly or explicitly, hold the practitioner responsible for the quality of the care he or she provides. Licensure of practitioners is not designed, however, to clearly demarcate their clinical competence and would, theoretically, allow practitioners to do specialty services for which they have not been trained. An individual's clinical competence to provide services in the hospital is defined by the hospital's privilege delineation process, a response to obligations the second type of licensure law places on hospitals.

Hospital licensure holds each hospital responsible for the quality of the care provided under its authority. Thus, the hospital must be assured that each licensed practitioner has the education, training, and experience to deliver competently the services authorized by the hospital. Privilege delineation is, therefore, the most important mechanism for the two licensing processes to combine to provide high-quality care.

Medical staffs are asked to judge the clinical competence of practitioners because hospital governing bodies lack the necessary expertise. Medical staffs have, in turn, needed support from the governing body and management to create systems for defining and monitoring the quality of care the staff provides and to use this and other essential information to make recommendations for clinical privileges. The privilege delineation process epitomizes the essential interdependency that characterizes the best hospitals.

Our hospitals are changing fundamentally and rapidly. The factors that will influence day-to-day patient care in the years ahead are changing dramatically. These changes, the most important features of which we describe in the following section, will profoundly affect hospital operations in general and privilege delineation in particular.

## The Transformation of Hospitals and Care

From a position of relative tranquility, hospitals have been vigorously shaken by the hands of competition, cost control, and public accountability. Once the recipients of unquestioning public trust, hospitals must suddenly begin to prove their efficiency and effectiveness. A recent sign of this change is the release by the Health Care Financing Administration (HCFA) of hospital-specific mortality data.[1] Although properly criticized for their imprecision, such data have been welcomed by consumer groups and by many in the business community, and they will undoubtedly continue to be released. The business community needs to better understand and differentiate among the organizations to which they are providing a growing proportion of their revenue, and are using clinical and financial performance data to make judgments about the health care organizations their employees use.[2] Government and business leaders have riveted their attention on major components of a cost-control strategy: prospective pricing, competition, cost-shifting to consumers, and movement of care to lower cost settings.

Concern about cost control has, in turn, prompted concern about the quality of care. Has the use of diagnosis-related groups (DRGs) harmed quality? Are patients being discharged too early from hospitals? Is the rate of surgery too high or too low? Is endoscopy done too frequently? How much unnecessary care is being provided? How should hospitals respond? The answer is simple to state but difficult to achieve. Each hospital must improve understanding of the current and future needs of their patients, what the hospital is doing and will need to do to meet these needs efficiently, and the degree to which the care provided comports with contemporary standards of quality and appropriateness.

The challenge a hospital faces is similar in type (although more complex) to that of a large, financially comfortable family faced with a sudden and persistent decline in income. From a position of assured comfort, such a family must scale down its expenditures by focusing on what is truly needed. Key questions arise. What is needed by each member of the family and by the family as a unit? What are the family expenditures buying, how much is being spent, and how do these expenditures compare to the family's most important priorities? How does the family reconcile the differences in priorities among family members? Are new sources of revenue needed, and what skills do family members have to pursue additional income? To answer these questions the family must plan better, monitor expenditures most closely, decide how well spending is meeting goals, and change behavior where needed. If the family takes these steps, it will probably withstand the shock.

Faced with a similar shock, hospitals must also improve their ability to plan, monitor, and make decisions and improve their governance, clinical, and managerial activities. Leaders of the governing bodies, management, and clinical staffs of hospitals have become energized and are examining tools for meeting the rigorous demands of this new environment. As we might suspect, they are finding that many of these tools are dull—especially their ability to judge and match a practitioner's capabilities with the hospital's current and future needs.

The weaknesses being found in the privilege delineation processes include difficulty in obtaining complete past histories for a practitioner seeking the right to practice at the hospital; the inability of most hospital data systems to provide the information needed to judge the clinical competence of individual practitioners; difficulty assuring that the hospital's judgment is free of significant legal risk; and difficulty obtaining data to compare the clinical performance of a practitioner with that of others inside and outside the hospital.

## Variation in Individual Practices

The transformation in individual practices has equaled that of hospitals. Research shows wide variations in the patterns of clinical practice and an association of volume and quality for some clinical activities; a demand for rapid movement of patients across settings of care; continued specialization of care and the resulting need to coordinate care among multiple practitioners; and the growing importance that technologic improvements and cost controls have placed on ethical considerations in clinical decision making.

Practice variation, which surfaced several decades ago,[3,4] exists across national,[5] regional,[6] and community[7] areas, and includes rates of admission,[8] use of specific procedures,[9] and mortality.[10] Although these variations appear related, at times, to differences in the severity of illness among the comparison groups[11] and to differences in the appropriateness with which services are used,[12] much of the variance remains unexplained.[13] Because of evidence, however, that some of the difference is caused by the provision of clinically nonindicated care, practice variation has captured the attention of those deeply concerned about health care costs. Business and governmental leaders have demanded explanations for variations and have used the incentives created by prospective pricing systems and the peer judgments in second-opinion and prior-approval programs to attempt to reduce the inappropriate use of services. Evidencing equal concern, professional societies have studied proper uses of diagnostic and therapeutic services[14] and have developed foresighted collaborative efforts with insurers to prompt more rational use of services.[15]

At a more fundamental level, significant practice variations have highlighted research showing that many clinical decisions are not supported by solid scientific studies.[16] This reality, surprising to many clinicians and to those who finance and receive care, has prompted long-overdue interest in clinical trails targeted to investigate the most effective use of high-volume, expensive diagnostic and therapeutic procedures.[17]

Hospital privilege delineation programs must change in response to variations in practice and must respond to the research that practice variation will continue to prompt. Although information useful to the clinician is available, it does not appear to reach the practice setting[18] nor will it until the unique characteristics of these two "cultures" (research and practice) understand each other and learn to work together more closely.[19]

Thus, it is particularly important that hospital data systems and quality assurance programs be improved by 1) developing the capability to monitor key process and outcome indicators to show variation in patterns among departments providing the same services (anesthesia, obstetrics) and among practitioners for the same type of care; 2) using the best clinical standards to detect undercare and overuse of services; 3) continuing to improve internal capabilities to account for differences in severity of illness; and 4) developing the capacity to compare a hospital's performance with that of other hospitals with clinically similar patients. None of these improvements will be made quickly, and each will become more effective over the next 10 years, but all are essential for accurate delineation of clinical privileges.

## Continuity of Care

Another area of growing importance to effective privilege delineation is assuring that a patient's care among practitioners is effectively coordinated within a hospital and between the hospital and other care settings. Pressures for cost-control have prompted hospitals to shift some care previously provided in inpatient settings to ambulatory, nursing home, and home care settings. This shift means that patients receiving inpatient care are, in the aggregate, either more intensely ill than in the past or require more complex or risky procedures than previous inpatient populations. Thus, a higher proportion of the inpatients will be cared for by several medical specialists and expert support teams, rather than by a single physician and staff nurses. Practitioners who can effectively care for all of their patients without the active, coordinated involvement of other specialists and skilled support teams will become even rarer. Thus, as medical staffs attempt to judge individual clinical competence, they will need to assess the ability of the practitioner to seek the services of consultants and to work smoothly with and integrate into teams of practitioners. Likewise, pressures for rapid movement of patients from inpatient to outpatient and nursing home care, and the potential legal liability associated with premature discharge, should prompt hospitals to give greater attention to the ability of practitioners to judge when the patient should be discharged and the ability of a family, nursing home, or home care agency to receive and care for the patient.

## Volume of Services

A growing body of literature seems to link volume of services to the quality of care. Careful analyses have shown that, although not in every instance will practitioners or institutions with low volumes predictably provide poor quality care,[20] the association does exist. Evidence for such an association is strong enough to prompt hospitals to consider the volume of services of a practitioner seeking clinical privileges for the first time (whether the person is new or is a current staff member requesting new privileges after training outside the hospital). Specifically, it is wise to obtain verified information on how often the practitioner treated patients with specific diagnoses or clinical problems and how often he or she did the specific service. While low volumes may not justify denial of specific privileges, they should lead to caution, especially if data show moderate or high complication rates or apparently poor levels of patient improvement. Low volume could, for example, result in specific monitoring of a practitioner's performance until acceptable levels are shown.

The association between volume of service and the quality of performance is strong enough that hospitals should seriously question whether privileges should be granted for services that its patient population will not need in significant volume. If these services are not available from other organizations and they are essential, are there sufficient data available to determine who are the most skilled practitioners in these services? Adding new services may be tempting, but is unwise when demand will not be sufficient to maintain competence. The risks to patients, the practitioner, and the hospital are too great.

## Ethical Issues and Day-To-Day Practice

The growing importance of ethical issues in day-to-day clinical decision making will also alter the face of privilege delineation. Life can be prolonged with artificial support systems; new technology engenders discussion of the interface between moral, religious, and scientific perspectives and values; judicial and legislative mandates call for changes; and more consumers wish to participate in important decisions. Thus, in health care we are faced with the difficult task of integrating complex and controversial ethical considerations into the decisions that a clinician makes about patients. To do so effectively, clinicians must be able to recognize when such issues have arisen in patient care. They must know how to consult with people within the hospital, the community, the family, and the family's support systems to explore ethical issues. They must be able to integrate a frequently diverse set of views with legal requirements and reach a rational decision. This complex set of skills is matched by the duty of the hospital to support the clinician with resources to help in making appropriate decisions. Lacking such capability, the hospital either should not voluntarily enter into providing services that predictably raise these ethical issues or it should develop the ability to meet these needs.

## Information Needs

Some basic questions must be answered when evaluating practitioners for clinical privileges (Table 1). Clinical competence is the product of initial education and training, subsequent clinical experience, the willingness to stay current with the evolving state of the art, and the physical and mental health needed for sound clinical judgment and proper dexterity in technical skills. Our society has properly decided that judgment of a practitioner's competence to provide care in a hospital will not be made by the practitioner or, except in extreme cases, by governmental licensing agencies. Licensure confers the right to practice but it is insufficient to identify the specific types of services a practitioner can do competently.

Given this limitation of licensure, the increasing specialization of knowledge and skills in health care, and the differences in practitioners' capabil-

---

**Table 1. Key Questions for Evaluating Clinical Privileges**

1. Is practitioner clinically competent to do the services for which privileges are sought?
2. Does the law allow the practitioner to do the services for which privileges are sought? What special conditions does the law place on providing such services?
3. Does the hospital want to provide such services or, if already provided, can it adequately support such services?
4. Will the person contribute to and integrate well into hospital routines?

ities, each practitioner must be able to show the hospital that he or she possesses clinical competence to do the services it provides. The hospital must assess clinical competence carefully and match the practitioner's competence with the hospital's capabilities and plans.

The information necessary to judge clinical competence includes: education and training (where, what type, how much, and how well); certification (board certification and recertification); clinical experience (where, what type, how much, and how well); previous actions regarding the practitioner's licensure (suspensions, revocations, surrenderings) or clinical privileges (reductions, temporary suspensions, and removal from a hospital staff [voluntary or involuntary]; and experience with professional liability (number and type of actions against the practitioner and the results [settlements, final judgments, dismissed from the action]). Gathering and verifying this information is becoming routine in many hospitals. County medical societies often gather much of the necessary information for use by several hospitals in their area.[21] The American Medical Association's Physician Masterfile provides information on a physician's (M.D.s, not D.O.s) education, residency training, and board certification status that the hospital can compare with the practitioner's application. The Federation of State Medical Board's Physician Disciplinary Action Data Bank contains information on actions taken by any of the state medical licensing boards concerning a physician's licensure.

A final source of potentially useful information is the national clearinghouse of physician data mandated by the PL 99-660, the Health Care Quality Improvement Act of 1986.[22] Although it is not yet in operation (or even funded), the clearinghouse could both protect good-faith quality assurance and provide physician-specific information to help health care organizations judge the competence of physicians.

Information that would be available from the clearinghouse includes the dollar amounts of settlements or judgments in professional liability actions and the reasons for them; actions of a state medical licensure board including licensure revocation or suspension and censure, reprimand, or probation actions; instances of voluntary surrendering of a license and the causes; and restrictions by a health care organization of the clinical privileges of a physician for 30 days or more.

The experiences to which residents are exposed vary among training programs. A resident in a large urban hospital teaching program is likely to encounter a substantially different set of patient problems than the resident in a medium-sized hospital. Therefore, certifying boards such as the American Board of Internal Medicine have established minimum standards and a review of trainee practice competence.[23]

Fellowship programs and short-course programs designed to teach new skills to practicing physicians also differ. Because of these uncertainties, the applicants must provide the hospital-specific information on the content of their training program, including the number of patients seen with specific problems; how often the practitioner did specific procedures; and the quality of the performance.

The availability of such detail varies among specialties, programs, and hospitals; however, it is important for the hospital granting privileges to seek such information. This information should be more uniformly available as hospitals increase the sophistication of their clinical data systems and as specialty boards require or encourage the use of log books during training.[24]

Interpreting professional liability actions against a practitioner is complex. Some object to hospitals obtaining information on professional liability actions because such liability actions may be groundless. Some specialties (for example, radiology and pathology) are routinely captured in the broad net thrown by plaintiffs' attorneys, and some or all of the defendants are eventually dismissed.

These considerations call for caution by hospitals in using such information. A possible problem could be reflected, however, either in individual actions or in patterns of involvement, and the hospital must explore these carefully with the practitioner.

The physical and mental health of practitioners is important in granting clinical privileges. Impairments do not, by definition, disqualify a practitioner from being granted clinical privileges. A decision requires clear understanding of the physical and mental demands of the practice privileges being sought and a judgment on the degree to which a practitioner can consistently meet the demands. The range of most practitioners' clinical capabilities is broad enough that a hospital can tailor individual privileges to these capabilities.

When the impairment is serious (use of alcohol or drugs), it poses a threat to patients and to the hospital. Decisive, yet sensitive, action is needed; the growing number of impaired practitioner programs[25] can help.

Hospital medical staffs are no longer composed exclusively of physicians and dentists. Expanded clinical capabilities, modification of state laws governing practitioner licensure, and a broadened scope of hospital services have led to a larger group eligible for hospital privileges. The laws governing practice of these groups vary greatly among states and are evolving in many states. Laws sometimes define the nature of hospital practice for the group and the relationship of its practice to that of physicians, and hospitals must reflect these laws in the privileges granted individual practitioners.

Until recently, it was assumed that hospitals would and could accommodate new practitioners and new services. The situation is now more complex. Many hospitals have scaled-down services or have seen inpatient services shrink under utilization control programs and care shift to other settings. Hospitals now target expansion. Alcohol and drug programs and physical rehabilitation services expand because they are exempt from prospective pricing. Imaging services enlarge to accommodate new technology and to capture new market opportunities. Most hospitals have a powerful incentive to concentrate on services that are most needed and that the hospital can provide well in the marketplace.

A hospital's success depends in part on its ability to forecast the needs of the community and the evolution of technology, and to modify services to meet these needs and advances. Improved understanding of current capabilities and future service needs will allow more rational consideration of staff expansion. Such reasoned consideration is also vital to the legal defense of a hospital's decision to close its medical staff, or a department within the staff, to admission of new members.

A practitioner must work well with others and be able to call for other specialists when needed and coordinate care among several providers.

How well a practitioner will contribute to the work of the medical staff must also be assessed. Hospitals depend on their medical staff to monitor and improve the quality and appropriateness of care, to make objective recommendations for staff membership and clinical privileges, and to contribute clinical expertise to the hospitals' decisions on current and future resource needs and allocations. Thus, another important consideration is judging the practitioner's past contributions.

## The Importance of Effective Leadership

Challenging times call for effective leadership. The demands for efficient, high-quality care are great, and how a hospital and, eventually, a physician perform will be public record. Added to this demand are the uncertainties of clinical decision making created by a litigious environment, the limited scientific base of medical care, and difficult ethical issues.

Leadership is a complex notion, about which volumes have been written.[26] Leadership is defined as the ability to use vision and information to transform responsibility into reality and to sustain that transformation. If a hospital is to succeed, key hospital leaders must truly lead.

The leaders needed to assure the effectiveness of privilege delineation are the chairman of each medical staff clinical department or service, the chairman of the medical staff executive committee, the person responsible for direction of the quality assurance program, the hospital's chief executive officer, and the chairman of the hospital's governing body. Directors of clinical training programs must be willing to collect and provide the information necessary for judgments about the clinical knowledge, skills, and potential contributions of an applicant for clinical privileges.

## Chairman of a Clinical Department

As the inpatient component of hospital care becomes more intense it becomes more specialized. To compensate for lost inpatient revenues, many hospitals are expanding ambulatory care and, especially in the mental health field, developing residential and day-hospital services. Likewise, hospitals are expanding oncologic care into comprehensive hospice services and creating new and expanded home care capabilities. This expansion has prompted most hospitals to create clinical departments or services and to realize that effective leadership of these departments is vital for the hospital's success.

Many hospitals have traditionally viewed departmental chairmanship as a relatively pro forma, honorary duty, but persons holding such positions must be able to handle their many responsibilities well. Chief among these duties is to implement and oversee the department's participation in quality assurance and privilege delineation activities.

Specialty peers are the best judges of clinical competence. In a departmentalized or service-structured hospital, the principal responsibility for peer judgment rests with the department chairmen or service chiefs who must define the information needed and the criteria for evaluating the competence of new applicants and those seeking reappointment. They must also judge the degree to which a practitioner will or has participated appropriately in meeting internal and interdepartmental responsibilities. The chairman also depends on sources outside the hospital and on an internal program[27] for monitoring the quality and appropriateness of patient care. Internal programs depend on incorporating state-of-the-art clinical concepts into daily practice and contemporary methods into the data collection, analysis, and peer review activities of the quality assurance program.

The chairman must apply information about the hospital's current and projected support capabilities in considering a practitioner for clinical privileges. If the hospital cannot support a service or it is saturated, privileges should not be granted.

## Chairman of the Medical Staff Executive Committee

The medical staff executive committee serves a vital role as the final common pathway between the medical staff and the hospital governing board. The executive committee makes formal recommendations to the board for appointments to the staff and specifies the clinical privileges that should be granted. The chairman must verify that these recommendations are appropriate.

Although the executive committee may not be able to make an independent judgment of a practitioner's clinical competence, it must be sure the recommendations from the department chairman (or from the credentials committee) were developed through effective mechanisms for monitoring individual clinical performance, gathering information from external sources, and analyzing requests for privileges in the context of hospital and departmental capabilities.

## Chief Executive Officer

The chief executive officer is the linchpin of the hospital, with responsibilities for identifying needed resources; identifying current capabilities and projecting future hospital service needs; providing adequate staff and information for quality assurance, risk management, and privilege delineation systems; and maintaining information about the local, state, and federal legal determinants that affect and must guide the privilege delineation process.

## Chairman of the Governing Body

The unique organizational structure of U.S. hospitals is evident in the role that hospital governing bodies play in the assignment of clinical privileges. In most corporations, the governing body or board is responsible for employing only the chief executive officer who is, in turn, responsible for selecting senior managers and, through them, for hiring all employees and consultants. In contrast, the hospital board appoints not only the chief executive officer but the entire medical staff; the board also makes final assignment of clinical privileges. The specific duties of the governing body include assuring the following:

1. The hospital's quality assurance and risk management activities are adequately funded, objective, and designed to improve the quality of care;
2. The privilege delineation process has access to and bases recommendations on objective information on an individual's clinical com-

petency, contribution to the hospital, and ability to work cooperatively with others;
3. Judgments made by various departments concerning the same type
of clinical care are guided by comparable professional criteria;
4. Recommendations for clinical privileges are free from economic or
anticompetitive motivations;
5. The information about current capabilities and future plans is incorporated into the process of privilege delineation;
6. Adequate resources are provided to support effective quality assurance, risk management, and privilege delineation.
7. Adequate financial protection for the department chairman and others
who organize or participate in good faith, quality assurance, and privilege delineation.

Because these responsibilities are unique and often require decisions that
involve clinical knowledge beyond the expertise of its members, the chairman of the governing body has a special responsibility to guide and assist
the other members.

### Residency Program Directors

Directors of training programs are critical in helping hospitals accurately
delineate clinical privileges. Directors must certify that trainees are able
to sit for board examinations and attest to the behavior and moral integrity
of candidates before the board. They now maintain and endorse procedural logs that document a candidate's technical proficiency. Program directors must be honest in evaluating trainees so weaknesses can be corrected
and patients will receive high-quality care. Unfortunately, many personal
references program directors write about trainees suffer from over-
zealousness. Program directors' evaluations are the critical first step in helping a hospital assess a physician applying for privileges. Much work in
this area is now being done by the Association of Program Directors in
Internal Medicine (APDIM) through its newsletter.[28]

### Conclusion

Accurate assessment of a practitioner's clinical competence is one of the
cornerstones of effective hospital quality assurance. The first eight papers
from the American College of Physicians specifying minimum competence
necessary to perform certain procedures should help in that assessment.
Concepts such as time-limited certification and recertification have not been

discussed in these concluding comments, and other critical policy issues must also be left for another forum. How has the introduction of prospective payment and more accurate tracking of physician-generated costs influenced the delineation of privileges?[29] As more young physicians join salaried group practices, essentially as employees, will hospital privilege decisions increasingly reflect economic concerns of the employer?[30] Will hospitals actively limit referrals once their true costs are recognized,[31] and what impact will this limitation have on the privilege delineation process?

Physicians must play an active role in ensuring the delivery of high-quality medical care. A thorough and well-reasoned privilege delineation process helps to safeguard this public trust.

## Acknowledgements

This paper was encouraged by the Clinical Privileges Project Steering Committee, but its content does not reflect official policy of the American College of Physicians, the Joint Commission on Accreditation of Healthcare Organizations, or the Leonard Davis Institute of Health Economics, and solely represents the opinions of the authors.

## References


1. HEALTH CARE FINANCING ADMINISTRATION. *Medicare Hospital Mortality Information.* Washington, D.C.: 1987.
2. Honeywell will demand that insurers submit provider-specific data. *American Hospital Association News.* 1988;March 7:3.
3. LEWIS CE. Variations in the incidence of surgery. *N Engl J Med.* 1969;281:880-4.
4. MOSES L., MOSTELLER F. Institutional differences in postoperative death rates: commentary on some of the findings of the National Halothane Study. *JAMA.* 1968;203:492-4.
5. VAYDA E. A comparison of surgical rates in Canada and in England and Wales. *N Engl J Med.* 1973;289:1224-9.
6. WENNBERG JE, GITTLESOHN A. Small area variations in health care delivery. *Science.* 1973;182:1102-8.
7. WENNBERG JE. *The Medical Care Outcomes Problem: An Agenda for Action.* Washington, D.C.: National Leadership Commission on Health Care; 1987.
8. DEPARTMENT OF HEALTH CARE. *Confronting Regional Variations: The Maine Approach.* Chicago, Illinois: American Medical Association; 1986.

9. MERRICK NJ, BROOK RH, FINK A, SOLOMON DH. Use of carotid endarterectomy in five California Veterans Administration medical centers. *JAMA.* 1986;256:2531-5.

10. BLUMBERG MS. Measuring surgical quality in Maryland: a model. *Health Aff.* 1988;Spring:62-78.

11. POLLACK M, RUTTIMANN U, GETSON P. Accurate prediction of the outcome of pediatric intensive care. A new quantitative method. *N Engl J Med.* 1987;316:134-9.

12. CHASSIN MR, KOSECOFF J. PARK RE, et al. Does inappropriate use explain geographic variations in the use of health care services? *JAMA.* 1987;258:2533-7.

13. WENNBERG JE. Which rate is right? [Editorial]. *N Engl J Med.* 1986;314:310-1.

14. DEPARTMENT OF TECHNOLOGY ASSESSMENT. *Diagnostic and Therapeutic Technology Assessment; (DATTA) Program.* Chicago, Illinois: American Medical Association.

15. AMERICAN COLLEGE OF PHYSICIANS. A new series of papers on diagnostic tests. *Ann Intern Med.* 1986;104:117.

16. EDDY DM, BILLINGS J. The quality of medical evidence: implications for quality of care. *Health Aff.* 1988;Spring:19-32.

17. WENNBERG JE. Improving the medical decision-making process. *Health Aff.* 1988;Spring:97-106.

18. KOSECOFF J, KANOUSE DE, ROGERS WH, McCLOSKEY L, WINSLOW CM, BROOK RH. Effects of the National Institutes of Health consensus development program on physician practice. *JAMA.* 1987;258:2708-13.

19. GREER AL. The two cultures of biomedicine: can there be consensus? [Editorial]. *JAMA.* 1987;258:2739-40.

20. LUFT HS, HUNT SS. Evaluating individual hospital quality through outcome statistics. *JAMA.* 1986;255:2780-4.

21. HENNEPIN COUNTY MEDICAL SOCIETY. *Central Credentialing Program.* Minneapolis, Minnesota; 1987.

22. IGLEHART JK. Congress moves to bolster peer review: the Health Care Quality Improvement Act of 1986. *N Engl J Med.* 1987;316:960-4.

23. AMERICAN BOARD OF INTERNAL MEDICINE. *A Guide to Evaluation of Residents in Internal Medicine.* Portland, Oregon: 1987.

24. AMERICAN BOARD OF INTERNAL MEDICINE. *Evaluation of Clinical Competence.* Portland, Oregon: 1986.

25. DIVISION OF MEDICAL AFFAIRS. *Selected Bibliography—Physician Impairment.* Chicago, Illinois: American Hospital Association; 1986.

26. BENNIS W, NANUS B. *Leaders: The Strategy for Taking Charge.* New York: Harper and Row; 1985.

27. ROBERTS JS. Reviewing the quality of care: priorities for improvement. *Health Care Financ Rev.* 1987;(Suppl):69-74.
28. HILDRETH EA. A practical approach to teaching medical residents procedural skills. Careers. 1987;3:9-14.
29. HERSHEY N. Applying utilization review findings in medical staff appointment and reappointment decisions. *Qual Assur Util Rev.* 1986;1:109-12.
30. SCHROEDER SA, MITCHELL T. Employment choices in conditions of physician oversupply: a study of graduates of San Francisco internal medicine programs, 1979-1984. *J Gen Intern Med.* 1988;3:25-31.
31. GLENN JK, LAWLER FH, HOERL MS. Physician referrals in a competitive environment: an estimate of the economic impact of a referral. *JAMA.* 1987;258:1920-3.

# ACP/ACC/AHA Task Force Statement: Clinical Competence in Exercise Testing

A STATEMENT FOR PHYSICIANS FROM THE ACP/ACC/AHA TASK FORCE ON CLINICAL PRIVILEGES IN CARDIOLOGY

The granting of clinical staff privileges to physicians is one of the primary mechanisms used by institutions to uphold the quality of care. The Joint Commission on Accreditation of Healthcare Organizations requires that the granting of initial or continuing medical staff privileges be based on assessments of applicants against professional criteria specified in medical staff bylaws. Physicians themselves are thus charged with identifying the criteria that constitute professional competence and with evaluating their peers accordingly. But the process of evaluating a physician's knowledge and competence is often constrained by the evaluator's own knowledge and ability to elicit the appropriate information, a problem that is compounded

Writing Group: Robert C. Schlant, MD, FACP, FACC, Chairman; Gottlieb C. Friesinger II, MD, FACP, FACC; James J. Leonard, MD, FACP, FACC

TASK FORCE MEMBERS: Sankey V. Williams, MD, FACP, *Chairman*; James L. Achord, MD, FACP; Gottlieb C. Friesinger II, MD, FACP, FACC; Francis J. Klocke, MD, FACP, FACC; James J. Leonard, MD, FACP, FACC; Richard L. Popp, MD, FACP, FACC; William A. Reynolds, MD, FACP; Thomas J. Ryan, MD, FACP, FACC; Robert C. Schlant, MD, FACP, FACC; William L. Winters, Jr., MD, FACP, FACC.

*Clinical Competence in Exercise Testing* was approved by the American College of Physicians Board of Regents, the American College of Cardiology Board of Trustees and the American Heart Association Steering Committee.

*Address for reprints:* David J. Feild, Associate Executive Vice President, American College of Cardiology, 9111 Old Georgetown Road, Bethesda, Maryland 20814.

Reprinted by permission of JOURNAL AMERICAN COLLEGE OF CARDIOLOGY, Volume 16, Page 1061, 1990. Copyright American College of Cardiology.

**437**

by the growing number of highly specialized procedures for which privileges are requested.

This guideline is one of a series developed by the American College of Physicians, the American College of Cardiology and the American Heart Association to assist in the assessment of physician competence on a cardiovascular procedure-specific basis. The minimum education, training, experience and cognitive and technical skills necessary for the competent performance of exercise testing are specified. These are based, when possible, on published data linking these factors with competence in certain procedures or, in the absence of such data, on consensus of expert opinion. They are applicable to most practice settings and can accommodate a variety of ways physicians might substantiate competence in the performance of specific cardiovascular procedures (see also "Guide for the Use of American College of Physicians Statements on Clinical Competence," *Ann Intern Med* 1987;107:588-9).


## Overview of the Procedure

Exercise testing has been used in clinical practice for many years and its use has contributed significantly to the management of many patients. In its current form clinical exercise testing consists of the continuous monitoring of an electrocardiogram (generally a 12-lead system) with frequent 3-lead or 12-lead recordings taken according to clinical circumstances, frequent blood pressure determinations and continuous patient observation before, during and after exercise of progressively increasing intensity (usually with a treadmill or cycle ergometer) to any of a number of test end points. Arm exercise is occasionally used in selected patients, although it is seldom as satisfactory. Ventilatory gas exchange measurements, such as oxygen consumption or respiratory exchange ratio, may also be measured. The patient is also observed and monitored for 5 to 10 min after exercise ends.

In many instances exercise testing may be combined with other procedures, such as myocardial perfusion imaging, radionuclide ventriculography, echocardiography or other imaging procedures. If a physician is responsible for both exercise testing and imaging, clinical competence in both areas is required. In other cases one physician may be responsible for the exercise test and another for imaging. In such cases staff privileges are granted accordingly. The guidelines in this document pertain only to exercise testing.

Since the procedure entails a very small but definite risk, it should only be performed under the following conditions: with appropriate indications and careful consideration of contraindications, under the supervision of a properly trained physician and with appropriate technique and safety measures. The supervising physician should know that specificity, sensitivity and diagnostic accuracy of the test can vary considerably according to the prevalence of the condition in the population being tested (Bayes theorem) and according to the criteria used to determine a "positive," "negative" or "indeterminate" result. The physician must understand the many factors that can result in false positive, false negative or indeterminate results.

The clinical indications for exercise testing are broad and varied. In general, the procedure is used to answer a specific question and should not be performed if the information gained may be obtained with other techniques that have been or will be performed. Exercise testing should be conducted when it is anticipated that the results will affect patient management. It is important that the physician performing an exercise test know the indications for and diagnostic accuracy of other tests used in the evaluation of patients with known or suspected cardiovascular disease. Such tests include radionuclide ventriculography, nuclear magnetic resonance imaging, other imaging methods, ambulatory electrocardiography, cardiac catheterization and exercise testing combined with myocardial perfusion imaging, first pass or equilibrium radionuclide angiography or echocardiography.

For the purpose of this statement, performance of exercise testing includes knowing indications for and contraindications to the test, recognizing normal end points and abnormal responses or complications that may require that the test be discontinued, managing complications of the test and interpreting the test results. In selected patients exercise testing can be safely performed by properly trained nurses, exercise physiologists, physical therapists or medical technicians working directly under the supervision of the physician who should be in the immediate vicinity and available for emergencies. However, the physician should be present to observe the patient continuously when the test is performed on a patient with severe angina pectoris, possible unstable angina pectoris or exertional left ventricular dysfunction or arrhythmia. In all instances, the patient should be screened for contraindications immediately before the test.

Competent performance of exercise testing requires significant cognitive knowledge including clinical evaluation of the patient, knowledge of the pathophysiology of the disease or condition for which the test is performed and knowledge of electrocardiography, cardiac arrhythmias and exercise physiology including normal and abnormal responses to different types and levels of exercise.

### Justification for Recommendation

The number of procedures that must be performed under supervision and the duration of training vary depending on the individual's aptitude and other training. The following recommendations for minimum criteria for competence are based on the American College of Cardiology's 17th Bethesda Conference on Cardiology Training[1] and the expert opinion of cardiovascular consultants, as well as the expert opinion of the Subcommittee on Cardiology of the American College of Physicians Committee on Clinical Privileges.

### Indications, Contraindications and Complications

Individuals who perform or supervise exercise testing must understand the indications for and contraindications to the test.

General indications for exercise testing in cardiology patients are listed in Table 1 and categorized as class I, which comprises conditions for which there is general agreement that exercise testing is justified, and class II, which comprises conditions for which exercise testing is frequently used but in which there is a divergence of opinion about its value and appropriateness[2].

---

**Table 1. General Indications for Exercise Testing**

Class I: Conditions for which there is general agreement that exercise testing is justified
- To assist in the diagnosis of coronary artery disease (CAD) in male patients with symptoms that are atypical for myocardial ischemia
- To assess functional capacity and to aid in assessing the prognosis of patients with known CAD
- To evaluate the prognosis and functional capacity of patients with CAD soon after an uncomplicated myocardial infarction (before discharge or early after discharge)
- To evaluate patients after coronary artery revascularization by surgery or coronary angioplasty
- To evaluate patients with symptoms consistent with recurrent, exercise-induced cardiac arrhythmias
- To evaluate functional capacity of selected patients with congenital heart disease
- To evaluate patients with rate-responsive pacemakers

---

**Table 1. General Indications for Exercise Testing, continued**

Class II: Conditions for which exercise testing is frequently performed but in which there is a divergence of opinion with respect to its value and appropriateness

- To evaluate asymptomatic male patients over the age of 40 with special occupations (pilots, air traffic controllers, fire fighters, police officers, critical process operators, bus or truck drivers and railroad engineers)
- To evaluate asymptomatic males over the age of 40 with two or more risk factors for CAD
- To evaluate sedentary male patients over the age of 40 who plan to enter a vigorous exercise program
- To assist in the diagnosis of CAD in women with a history of typical or atypical angina pectoris
- To assist in the diagnosis of CAD in patients who are taking digitalis or who have complete right bundle branch block
- To evalute the functional capacity and response to therapy with cardiovascular drugs in patients with CAD or heart failure
- To evaluate patients with variant angina
- To follow up serially (at 1-year intervals or longer) patients with known CAD
- To evaluate patient with a class I indication who have baseline electrocardiographic changes or coexisting medical problems that limit the value of the test (in some of these patients exercise testing may still yield clinically useful information, such as duration of exercise, blood pressure response and production of chest discomfort)
- To evaluate patients who have sustained a complicated myocardial infarction but who have subsequently "stabilized" (before discharge or early after discharge)
- To evaluate on a routine, yearly basis patients who remain asymptomatic after a revascularization procedure
- To evaluate the functional capacity of selected patients with valvular heart disease
- To evaluate the blood pressure response of patients being treated for systemic arterial hypertension who wish to engage in vigorous dynamic or static exercise
- To evaluate selected children and adolescents with valvular or congenital heart disease

From Subcommittee on Exercise Testing.[2] Adapted with permission.

It is important to note that approximately 90% of men with a history consistent with typical angina pectoris have significant coronary artery disease when studied by coronary arteriography.[3] In such patients an exercise test adds only slightly to the diagnostic accuracy of the clinical impression, although it may provide other important information. In contrast, the prevalence of significant coronary artery disease, as measured by angiography in women with a history of typical angina pectoris, may be as low as 60% to 70%. Since a false positive exercise ST segment response is much more frequent in women than in men, an abnormal ST segment response in this group of women does not greatly enhance the predictive accuracy of the clinical diagnosis based only on clinical history. As a result, exercise testing alone without radionuclide imaging in women with atypical chest pain is of limited value when performed for diagnostic purposes.

General contraindications to exercise testing are listed in Table 2 and together with indications for exercise testing are representative of the cognitive material that the individual performing or supervising the test should know. The common causes of electrocardiographic false positive (or, in some instances, indeterminate) exercise tests are listed in Table 3. The major complications of exercise testing are listed in Table 4. More detailed discussions of indications, contraindications and complications of exercise testing are available elsewhere.[2,4-13]

---

**Table 2. General Contraindications to Exercise Testing to Evaluate Myocardial Ischemia**

- Very recent acute myocardial infarction (generally <6 days)
- Angina pectoris at rest
- Severe symptomatic left ventricular dysfunction
- Potentially life-threatening cardiac dysrhythmias
- Acute pericarditis, myocarditis, or endocarditis
- Severe aortic stenosis
- Severe arterial hypertension (generally >200 mm Hg systolic or 120 mm Hg diastolic)
- Acute pulmonary embolus or infarction
- Acute thrombophlebitis or deep vein thrombosis
- Acute or serious general illness
- Neuromuscular, musculoskeletal, or arthritic condition that precludes exercise
- Uncontrolled metabolic disease, such as diabetes, thyrotoxicosis, or myxedema
- Inability or lack of desire or motivation to perform the test

---

**Table 3. Possible Causes of False Positive or Indeterminate Electrocardiographic Exercise Test for Coronary Artery Disease**

- Female gender
- Hyperventilation
- Nonfasting state
- Mitral valve prolapse syndrome
- Vasoregulatory abnormality
- Systemic arterial hypertension
- Left ventricular hypertrophy
- Drug administration (digitalis and others)
- Anemia
- Hypoxemia
- Electrolyte abnormalities, such as hypokalemia
- Sudden excessive exercise
- Excessive double product
- Cardiomyopathy
- Congenital heart disease
- Valvular heart diease
- Pericardial disorders
- Bundle branch block, especially left bundle branch block
- Ventricular pre-excitation (Wolff-Parkinson-White syndrome, pre-excitation variants)
- Ventricular pacemaker
- Advanced age
- Improper lead system
- Inadequate recording equipment
- Incorrect criteria
- Improper interpretation

---

## Minimum Training Necessary for Competence

The role of the credentials committee is critical because of the varied training backgrounds of physicians performing exercise testing, and individual consideration is important. Many physicians acquire the skills necessary for exercise testing during a fellowship in cardiovascular disease. Some internal medicine residency programs provide training in exercise testing, often as an elective. A minimum of 4 weeks should be devoted to this training to achieve competence.

---

**Table 4. Complications of Exercise Testing**

- Hypotension
- Congestive heart failure
- Severe cardiac dysrhythmia
- Cardiac arrest
- Acute myocardial infarction
- Acute central nervous system events such as syncope, stroke
- Accidental physical trauma (falls, etc.)
- Death

---

Because of the variable backgrounds of physicians and the diversity of their training experiences, multiple pathways to acquire competence are possible. The clinical and institutional setting in which the training occurs, the case mix, backup and collaboration available to trainees performing the procedures and the number of procedures performed under supervision must all be considered when granting privileges.

The number of procedures necessary to ensure competence has not been established by objective criteria. The majority opinion of this committee and its consultants is that the trainee should participate in at least 50 exercise procedures during training. However, it is recognized that not all training or practice environments are the same and a greater or smaller number of procedures may be deemed appropriate by a local credentials committee. Since survey data[14,15] indicate that some programs do not currently provide adequate training to fulfill the requirements of these guidelines, internal medicine program directors will need to plan with individual trainees to obtain appropriate experience.

Physicians who did not receive formal training during a residency or fellowship but who are currently performing exercise testing should have gained appropriate experience under the supervision of a physician qualified in exercise testing. Such postgraduate training may have included didactic courses and workshops, personal tutorials and, importantly, exercise testing performed under the supervision of a qualified physician. For physicians who finish training before 1992 without the opportunity for such formal training but who have performed exercise testing on a regular and substantial basis for more than 3 years, experience may be individually considered in lieu of formal training. Training in any setting must result in the acquisition of the cognitive skills outlined in Table 5.

While acquiring the knowledge and skills of exercise testing as part of a formal training program or subsequently, the physician should be super-

**Table 5. Cognitive Skills Needed to Perform Exercise Tests Competently**

- Knowledge of appropriate indications for exercise testing
- Knowledge of appropriate contraindications and risks of testing
- Knowledge to promptly recognize and treat complications of exercise testing
- Competence in cardiopulmonary resuscitation and successful completion of an AHA-sponsored course in advanced cardiac life support
- Knowledge of specificity, sensitivity and diagnostic accuracy of exercise testing in different patient populations
- Knowledge of how to apply Bayes' theorem to interpret test results
- Knowledge of various exercise protocols (Bruce, Naughton, Balke-Ware, USAFSAM and others) and indications for each
- Knowledge of basic cardiovascular and exercise physiology including blood pressure and heart rate response to exercise
- Knowledge of electrocardiography and changes in the electrocardiogram that may result from exercise, hyperventilation, ischemia, hypertrophy, conduction disorders, electrolyte disturbances and drugs
- Knowledge of cardiac arrhythmias and treatment of serious arrhythmias
- Knowledge of cardiovascular drugs and how they can affect exercise performance, hemodynamics and electrocardiogram
- Knowledge of conditions and circumstances that can cause false-positive, indeterminate or false-negative test results
- Knowledge of the effects of age and disease on hemodynamic and electrocadiographic responses to exercise
- Knowledge of principles and details of exercise testing including proper lead placement and skin preparation
- Knowledge of prognostic value of exercise testing
- Knowledge of alternative diagnostic procedures to exercise testing
- Knowledge of end points of exercise testing and indications to terminate exercise testing
- Knowledge of the concept of metabolic equivalent (MET) and estimation of exercise intensity in different modes of exercise
- Ability and commitment to communicate diagnostic accuracy, risks, and results of the test to the patient, the medical record, and other physicians so that appropriately informed patient consent can be obtained

Abbreviations as in Table 1.

vised by an effective teacher who is expert in the clinical use of the procedure and performs testing on a regular basis. The trainee's experience should be documented in writing and confirmed by the supervisor. The following information should be documented in a training log book for each test performed during training: Date of test, patient identification number, patient age, indications for test, duration and results of the test (both electrocardiographic and hemodynamic), reason for terminating the test, complications and signature of the supervisor.

The completion of a short course or workshop that offers a limited cognitive background in cardiology or inadequate hands-on experience with the procedure will not, by itself, result in competence.

## Maintenance of Competence

Continuing competence in exercise testing requires regular, continued performance of exercise testing. Performance of only a rare test can lead to missed or inappropriate diagnoses and may lead to a higher rate of complications. Twenty-five tests per year are suggested as the minimum number the physician should perform to maintain competence. Successful completion of a course in advanced cardiac life support and renewal on a regular basis is necessary.

## References

1. 17th Bethesda Conference: Adult cardiology training. J Am Coll Cardiol 1986;7:1195-1218.
2. Guidelines for Exercise Testing: a report of the American College of Cardiology/American Heart Association Task Force on Assessment of Cardiovascular Procreudres (Subcommittee on Exercise Testing). J Am Coll Cardiol 1986;8:725-38.
3. Weiner DA, Ryan TJ, McCabe CH, et al. Exercise stress testing: correlations among history of angina, ST-segment response and prevalence of coronary-artery disease in the Coronary Artery Surgery Study (CASS). N. Engl J Med 1979;301:230-35.
4. Erb BD, Fletcher GF, Sheffield LT. AHA Committee Report: Standards for cardiovascular exercise treatment programs. Report of the American Heart Association Subcommittee on Rehabilitation, Target Activity Group. Circulation 1979;59(suppl A):1084A-90A.
5. Council on Scientific Affairs. Indications and contraindications for exercise testing: Council report. JAMA 1981;246:1015-8.

6. Astrand P-O, Rodahl K, eds. Textbook of Work Physiology: Physiological Bases of Exercise. 3rd ed. New York: McGraw-Hill, 1986.
7. Ellestad MH, ed. Stress Testing: Principles and Practice. 3rd ed. Philadelphia: FA Davis, 1986.
8. Bardsley WT, Mankin HT. Exercise testing. In Brandenburg RO, Fuster V, Giuliani ER, McGoon DC, eds. Cardiology: Fundamentals and Practice. Chicago: Year Book Medical, 1987:369-402.
9. Froelicher VF. Exercise and the Heart: Clinical Concepts. 2nd ed. Chicago: Year Book, Medical, 1987.
10. Hanson P. Clinical exercise testing. In Blair SN, Painter P, Pate RR, Smith LK, Taylor CB, eds. Resource Manual for Guidelines for Exercise Testing and Prescription, American College of Sports Medicine. Philadelphia. Lea & Febiger, 1988:205-22.
11. Fletcher GF, ed. Exercise in the Practice of Medicine, 2nd ed. Mt. Kisco. NY: Futura, 1988.
12. Detrano R, Froelicher VF. Exercise testing: uses and limitations considering recent studies. Prog Cardiovasc Dis 1988;31:173-204.
13. Naughton J. Exercise Testing: Physiological, Biomechanical, and Clinical Principles. Mt. Kisco, NY: Futura, 1988.
14. Wigton RS, Nicolas JA, Blank LL. Procedural skills of the general internist: a survey of 2500 physicians. Ann Intern Med 1989;111:1023-4.
15. Wigton RS, Blank LL, Nicolas JA, Tape TG: Procedural skills training in internal medicine residencies: a survey of program directors. Ann Intern Med 1989;111:932-8.

# Preventive Risk Management Requires Objectivity, Consistency

Richard E. Thompson, MD, and David R. Thompson

Credentials: Hospital medical staff membership and/or specific clinical privileges, requested by an applicant, recommended through specified medical staff mechanisms, awarded, denied, restricted/reduced, updated/revised and/or revoked by the hospital board, and renewable every two years.

Regardless of any other "credentials" held by a practitioner, only the hospital board determines what a practitioner is allowed to do in the hospital. Anyone who does anything to patients in or under the auspices of the hospital must have a ticket from the board.

Hospital credentials represent a control over and above controls in other settings, such as office practice. This control is often resented and viewed with suspicion by physicians and others subject to hospital credentialing. Thus, "credentials" becomes the "war department" of the hospital/medical staff relationship.

## The patient-protective role of credentialing

Credentialing was conceived as a patient-protection activity. The patient-protection function of credentialing is necessary because:

- Medical care is now complex. So is medical training. These days, a doctor is not a doctor is not a doctor. For example: One pediatrician



**449**

may perform magnificently in the office setting with "behavioral problems" and child-raising advice to parents, but, another pediatrician might have subspecialty training in neonatology.

- Credentialing is necessary because no other mechanism distinguishes between two practitioners with different current competence, who hold the same degree, the same state license to practice "medicine and surgery in all its branches," and even the same specialty certificate.

In spite of its patient-protective intent, credentialing is sometimes distorted and "economically contaminated" so that it appears to be: a) union-type activity by medical specialties ('You can't do this type of procedure unless you have our kind of specialty certificate."), or b) based on the hospital's economic relationship with the physician, rather than on the physician's qualifications (picture new economic relationships such as HMOs and PPOs). When these distortions occur, the medical staff, the hospital, and individual physicians sometimes make themselves vulnerable to accusations of unfairness to the point of lawsuits based on restraint of trade.

## Who is involved in credentialing?

The most accurate and important recommendation on the applicant's qualifications theoretically should come from an individual with the combined attributes of authority, responsibility, and relevant clinical expertise.

In today's hospital organization, this individual is the clinical department chairman, or an officially selected representative of the credentials committee with the same clinical training, skills, and experience as the applicant.

This system made perfect sense when medicine was a profession. But now, hospitals and medical practice are businesses. So now, the spectre of possible anticompetitive behavior rears its ugly head. "His qualifications are impeccable," a department chairman might be tempted to say about a physician he has recruited to join his own practice. About a potential competitor, a department chairman might be tempted to say, "He doesn't look qualified to me."

So a complicated system of checks and balances is necessary, with the board making the final credentials decision.

In an effective credentialing system, each of the following players must understand and perform their designated roles: the applicant, the hospital board, the medical executive committee, the credentials committee, the relevant clinical department chairman, the medical staff coordinator or administrative secretary handling credentials applications, the chief executive officer (the ultimate coordinator and "head coach" in the credentialing process), legal counsel and consultant who presume to assist with credentials problems and related medical staff bylaws provisions.

## Causes for confusion

There are two major causes for confusion about credentialing: a) imprecise definition, and b) continuing evolution of credentials methods.

Presently, there are three parts to credentialing: initial appointment, initial granting of clinical privileges, and information-based reappraisal and reappointment.

The initial appointment is completed before the practitioner begins work at the hospital. (As recently as 15 years ago, this was all there was to credentialing.) Application forms and procedures for initial appointment are now mostly boilerplate and generally accepted. Familiar elements include the written application, the acceptance by the applicant of the burden to provide information in support of the application, three (or some other number) references, proof of state license, Drug Enforcement Agency number, appearance for an interview, etc.

Granting initial clinical privileges also is completed before the practitioner begins work at the hospital. Basic methods are now in place but are, so far, inadequate to solve several common credentialing problems. Basic methods include:

- The "laundry list"—an exhaustive, theoretically complete listing of medical conditions and procedures. The applicant checks off intended treatments/procedures. There are shortcomings to this method. A complete list of medical conditions and procedures is difficult to compile, and physicians tend to check off everything, because "they might want to do that some day."

- Group credentialing—granting privileges because an applicant holds a specialty certificate. While specialty certification is one of the many ways an applicant might support the claim that he is qualified, dependence on certificate-only may cause problems. This is because skills and competence in the certified specialty may vary widely from one physician to the next.

  Group credentialing poses the question "What kind of specialty certificate does the applicant have?" Currently required individual-specific credentialing asks, "How qualified is this applicant to perform these procedures or treat these conditions?" (Board certification is one way to provide evidence of qualifications, if formal training has been recent enough.)

- Defined categories—as defined in the relevant department procedure manual: Category I—emergency care; Category II—general care; Category III—specialty care; Category IV—the applicant has accepted the burden of providing additional evidence of qualifications in this subspecialty area.

In the granting of initial clinical privileges, the major need is to avoid the error of group credentialing and pay attention to the concept of individual-specific credentialing as required by the Joint Commission on Accreditation of Hospitals.

The required level of qualifications format (figure I) is a helpful adjunct to initial privilege mechanisms.

Information-based reappointment is performed every two years. Information-based reappointment should accomplish:

- Part I: Reconfirmation of basic information such as current state license to practice, Drug Enforcement Agency registration in effect, continued malpractice liability coverage, etc.
- Part II: Volume of hospital practice information, numbers of admissions, numbers of procedures performed, numbers of cases treated, numbers of consultations asked for/provided, etc.
- Part III: One-page summary of clinical performance based on ongoing review activities.

### Following the rules

Since the emergence of antitrust questions and the passage of the Health Care Quality Improvement Act of 1986, safeguards in credentialing are:

- Good faith efforts.
- Written procedures on file.
- Consistent application of written procedures.
- Documentation of the process.

In addition to hospital and medical staff bylaws, a medical staff membership and clinical privileges policy and procedure manual should be developed by medical staff leaders, the board, administration, legal counsel, and support personnel such as the medical staff coordinator. The manual should include interpretations of relevant bylaws provisions, as well as specific worksheets, forms, and letters used in implementing all phases of credentialing.

---

### Figure 1. "Required Level of Qualifications" Statement

Procedure/Condition _______________________________________________

Statement prepared by: _______________________ _______________________
                                  Department                    Name

                                  Department                    Name

                                  Department                    Name

Statement approved by: _______________________ _______________________
                            Medical Executive Committee,      Governing Body,
                                    Chief of Staff                        Chairman

---

The following evidence of qualifications and performance *are* or *are not* acceptable, as indicated.

1. Completed an approved residency in the broad specialty(ies) within which the procedure or case is ordinarily expected to be performed. ☐ Yes ☐ No

   Specifications: _______________________ ☐ Yes ☐ No

   But more than _____________ years ago. ☐ Insufficient alone

OR 2. Preceptorship (applicant was primary surgeon or attending, under supervision) ☐ Yes ☐ No

   Specific qualification of the preceptor ___ ☐ Yes ☐ No

   _______________________________________

   Only with written confirmation of competence from the preceptor. ☐ Yes ☐ No

OR 3. Attended a CME program and obtained a certificate of attendence. ☐ Yes ☐ No

OR 4. Confirmation, in writing of _________ procedures/medical cases within the past _________ months/years. ☐ Yes ☐ No

AND    Letter indicating satisfactory performance. ☐ Yes ☐ No

OR 5. Letter from chairman of clinical department of university residency program stating that the applicant is qualified in the clinical area(s) requested. ☐ Yes ☐ No

   But if more than _________ years ago. ☐ Insufficient alone

OR 6. Other _______________________________________

   _______________________________________

(Continue on back or attached sheet, if necessary)

### Five keys to effective credentialing

**Emphasize joint efforts.** The medical staff, board, and administration must work together to respond to today's critical credentialing dilemmas.

**Be objective.** Collect and use as much information as possible.

**Be consistent.** If it's the rule for one applicant, then it's the rule for all applicants.

**Separate "membership" from "privileges."** Medical staff appointment/ membership and category assignment (active, courtesy, etc.) relate only to placement on the staff and membership prerogatives such as voting and holding office. Delineation of clinical privileges separately provides a specific definition of the exact nature of each staff member's hospital practice.

**Follow written rules.** Medical staff bylaws must be updated, explained, followed, and supplemented.


### Credentials and risk management

Because the physician dictates the patient's hospital care, through "the order sheet," and performs potentially harmful invasive procedures, confirmation and reconfirmation of current physician competence through credentialing is an important facet of *preventive* risk management.

However, it is a fallacy to believe that credentialing is a solution to the malpractice problem. No matter how sophisticated a credentialing program is, individual mistakes will occur and people will be owed money because of them.


### Where is credentialing headed?

The biggest need right now is to resolve the dilemma of 1) needing peer judgments on applicants' qualifications while simultaneously 2) avoiding abuse by peers who allow economics to contaminate their conclusions, thus violating the patient-protection intent of credentialing.

If that dilemma cannot be resolved, then obviously credentialing is needed away from local hospital-medical staff control. Physicians would then be licensed by the state not to practice "medicine and surgery in all its branches," but by law, physicians would become limited-license practitioners.

We hope that objectivity and consistency in local hospital-specific, individual-specific credentialing activities will be sufficient to prevent such an unfortunate turn of events.

# Performance-Based Credentialing: What Does This New Buzzword Really Mean?

Richard E. Thompson, MD, and David R. Thompson

In general, "credential" means "something that gives title to credit or confidence; testimonials showing that a person is entitled to credit or has a right to exercise official power."

However, to doctors working in hospitals, "credentialing" has taken on a very special meaning:

> Hospital credentials = Hospital medical staff membership and/or specific clinical privileges requested by an applicant, recommended through specified medical staff mechanisms, awarded, denied, restricted/reduced, updated/revised and/or revoked by the hospital Board, and renewable every two years.

Regardless of any other "credentials" held by a practitioner, only the hospital's Board determines what a practitioner is allowed to do in that hospital. *Everyone* who does *anything* to patients in or under the auspices of the hospital or medical center must have a "ticket" from the *Board*.

This state of affairs has been much misunderstood. There are still physicians who feel that hospital membership and privileges are granted in one of the following ways:

---

Reprinted by permission of NORTH CAROLINA MEDICAL JOURNAL, Volume 48, page 459, 1987. Copyright North Carolina Medical Society.

as a result of discussion and vote at a general medical staff meeting—a definite "no-no" in today's antitrust and conspiracy-conscious era;

by award of the Credentials Committee of the medical staff. No. The Credentials Committee recommends to the Medical Executive Committee which recommends to the Board;

by award of the clinical department chairman. No. The clinical department chairman's recommendation to the Credentials Committee as part of preliminary work in processing the application is critical, but clinical departments do not grant membership and privileges.

This is not a new concept. In the statement which really created "the medical staff organization" in 1917 (one-page standard for hospitals of the American College of Surgeons), it is established that medical staff rules and regulations must be subject to Board approval.

Therefore, the real question is not "Does the medical staff grant membership and privileges or does the Board?" That question was answered long ago. It is the Board. The real question is "who is the Board and how is it acting?" One of the major challenges of the next few years is to solve the inherent dilemma of needing true peer recommendations and judgments on credentials qualifications, yet avoiding abuse by true peers who are in competition with the applicant. The solution is simple to describe, but not easy to implement: objective hospital-conscious, patient-conscious, and community-conscious physicians participating in good faith as hospital Board members.

For now, "credentials" may be the "war department" of your hospital/medical staff relationship. This is because hospital credentialing represents a control over and above controls in other settings, such as a physician's office practice. This control is often resented by physicians and is often viewed with suspicion by physicians and others who are subject to hospital "credentialing."

### The Patient-Protective Role of "Credentialing"

It must be remembered that "credentialing" was conceived as and continues to be a patient-protective activity, not a means of economic control. One must not deviate from this patient-protective function by making "credentials" decisions about applicants that can even be perceived as "economically contaminated": a true peer in a position of authority, using the credentials mechanism to take advantage of a competitor.

## Antitrust and Credentialing

Readers should become thoroughly familiar with the provisions of the Health Care Quality Improvement Act of 1986. In brief (check this interpretation with an attorney):

The Act requires a national data base containing information about physicians who have lost clinical privileges or state licenses to practice. Once this information base is available, hospitals will be expected to refer to it prior to awarding membership and privileges to physician applicants.

The most immediate provision of the law is some relief from antitrust complaints by an aggrieved denied applicant. Primarily related to credentialing actions based on peer review, the Act can be summarized as requiring good faith effort, action taken in the interests of patient care and based on confirmed information about practice problems, and compulsive attention to "due process."

## The Joint Commission's "Agenda for Change"

Another pressure on medical staff functions, including the function of "credentialing," is from the Joint Commission on Accreditation of Hospitals, whose thick accreditation manual is the great-great-great grandchild of the one-page standard for hospitals of the American College of Surgeons. Effective performance-based credentialing is now a major requirement of the Joint Commission on Accreditation of Hospitals medical staff standard.

## Public Watchdog Groups

Many newspapers, news magazines and TV news broadcasts have recently examined the public's dissatisfaction with the dependability and quality of services provided by "service industries," including airlines, hotels, hard goods industries such as the automobile industry, and *hospitals and physicians.*

Because of "the order sheet" (the physician "orders" the patient's care), hospital medical staffs will be in the thick of efforts to respond to these public demands for accountability, defined as data-based, objective evidence confirming consistent, effective and careful performance by practitioners in hospitals.

### Just Plain Old Patient Care

Pretend your family member is the patient. If you wanted to evaluate and know the current competence (not just the qualifications, as represented in diplomas and certificates) of the physician who just hospitalized your family member, what would you depend on?

At the present time, no credential held by the physician reflects:

* the exact nature of the physician's practice, and
* the physician's current competence

other than the physician's clinical privileges at the hospital which are assumed to be:

* based, initially, on careful evaluation of qualifications and current competence, and
* reappraised objectively every two years.

### The "Credentialing" Process

Hospital "credentialing" has three major parts:

1. Initial granting of medical staff membership
2. Initial granting of clinical privileges
3. Renewal, revision and/or updating of clinical privileges
   * routinely, every two years
   * by "corrective adjustments," which may be clinical department-level functions, and/or
   * corrective action—Medical Executive Committee and Board function.

### Initial Membership

Granting of initial membership on the staff has nothing to do with performance. It is based on general information about training, past experience, current state licensure, Drug Enforcement Agency (DEA) registration, liability insurance coverage, references, an interview, etc.

For a new staff member, assignment to a medical staff category and assignment to a clinical department also have nothing to do with performance. They are based primarily on:

* the individual's clinical specialty
* the individual's anticipated use of this hospital.

## Initial Clinical Privileges

This is the first of two applications of "performance-based credentialing."

*Once upon a time.* Up until twenty years ago, there was no such thing as delineating specific clinical privileges. A physician could pretty much treat whatever came his or her way, no questions asked. Active staff status was something like "tenure." Active staff status somehow implied more clinical privileges than courtesy staff status, even though there was no performance-based logic to that use of "categories."

*Delineation of clinical privileges based on board certification.* Until recently, clinical privileges were distributed according to board certification. That is, if a practitioner possessed a certain specialty certificate, then he or she was deemed (forever) to be qualified in all aspects of that clinical specialty. Conversely, if an individual did *not* hold a specialty certificate of a certain kind, then he or she was automatically deemed unqualified to treat certain medical conditions and/or perform certain surgical or invasive diagnostic procedures.

*Initial credentialing based on performance/training: subdividing the board certified.* The new approach—performance-based credentialing—can be best summarized as "pretend you're the patient" credentialing.

Example 1: You have an orthopaedic certificate, but if you wish to do total hip joint replacement, you must provide additional evidence of training and/or performance in this particular procedure.

Example 2: You are a board certified pediatrician. But if you wish to do intensive newborn care, you must provide additional evidence of training and/or performance in this clinical area.

Example 3: You are board certified in the specialty once known as "ENT," now named otolaryngology/head and neck surgery. But, if you are recently trained, you may be qualified for the privilege of thyroidectomy and treating laryngeal cancer. But if your training and experience do not include these conditions and procedures, then you *cannot* argue that you should have this privilege just because another doctor with the same specialty certificate does.

Example 4: You are a family physician. You have always been really interested in reading EKGs. You request this privilege because another family physician in your small hospital has the privilege to read EKGs, so you figure you should have it, too.

Wrong.

The other family physician has had a six-month preceptorship with a cardiologist for the express purpose of being competent in reading EKGs. You have not. You cannot expect to have this clinical privilege just because the hospital (defined in credentialing as medical staff department/Credentials Committee/Medical Executive Committee *plus* Board *plus* hospital executive/management staff) gave that privilege to the other family physician.

Consistency in credentialing does *not* mean "we let this doctor do it, so I guess we have to let that doctor do it." Consistency in credentialing means that we have a clear rule, and we followed it. The other doctor met it and you did not, that is why that doctor has the privilege and you do not.

For an example of how to establish such a performance-based rule for granting initial clinical privileges, see Table 1.

### Renewal of Clinical Privileges: Information-Based Reappointment

The youngest and, so far, least developed area of "credentialing" is "information-based reappointment." Information-based reappointment now has three parts:

1. Updating of general information. Examples: Reconfirmation of state license to practice, DEA registration, continued malpractice liability coverage, meeting requirements for attendance at medical staff meetings (if active staff), etc.
2. "Volume of hospital practice." Simple figures indicating numbers of admissions, numbers of procedures performed, numbers of cases treated, numbers of consultations asked for/provided, etc.
3. Performance summary. The volume of hospital practice plus performance summary data together might be referred to by some as a "practice profile." This can be a simple, one-page summary on clinical performance, based on ongoing review activities (see Tables 2 and 3).

### Five Keys to Effective Credentialing

1. *Emphasize joint efforts.* The medical staff, board and administration must work together to respond to today's critical "credentialing" dilemmas.
2. *Be objective.* Collect and use as much information as possible.
3. *Be consistent.* If it's the rule for one applicant, then it's the rule for all applicants.
4. *Separate "membership" from "privileges."* Medical staff appointment/membership and category assignment (active, courtesy, etc.) relate only to placement on the staff and membership prerogatives such as voting and holding office. Delineation of clinical privileges

## Table 1. "Required Level of Qualifications" Statement

Procedure/Condition _______________________________________

Statement prepared by: _____________________ _____________________
                                 Department                       Name

_____________________ _____________________
                                   Department                       Name

_____________________ _____________________
                                   Department                       Name

Statement approved by: _____________________ _____________________
                              Medical Executive Committee,    Governing Body,
                              Chief of Staff                         Chairman

The following evidence of qualifications and performance *are* or *are not* acceptable, as indicated.

    1. Completed an approved residency in the broad specialty(ies) within which the procedure or case is ordinarily expected to be performed.   ☐ Yes   ☐ No

       Specifications: _______________   ☐ Yes   ☐ No

---

       But more than __________ years ago.   ☐ Insufficient alone

OR   2. Preceptorship (applicant was primary surgeon or attending, under supervision)   ☐ Yes   ☐ No

       Specific qualification of the preceptor __   ☐ Yes   ☐ No

       Only with written confirmation of competence from the preceptor.   ☐ Yes   ☐ No

OR   3. Attended a CME program and obtained a certificate of attendence.   ☐ Yes   ☐ No

OR   4. Confirmation, in writing of ________ procedures/medical cases within the past ________ months/years.   ☐ Yes   ☐ No

AND   Letter indicating satisfactory performance.   ☐ Yes   ☐ No

OR   5. Letter from chairman of clinical department of university residency program stating that the applicant is qualified in the clinical area(s) requested.   ☐ Yes   ☐ No

       But is more than ________ years ago.   ☐ Insufficient alone

OR   6. Other _______________________________

## Table 2. Clinical Review Summary of Questioned Cases Only

SUBJECT OF REVIEW

General ________________________

________________________

Specific ________________

Total
Questioned _________

STUDY SAMPLE

| Physician | # Pt Records |
|---|---|
| (Code Nos.) | |
| ________ | ________ |
| ________ | ________ |
| ________ | ________ |
| ________ | ________ |
| ________ | ________ |
| ________ | ________ |

(Continue on additional pages)

• Ask why
• Evaluate the answer

| Physician (Code) | Pt. Record No. (Code) | Reviewer's Evaluation | | | | Abstractor's Few-Word Summary |
|---|---|---|---|---|---|---|
| | | 1* | 2* | 3* | 4* | Screening Physician's Brief Questions & Comments |
| | | | | | | |

*1 = Screening indicator not met, but clinical practice expected and acceptable. Reviewer comfortable.
*2 = Questioned practice not necessarily routine, but not totally unexpected. Reviewer still comfortable.
*3 = Questioned practice unexpected. Reviewer uncomfortable.
*4 = Questioned practice *very* unexpected. Reviewer displeased.

NOTE TO REVIEWER: Make your judgment • pretending you're the patient.
• knowing what you know clinically.

separately provides a specific definition of the exact nature of each staff member's hospital practice.

5. *Follow written rules.* Medical staff bylaws must be updated, explained, followed and supplemented.

## Where Is Credentialing Headed?

Believe it or not, the next big issue in credentialing will probably be credentialing of nurses. Example: Two RNs work in the nursery, but one works in the normal newborn nursery, and the other works in the pediatric inten-

---

### Table 3. Feedback Reappointment

Part III

Name ________________________________________________

Specialty ___________________________ Department ___________________________

Date appointed to staff ___________________________ Current staff category ___________________________

| QUALITY REVIEW | | | | | | |
|---|---|---|---|---|---|---|
| | | | | Number or % | | |
| Summary of Clinical Review | | 1* | 2* | 3* | 4* | |
| Surgical Case Review | | | | | | |
| Blood Use | | | | | | |
| Drug/Antibiotic Use | | | | | | |
| Medical Records Completion & Eligibility | | | | | | |
| Mortality | | | | | | |
| Complications | | | | | | |
| DRG/Financial/PRO Information | | | | | | |
| Incident Reports | | | | | | |
| Peer Complaints | | | | | | |
| Nursing Complaints | | | | | | |
| Patient Complaints | | | | | | |

Example of Part III: Dr. Blade is a general surgeon. His reappointment form might indicate:

**FEEDBACK/REAPPOINTMENT**

Part III

Name  Harold G. Blade, M.D. _______________________________________

Specialty  General Surgery ___________________ Department  Surgery _______________

Date appointed to staff  1971 ___________________ Current staff category  Active _______________

| QUALITY REVIEW | | | | | | |
|---|---|---|---|---|---|---|
| | | | | Number or % | | |
| Summary of Clinical Review | | 1* | 2* | 3* | 4* | |
| Surgical Case Review | | 71% | 29% | — | — | |
| Blood Use | | 63% | 23% | 5% | — | |
| Drug/Antibiotic Use | | 59% | 41% | — | — | |

sive care unit. What "credentialing" tests should be demanded of the nurse working in the area requiring more nursing skills?

With respect to physician credentialing, the biggest need is to resolve the dilemma of

- the necessity of true peer judgment of applicants' qualifications, but
- the temptation by true peer competitors to abuse the system by "economically contaminating" their evaluation of an applicant's qualifications.

If that dilemma cannot be resolved, then obviously credentialing is headed away from the present "hospital-specific" system. Physicians would then not be licensed by the state to practice "medicine and surgery in all its branches," but by law, physicians would become limited license practitioners! Hopefully, objectivity and consistency in performance-based "credentialing" will prevent such an unfortunate occurrence.

# Medical Staff Privileging:
# How To Avoid Pitfalls in the
# Administrative Process

Danielle Lombardo Trostorff, JD, MSW

Medical staff privileging has become particularly important to both health care practitioners and hospitals. For the practitioner, privileging provides a powerful mechanism for preserving high standards of practice in medicine. At the same time access to privileges on a hospital's medical staff is an integral part of a practitioner's professional practice. For the hospital, privileging is fundamental to the ability to maintain high standards of care while containing costs. Furthermore, strong practitioner support of the hospital will attract patients to the hospital.

A hospital's medical staff bylaws are its guide to the privileging process and to dealing with quality of care and utilization issues as they arise. Medical staff bylaws should encompass the most pressing concerns of the hospital and medical staff. Historically, medical staff bylaws focused primarily on practitioners' qualifications for privileging; today they also address such concerns as proximity to the hospital; resource utilization patterns; the practitioners' allegiance to the facility, as reflected in their use of the facility; exclusive contracts with the hospital; and the ability of hospital facilities to support practitioners and their patients.[1] Advanced qualifications may also be required before practitioners can be granted privileges; board certification or specialization is accepted as a criterion for medical staff membership by both the courts and the Joint Commission on Accreditation of

Reprinted by Permission of QRB, June 1987, page 198. Copyright JCAHO

Hospitals, although the Joint Commission does not recognize board certification as a sole criterion for privileging.[1,2] Although refining the standards for privileging serves to improve the quality and cost-effectiveness of patient care, it also makes obtaining privileges more difficult for physicians. One result of this competitive environment has been an increase in litigation by practitioners who have been denied staff privileges, either as applicants for appointment or reappointment or through the disciplinary process.

Practitioners denied staff privileges have sued not only the hospital but also its medical staff on a number of grounds, including violation of bylaws, faulty substantiative grounds, or antitrust violations. Historically, the courts have refused to hear cases brought by disgruntled applicants without a clear showing of error.[3] Privileging decisions are generally not reviewed unless the hospital's action is in violation of the bylaws or is arbitrary and capricious. Although exceptions have been made to this standard (ie, courts have permitted practitioners to bring actions based on antitrust violations, due process violations, and discrimination), the premise that courts will not "second guess" hospital decisions remains largely intact.[4] However, because of the increasing competitive pressures and the trend toward seeking court intervention, it is imperative that the hospital's administration, governing body, and medical staff understand the importance of the privileging process within the hospital and adhere to the procedural and substantive requirements contained in the medical staff bylaws.

This article will address the requirements in medical staff bylaws that should be observed, during the privileging process, to avoid litigation. It will also highlight the key provisions of the recently enacted Health Care Quality Improvement Act (HCQI Act) that relate to privileging and other peer review activities.

### The HCQI Act

The HCQI Act of 1986 (PL 99-660), §401 *et seq* is a federal law that, in part, provides peer review protection and limited immunity for peer review activities. It is intended to encourage peer review by limiting the threat of litigation. The law provides immunity from damage suits, including antitrust suits, brought under federal law for peer review undertaken in good faith after November 14, 1986; this immunity is provided to medical staff, health care organizations, and persons who give information to professional review bodies. The immunity provision will also apply to damage suits brought under state laws that are effective on or after October 14, 1989, unless a state passes legislation before that date exempting it from the HCQI Act. A state can also pass legislation making the act effective sooner.

The HCQI Act sets forth standards for peer review activities. The peer review actions must be taken

- in the reasonable belief that the action would improve the quality of patient care;
- after reasonable effort to obtain the relevant facts;
- after adequate notice and hearing procedures, or other procedures deemed fair under the circumstances, have been afforded to the physician involved; and
- in the reasonable belief that the action is warranted by the facts known.

The HCQI Act requires a health care organization or insurer to report any payment made to settle or satisfy a judgment or claim in a medical malpractice action. Under threat of a fine, the organization is required to report the following information to a national clearinghouse designated by the secretary of the U.S. Department of Health and Human Services:

- The name of the practitioner involved;
- The hospital with which the practitioner is affiliated or associated;
- A description of the malpractice; and
- Such other information that the secretary deems appropriate.

These reporting requirements apply to physicians and nonphysicians who are providing health care services.

In addition the health care organization is required to notify the state board of medical examiners of any privileging sanctions imposed that relate to a physician's professional competence or conduct. Under this reporting requirement, a health care organization must report any "nonaction" taken in return for accepting the resignation of a physician to whom it has already granted privileges. "Nonaction" means that the organization has chosen not to take peer review action in return for accepting the physician's resignation or surrender of clinical privileges. The requirement will certainly affect informal resolution of problem cases and will alert health care organizations to problems that other organizations have encountered. Reporting privileging sanctions is not mandatory in regard to nonphysician health care practitioners.

The law also provides guidelines for giving notice and conducting hearings when a physician is being sanctioned or denied privileges. The notice and hearing guidelines are not mandatory; however, if these guidelines are followed, a peer review body is presumed to have met the Act's standards. The reporting requirements will become effective November 14, 1987.

## Important Considerations for Privileging

The most important considerations for the hospital and its medical staff when granting or reviewing privileges are to be familiar with and to follow the medical staff bylaws; to observe time requirements; to assure that the committee is impartial; and to document the reasons for actions taken. The reasons for the committee's actions should be related to patient care and the efficient and smooth operation of the hospital.[5] Denial of privileges based on criteria not relevant to patient care has been subject to attack. For instance, tying privileges to medical society membership has been found to be discriminatory.[6] A bylaw provision that requires the medical staff to live within the hospital's county has been attacked as "a classification without rationality,"[7] although a provision requiring a practitioner to live within a certain distance of the hospital to ensure continuous patient care has been upheld.[8] A bylaw criterion regarding personality—the ability to work with others—has been upheld as a legitimate consideration related to patient care.[9] A bylaw provision should be the foundation for the action taken. Once an individual or a group begins a procedure prescribed by the bylaws, it must adhere strictly to that procedure in order to avoid a future allegation of unfairness.[10]

## The Application for Appointment or Reappointment

Adherence to the bylaws begins at the initiation of the application process. All applicants must be treated consistently.[1] Once practitioners seek hospital privileges, they are bound by the requirements of the bylaws.[1,11] The practitioner must abide by the medical staff bylaws by completing the application and providing accurate information; failure to adhere to the requirements may be grounds for denial of privileges.[12]

The hospital, through its medical staff, which is responsible for reviewing an applicant's credentials, should thoroughly investigate the information provided. The HCQI Act requires the hospital to obtain information about the practitioner applying or reapplying for privileges. To do this the representatives of the hospital must contact organizations and individuals who have information pertaining to the practitioner's credentials and practices. As explained previously, the law permits the medical staff to obtain certain credentialing and privileging information from the state board of medical examiners and the national clearinghouse.

If a malpractice action arises against a practitioner—and the hospital has failed to obtain necessary information—the hospital is still presumed to have knowledge of any information reported to the clearinghouse. If obtaining this information would have precluded the hospital from granting privileges to the practitioner, the hospital may be liable in the malpractice action.

## Medical Staff Recommendation

Each department or committee making a recommendation during the privileging process should base its recommendation on patient care concerns. The basis for the recommendation should be documented, and this documentation may include minutes of department and privileging committee meetings, including the names of committee members in attendance; any medical staff records reviewed; resource utilization data; and recommendations.

Minutes of department or committee meetings should not include extraneous information, an account of the deliberations, or the votes of individual committee members; and the meetings should not be tape recorded. The deliberations contain extraneous information that may not reflect the body's ultimate conclusion; information concerning the debate during the meetings about the pros or cons of the action could only be used to fuel an attack on the privileging process.

When the recommendation is adverse, the practitioner should be notified according to the time and notice requirements of the bylaws.[13] The notice should refer to the practitioner's right to an appeal, when applicable, and the time requirement for requesting an appeal. The notice does not have to set forth every right practitioners have or every procedure they must follow; it can refer them to the bylaws to obtain that information. However, because the right to appeal is critical, written notice should be given of this right.[14] The notice should also state the reasons for the adverse recommendation.

Under the HCQI Act, the health care organization has the responsibility to provide notice. The Act states that the following notice information is considered adequate:

- The fact that a professional action is recommended against the physician;
- The reasons for the action;
- The right to a hearing;
- Any time limit for requesting a hearing (but not less than 30 days); and
- A summary of hearing rights.

The notice should be given by the individual required to do so by the bylaws. If the bylaws do not set forth a time requirement for notice, the notice should be sent as soon as is reasonably possible after the recommendation is made.[15]

Once notice of the adverse recommendation has been given, it is the affected physician's responsibility to request a hearing within the time limits. When a practitioner requests a hearing, the HCQI Act requires that the health care organization give him or her at least the following information: notice of the time, place, and date of the hearing, which is scheduled not less than 30 days after the date of the notice, and a list of witnesses expected to testify on behalf of the body making the adverse recommendation. An untimely request made by the practitioner usually activates the hearing waiver provision of the bylaws. When a hearing is waived, an adverse recommendation is submitted directly to the board of directors of the health care organization for final action.

Often the medical staff wants to implement its adverse recommendation (ie, not grant privileges to the practitioner) before the board of directors makes its decision. However, because the medical staff's recommendation is not final until it has been approved by the board, it cannot be implemented prematurely. In cases of reapplication for privileges, the effect of premature implementation of an adverse action would be a summary suspension, which the bylaws allow to occur only for special reasons and according to specific procedures. Some bylaws, however, permit implementation of a medical staff recommendation pending the board's decision when a practitioner has waived a hearing. If the practitioner is on notice that this practice is an effect of a waived hearing, the procedure may be considered fair. State and case law should be reviewed and an attorney consulted before specific procedures are implemented.

**Appointment of Hearing Committee**

The composition and impartiality of the hearing committee have been the targets of much of the litigation concerning privileging. The hearing committees of both the medical staff and the board of directors should exclude those who participated in the deliberations leading to the adverse recommendation.[16] As the court commented in *Applebaum v Board of Directors of Barton Memorial Hospital*, "having served on one committee and having formed an opinion in the matter, the person could hardly be expected to exercise impartial judgment in subsequent proceedings."[16] Also, the committee that made the adverse recommendation cannot act as the impartial hearing body. If a medical staff committee were to make a recommendation and then conduct a hearing on that recommendation, the committee could be acting as a judge of its own recommendation. This practice allows for bias, partiality, and conflict of interest. Inherent conflict of interest is also obvious in provisions that permit a board of directors to make its decision and then permit the practitioner to present his or her position in a hearing, before the decision is finalized.

In addition, the HCQI Act prohibits an individual who is in direct competition with the practitioner being considered for privileges from serving on the hearing committee.[17]

The hearing officer or committee recommended by the HCQI Act may be an arbiter chosen by both parties; a hearing officer, chosen by the hospital, who is not in direct competition with the practitioner; or a panel of individuals who are not in direct competition with the practitioner.

According to most medical staff bylaws the practitioner affected by the decision is entitled, prior to the hearing, to the records forming the basis for the adverse recommendation. The failure to produce records to which the practitioner is entitled, and which the practitioner needs to refute the allegations against him or her could be grounds for an attack on the entire process.[18] Disgruntled practitioners could contend that they have been denied proper notice of the basis for adverse recommendations and, thus, the tools to properly defend their positions.[19]

The documentation forming the basis for the adverse recommendation may include department and privileging committee minutes, any medical staff records reviewed, utilization review data, and adverse recommendations. As explained previously, the documentation should not include extraneous information, an account of deliberations, vote counts, or dissenting opinions.

Bylaw provisions for dissenting opinions can only be divisive to the committee system and privileging process. The committee structure provides for a diversity of input, but the recommendation is based on consensus after appropriate deliberation. The individuals and groups who have contributed to the privileging process should not feel as though they must protect themselves by recording their dissents as long as the procedures outlined in the bylaws have been followed and the groups' records include the recommendation made and the reasons for it, based on bylaw requirements. Privileging committees become vulnerable to criticism when bias or an anticompetitive rationale is the basis for the decision.[20] Care must be taken to make the right recommendation for the right reason.

## The Hearing Process

The hearing process itself must focus on the reasons given for the adverse recommendation.[21] The committee making this adverse recommendation may present witnesses and documentation to support its action. The practitioner affected by the recommendation must refute the grounds for the adverse action. The hearing committee may ask its own questions.

Generally, the practitioner has the right to confront and examine persons who have made statements supporting the negative action.[22] Those persons may be called either by the committee who made the adverse recommendation or by the practitioner. The HCQI Act also permits the practitioner to call, examine, and cross-examine other witnesses.

There is considerable debate over whether legal counsel may be present and represent either party in the hearing. The courts have generally not held the right to counsel to be essential to the fair hearing process.[23] The bylaws may dictate the approach to be followed. For example some bylaw provisions permit the parties to be represented by counsel; a denial of counsel would then be in violation of the bylaws. Most bylaws, however, stress the intraprofessional nature of the privileging process and allow only peer representation, although practitioners are not denied legal counsel when preparing their positions.

The bylaws may permit representation by counsel at the sole discretion of the hearing committee. If discretion is properly exercised, the courts should uphold the committee's decision. The requirement for fair procedure will be satisfied if the hearing is conducted in accordance with the bylaws, testimony by witnesses and documents are limited to the issues that form the basis for the adverse recommendation, and the committee makes a fair and thorough consideration of the matter.[24] The privileging hearing does not need to have all the elements of a formal judicial hearing.[25] When in doubt, however, it is better to err on the side of fairness and allow legal counsel to assist the practitioner at the hearing. Furthermore the debate may now be academic because the HCQI Act permits physicians to be represented at hearings by an attorney or person of their choice. When counsel is present for one party, all parties should be represented by counsel.

Some bylaws permit the hearing committee to recess the hearing while gathering additional evidence. This does not mean that the hearing committee is permitted to conduct its own investigation or discover its own evidence for the adverse recommendation. The role of the hearing committee is to decide whether the recommendation, which was made by another committee, is supported by the facts. Except in unusual circumstances, the committee's power to gather additional information is limited to clarifying the issues that have been raised. A hearing committee that does not confine its inquiries to matters referred to in the adverse recommendation may jeopardize the fairness of the entire process.[26]

The HCQI Act permits physicians to submit a written statement of their positions at the conclusion of the hearing.

## Hearing Committee Recommendation

Once it has made its recommendation, the hearing committee should submit the recommendation along with the record of the hearing, prior recommendations, and documentation directly to the board of directors of the health care organization for its final determination. The HCQI Act states that physicians are entitled to a record of the proceedings at their own cost and that they must be given timely notice of every recommendation, as well as of the final decisions and supporting reasons.

Some bylaws provide for referral back to the committee that originally made the adverse recommendation (for its final recommendation) or to the medical staff for a full vote before submission to the board of directors. Serious flaws can be found in both approaches.

The first provision—permitting referral back to the original committee— allows that committee to have two opportunities to make a decision. If the bylaws permit the original committee to modify or reverse the hearing committee's recommendation, the hearing process becomes meaningless.[27]

The second provision—permitting a vote by the medical staff as a whole— raises the question of bias and the potential for a conspiracy by the medical staff to protect its own interest and exclude a competitor. Not only are the medical staff members who participated in a prior recommendation and formed a previous opinion able to vote again, but they could influence other members of the staff to vote with them. In addition, when this practice is allowed, the medical staff usually votes only pro or con, without deliberating on the merits of the reasons for denial, which further contributes to the conspiracy theory and the lack of fair consideration of the matter.

Some courts have held that the medical staff is a "walking conspiracy capable of imposing its economic interest to exclude competitors from its staff."[28] Regulatory agencies have ruled that medical staff members, as competitors of a physician, could conspire with the hospital.[29] Both scenarios raise serious antitrust implications that could be challenged in court.[30]


## The Decision of the Board of Directors

The board of directors of the health care organization, which is ultimately responsible for the quality of patient care provided in the hospital,[31] makes the final decision in medical staff privileging matters.[32] The hospital is held responsible for any negligent decisions made by its staff.[33]

The board reviews the recommendations made by the various medical staff privileging committees, the documentation on which the recommendations were based, and the records of hearings, if any. The board's decision is based on the information submitted and must be guided by legitimate patient care considerations, the bylaws, and concern for the effective and efficient operation of the hospital. The board may take into consideration the economic well-being of the hospital in reaching its decision: In a recent New Jersey case, the court upheld the decision of the board of directors to deny staff privileges based on the practitioner's pattern of overutilization of resources.[34]

The board is not bound by the medical staff's recommendations. It may choose to overturn all medical staff recommendations and reach its own conclusions,[35] or it may reject a hearing committee recommendation in favor of the original executive committee recommendation.[36] The board has the ultimate authority, under the bylaws, as long as the decision is not arbitrary, capricious, or in excess of the authority conferred on it by the bylaws.[37] From a practical standpoint, however, the board relies on the medical staff's expertise in privileging matters and will uphold its recommendation unless the board has good cause not to do so.

Notice of the board's decision is sent to the practitioner, according to the requirements of the bylaws. The HCQI Act requires that the notice state the decision and the reasons for the decision.


## Conclusion

The medical staff bylaws serve as the blueprint for all privileging actions taken by health care organizations. The bylaws should clearly reflect not only the current practices of the hospital, but also the practices prepared by the health care organization's administration and medical staff for proper privileging of practitioners. Bylaws that clearly address the basic concerns of the hospital and its medical staff and set forth the substantive and procedural components of privileging will serve to insulate the process from attack. Potential litigation will be deterred by medical staff and administrators who are familiar with the organization's bylaws and who apply them properly.


## References and Notes

1. Joint Commission on Accreditation of Hospitals: *Accreditation Manual for Hospitals*, 1987 ed. Chicago: Joint Commission, 1986.
2. Cameron v New Hanover Memorial Hosp., 293 S.E.2d 901 (N.C. Ct. App. 1982), *dismissed*, 297 S.E.2d 399 (N.C. 1982); Sarasota County Public Hosp. Bd. v Shahawy, 408 So.2d 644 (Fla. Dist. Ct. App. 1981); Khan v Suburban Community Hosp., 340 N.E.2d 398 (Ohio 1976).

3. Yarnell v Sisters of St. Francis Health Services, 466 N.E.2d 359 (Ind. Ct. App. 1983) (where the hospital follows the procedures set out in the bylaws, any decision reached by the hospital board shall not be subject to judicial review); *see also* Everhart v Jefferson Parish Hosp. Dist., 757 F.2d 1567 (5th Cir. 1985); Dutka v Sinai Hosp., 371 N.W.2d 901 (Mich. Ct. App. 1985); Bello v South Shore Hosp., 384 Mass. 770, 429 N.E.2d 1011 (1981); Tigua General Hosp. v Feuerberg, 645 S.W.2d 575 (Tx. Ct. App. 1982).

4. *See, eg*, Patrick v Burget, 800 F.2d 1498 (9th Cir. 1986) U.S. Court of Appeal for the Ninth Circuit reversed $2 million jury verdict against defendant physicians in direct competition with plaintiff finding that peer review activities were protected from antitrust scrutiny under the state action doctrine. However, the case was remanded to the lower court for review of other claims because the appeals court concluded that the defendants had acted in bad faith); Stern v Tarrant County Hosp., 755 F.2d 430 (5th Cir. 1985) (en banc), 778 F.2d 1052 (5th Cir. 1985), *cert. denied*, 106 S.Ct. 1957 (1986) (a hospital rule requiring osteopathic physicians to have completed two years of postdoctoral training in an alleopathic [sic.] medicine program is not a denial of equal protection); Jefferson Parish Hosp. v Hyde, 513 F. Supp. 532 (E.D. La. 1981), *rev'd*, 686 F.2d 286 (5th Cir. 1982), *rev'd*, 104 S.Ct. 1551 (1984) (denial of privileges based on an exclusive hospital contract is not an antitrust violation); Rao v St. Elizabeth's Hosp., No. 5-84-0585 (Ill. App. Ct. 5th Dist., Jan. 24, 1986) (court found that although bylaws were not strictly adhered to, the doctor was afforded all administrative review provided for in the hospital bylaws).

5. Dooley v Barberton Citizen's Hosp., 11 Ohio St.3d 216, 465 N.E.2d 58 (1984).

6. Hamilton County Hosp. v Andrews, 84 N.E.2d 469 (Ind. 1949); Ware v Benedikt, 225 Ark. 185, 280 S.W.2d 234 (1955); Griesman v Newcomb Hosp., 40 N.J. 389, 192 A.2d 817 (1963); Blende v Maricopa County Medical Society, 97 Ariz. 240, 393 P.2d 926 (1964); Foster v Mobile County Hosp. Board, 398 F.2d 227 (5th Cir. 1968).

7. State *ex. rel.* Sams v Ohio Valley General Hosp. Ass'n, 413 F.2d 826 (4th Cir. 1969).

8. Berman v Valley Hosp., 196 N.J. Super. 359, 482 A.2d 944 (1984).

9. Rao v Auburn General Hosp., 573 P.2d 834 (Wash. Ct. App. 1978); Theissen v Watonga Municipal Hosp. Bd., 550 P.2d 938 (Ok. 1976); State *ex. rel.* Bronaugh v City of Parkersburg, 148 W.Va. 568, 136 S.E.2d 783 (1964); Hagen v Osteopathic General Hosp., 232 A.2d 596 (R.I. 1967).

10. Smith v Vallejo General Hosp., 170 Cal. App. 3d 450, 216 Cal. Rptr. 189 (1985); Tiholz v Northridge Hosp. Found., 151 Cal. App. 3d. 1197 (1984).

11. Pick v Santa Ana Tustin Community Hosp., 130 Cal. App. 3d. 970 (1982) (the hospital may deny a practitioner staff privileges on the basis of criteria in the bylaws related to the quality of patient care. Practitioner has the burden of showing that the criteria are not applicable).

12. Dunbar v Hospital Auth. of Gwinnett County, 227 Ga. 532, 182 S.E.2d 89 (1971); Pariser v Christian Health Care Systems, Inc., No. 84-293C(5) (E.D. Mo. Jan. 17, 1986) (the executive committee summarily curtailed a physician's privileges, after it discovered he had provided false answers on his application. The court upheld the action, finding that the hospital properly followed bylaws).

13. Miller v Eisenhower Medical Center, 27 Cal. 3d 614, 614 P.2d 253, (1980); Marin v Citizens Memorial Hosp., No. V-84-7 (S.D. Tex. Oct. 18, 1985) (court found due process violation where physician's surgical privileges were summarily suspended without notice and an opportunity to be heard in contravention of the hospital bylaws).

14. Silver v Castle Memorial Hosp., 53 Haw. 475, 497 P.2d 564, 571-75 (1972) *cert. denied*, 409 U.S. 1048, *reh'g denied*, 409 U.S. 1131 (1973) (the court set forth some fair procedure guidelines for notice: The physician should be on notice that a hearing is available to him or her and be given timely notice sufficiently prior to the hearing for him or her to adequately prepare a defense. In addition the physician should be provided with written statement of the specific charges).

15. Bock v John C. Lincoln Hosp., 702 P.2d 253, 257 (Ariz. Ct. App. 1985) (the court determined that one day's notice of the meeting of the executive committee was too short).

16. Applebaum v Board of Directors of Barton Memorial Hosp., 104 Cal. App. 3d 648, 660, 163 Cal. Rptr. 831 (1980); *cf.* Richards v Emanuel County Hosp. Auth., 603 F. Supp. 81, 84 (S.D. Ga. 1984) (due process was not violated because the members of the credentials committee were also members of the medical staff, some of whom requested a hearing on the staff member's privileges. The staff member failed to show actual prejudice).

17. The HCQI Act is a federal response to the Patrick v Burget case (see note 4). The defendants in Patrick v Burget were partners in a medical clinic in direct competition with the plaintiff. The plaintiff had been in practice with defendants but decided not to become a partner in their clinic and started an independent practice. Conflict arose between

the two groups, and one of the clinic doctors, who was in competition with the plaintiff, actively participated in the peer review process. The defendants' actions were attacked by the court.

18. Guild v Coliseum Medical Center, No. 82-15254 (La. CDC Orl. Parish, Oct. 26, 1982), *writ denied* (La. Dec. 21, 1982) (the court compelled discovery of documents finding "that a doctor suspended or terminated from the staff of a hospital is entitled to have all the information available which may show that the action was proper or improper").

19. Bock v John C. Lincoln Hosp. (see note 15); Silver v Castle Memorial Hosp. (see note 14); Anton v San Antonio Community Hosp., 19 Cal. 3d 802, 140 Cal.Rptr. 442, 567 P.2d 1162, 1168 n.12 (1977).

20. Weiss v York Hosp., 745 F.2d 786 (3d Cir. 1984), *cert. denied*, 105 S.Ct. 1777 (1985); Patrick v Burget (see note 4).

21. Silver v Castle Memorial Hosp. (see note 14).

22. Marin v Citizens Memorial Hosp. (see note 13).

23. Anton v San Antonio Community Hosp. (see note 19); Silver v Castle Memorial Hosp. (see note 14); Sussman v Overlook Hospital Ass'n, 95 N.J. Super. 418, 231 A.2d 389 (Ct. App. 1967); *contra*, Garrow v Elizabeth General Hosp., 79 N.J. 549, 401 A.2d 533 (1979).

24. Ascherman v San Francisco Medical Society, 39 Cal. App. 3d 623, 114 Cal.Rptr. 681 (1974); Silver v Castle Memorial Hosp. (see note 14).

25. Miller v Eisenhower Medical Center (see note 13); Peterson v Tucson General Hosp., Inc. 559 P.2d 186, 189 (Ariz. Ct. App. 1976).

26. Bock v John C. Lincoln Hosp. (see note 15; the hearing committee did not confine its inquiry to matters referred to in the notice to the affected practitioner. The court held, "to depart from the matter as to which notice has been given leaves the subject physician totally unprepared to meet the accusations. This, too, is fundamentally unfair.")

27. Applebaum v Board of Directors of Barton Memorial Hosp. (see note 16).

28. Weiss v York Hosp. (see note 20); Quinn v Kent General Hosp., Inc., 617 F.Supp. 1226 (D.Del. 1985); *cf.* Copperweld Corp. v Independence Tube Corp., 467 U.S. 752 (1984).

29. *In the matter of* Health Care Management Corp. 50 Fed. Reg. 41,693 (Oct. 15, 1985); in re Medical Staff of John C. Lincoln Hosp. and Health Care Center 3 TRADE REG. REP. (CCH) ¶22,271 (July 16, 1985).

30. Robinson v Magovern, 521 F.Supp. 842, 906-07 (W.D. Pa. 1981), *aff'd mem.*, 688 F.2d 824 (3d Cir.), *cert. denied*, 459 U.S. 971 (1982); Williams v Kleaveland, 534 F. Supp. 912 (W.D. Mich. 1981).

31. Darling v Charleston Community Memorial Hosp., 33 Ill. 2d 326, 211 N.E. 2d 253 (1965), *cert. denied*, 383 U.S. 946 (1966).

32. Moore v Board of Trustees of Carson-Tahoe Hosp., 88 Nev. 207, 495 P.2d 605 (1982). 33. Elam v College Park Hosp., 132 Cal. App. 3d 332, 183 Cal.Rptr. 156 (1982).

34. Edelman v J.F. Kennedy Hosp., No. C-2104-80 (N.J. Super Ct. June 25, 1982), *cert. denied*, 475 A.2d 585 (1984); *see also*, Rosenberg v Holy Redeemer Hosp., 351 Pa. Super. 399, 506 A.2d 408 (1986) (court will not review hospital decision denying privileges on the basis of a moratorium on new appointments when hospital had "complied with necessary procedural requirements in making its decision").

35. The Ad Hoc Executive Comm. of the Medical Staff of Memorial Hosp. v Runyan, et al, No. 84SA10 (S.Ct.Colo. Mar. 31, 1986).

36. Siqueira v Northwestern Memorial Hosp., 477 N.E.2d 16 (Ill. Ct. App. 1985).

# Credentialing for Technology Use: An Important Issue for Hospitals

A patient undergoes three surgical operations at a North Carolina hospital as part of a subcutaneous mastectomy. Subsequently, the patient sues the hospital, alleging that she has suffered permanent injuries from the surgery and that, among other things, the hospital was negligent in granting clinical privileges to a physician unqualified to perform the procedures. The trial court grants the hospital's motion to dismiss the complaint, but the appeals court rules that the patient has a cause of action, under the doctrine of corporate negligence.*

Rulings such as this one underscore the necessity for hospitals to take very seriously the granting of clinical privileges to the medical staff. More than two decades have passed since the celebrated Darling** case was decided, and since then both the courts and the Joint Commission on Accreditation of Hospitals (JCAH) have made it clear that the hospital has a corporate responsibility for the quality of care delivered to its patients.

Reprinted by permission of HEALTH TECHNOLOGY, Volume 1, Page 3, 1987. Copyright Health Technology ECRI.

*Blanton v. Moses H. Cone Memorial Hospital, Inc., 337 S.E. 2d 200 (N.C. Ct. of App., 1985).

**Darling v. Charleston Community Memorial Hospital, 33 Ill. 2d 326, 211 N.E. 2d 253 (1965). This case concerned, in part, the hospital's liability for allowing a physician not proficient in orthopedics to treat the plaintiff, who had broken his leg playing football. Because of inadequate care, Mr. Darling's leg eventually had to be amputated.

**479**

The courts have established that a hospital has the duty to determine a physician's professional competence both before privileges are granted and before they are renewed; it has also been determined that hospitals must continually assess a physician's competence.[1] In *Elam v. College Park Hospital*,[2] for example, the court found the hospital negligent in failing to ensure the quality of care rendered by a podiatrist member of the medical staff. The hospital did have a medical care evaluation committee, but this committee never informed hospital administration that it considered the podiatrist incompetent or unqualified, or had reason for such a belief.[1]

These decisions have established that a hospital can be found directly—not just vicariously—liable for failing to control the standard of medical care offered at its facility.[1][Vicarious, or indirect liability, often takes the form of *respondeat superior*, in which the hospital is sued on the theory that it is liable for the actions of its employees.] Generally, direct liability suits have a longer statute of limitations than do actions asserting vicarious liability; they may also give the plaintiff a well-insured target (the hospital) in cases where the physician is inadequately covered. In addition, a direct liability suit may avoid the difficulty of the patient's having to prove that he or she thought the physician had some connection to the hospital (e.g., as its employee or agent).[1]

The 1987 JCAH Manual states that "Professional criteria specified in the medical staff bylaws and uniformly applied to all applicants for delineated clinical privileges constitute the basis for granting clinical privileges . . . . The criteria include, at the least, evidence of current licensure, relevant training and/or experience, current competence, and health status."[3] The process actually has two steps—first, a physician or other practitioner seeks appointment or reappointment to the medical staff and, second, the applicant seeks clinical privileges to perform certain procedures or treat specific kinds of disease. The board of trustees makes the decision on both steps, but in practice it does this by responding to the recommendations of the medical staff's credentials committee (which often serves as a conduit for the recommendations of the chiefs of the clinical services).

Although the importance of credentialing and privilege delineation is well understood and, indeed, has received considerable publicity lately—not just because of malpractice considerations but also because some hospitals are excluding physicians for economic reasons—it is likely that the process of privilege delineation is still inadequate at many U.S. hospitals. Areas where there may be particular problems include (1) the performance of "surgery-like" procedures by radiologists, cardiologists, gastroenterologists, and other non-surgeons; and (2) the use by surgeons of new technologies in which they have not been adequately trained.

## The Credentialing and Privileging Process

Procedures for credentialing physicians and delineating their privileges vary widely from hospital to hospital. The JCAH guidelines state that, "As long as the delineation of clinical privileges is performed adequately, considerable flexibility exists in the approach selected by the medical staff."[4] But, it is likely that many hospitals have not been sufficiently specific in this area, and would be better served by a more stringent process.[5]

According to the JCAH, "Specialty board certification is an excellent benchmark for the delineation of clinical privileges."[4] But the Joint Commission also notes that each clinical department should develop its own criteria for recommending privileges, and lists criteria other than board certification (e.g., training, experience, and competence) that should be considered when clinical privileges are being delineated.

### Internists and Radiologists

Today, many internists and radiologists are performing invasive, complex, and risk-bearing procedures on both inpatients and outpatients, in most cases outside of the operating room. These include percutaneous transluminal coronary angioplasty (PTCA), renal and peripheral vascular angioplasty, various sophisticated endoscopies (some using lasers), embolotherapy (therapeutic introduction of a substance, generally to occlude a blood vessel), percutaneous biopsies, insertion of prostheses, and many other "surgery-like" procedures. Thus, the lines separating the functions of surgeons and internists, and surgeons and radiologists, have been blurred.

These revolutions in internal medicine and in radiology offer great hope for improved diagnosis and therapy; many permit economic savings as well. However, they may also pose a threat to good patient care and be a potential source of liability for the hospital as well. First, because these practitioners are not surgeons, the hospital may not have delineated privileges specifically, thereby possibly permitting physicians to practice beyond their levels of competence. [Historically, delineation of privileges was applied only to surgeons.]

Second, because these procedures are generally performed outside the operating room or obstetrical suite (e.g., in the cardiac catheterization laboratory, the radiology department, the gastroenterology suite, at the bedside), the physicians involved will often avoid the processes (e.g., monthly surgical case review, oversight by anesthesiologists and nurses, posting of up-to-date privilege lists outside the OR and obstetrical suites) that ensure quality in the OR and delivery areas.

Third, the training of internists and radiologists does not prepare them, in many cases, to perform invasive procedures. While this can be overcome through continuing education, it is important to understand the limits of graduate medical education. In some radiology programs, for example, senior residents have never worked with a catheter.[6] In addition, rapid technological change may leave some physicians ill-prepared to perform new procedures. It was recently estimated, for example, that 71% of current U.S. radiologists did not receive primary training in CT scanning, while more than 99% did not receive such training in magnetic resonance.[7] Similarly, although well trained in the diagnosis and management of gastrointestinal disease, physicians who completed gastrointestinal fellowships before 1967 had no formal training in colonoscopy.[8]

## Surgeons and New Technologies

The need to delineate privileges for surgeons is well understood. Not so well understood, but just as important, is the need to delineate the surgical staff's privileges in a way that reflects the changes in the technology of surgery. Laser procedures, for example, require different kinds of skills than those needed for conventional surgery. In traditional approaches, the surgeon is guided by tactile feedback; this is generally not available in laser surgery.

The development of other new surgical technologies, whether these be sophisticated biopsy techniques, the introduction of prosthetic devices and implants, CT-assisted surgery, microsurgery, or other new procedures, raises the question of whether surgeons trained in the past can effectively perform in the current surgical environment. Specifically, there is a danger that some long-time members of the hospital staff, whose privileges are routinely renewed intact with little or no requalification, may be using technologies that are beyond their capabilities.

## Specialty Board Certification and Its Limitations

Although the idea of specialization has met with considerable resistance in American medicine and specialty certification was actually slow to take hold (for example, in cardiology fewer than 34 physicians per year were certified *nationally* before 1965[9]), specialization is a fact of life today. Indeed, in 1983 there were 7,719 certified cardiologists,[9] whose certification status reflects both broad and intensive experience in the discipline of cardiovascular disease. Yet, certification in cardiology does not guarantee competency in performing invasive cardiologic procedures. For example, rather than mandating that all trainees learn cardiac catheterization techniques, the standards for training programs in cardiology specify that the program should be structured so that *some* individuals may develop skills essential to one or more invasive cardiac diagnostic studies.[10]

In diagnostic radiology, also, completion of residency training does not guarantee competence in invasive procedures such as angioplasty, embolotherapy, biopsies, etc., as these are not mentioned in the training program standards.[10] And, while in recent years approximately 40-60% of graduates of diagnostic radiology programs have taken additional fellowship training, their extra training and study have not been formally recognized by certification.[11] Thus, it is impossible to determine, through inspection of a radiologist's board certification status alone, whether he or she is qualified to perform interventional procedures.

At present, 23 specialty boards are recognized by the American Board of Medical Specialties; 15 of these award subspecialty certificates.[12]* Still, several dozen specialty organizations (e.g., those representing maxillofacial surgery, hypnosis, abdominal surgery, nutrition, and lasers) are not recognized by the ABMS. Since "board certification" is overwhelmingly interpreted to mean certification by an ABMS-recognized specialty, certification by these other organizations is generally not recognized.[13] Thus, when an entity such as the American Board of Laser Surgery (Milwaukee, WI) gives an examination, as it did in October 1986, with the intent of offering certification, it embroils itself in controversy and causes confusion among physicians seeking to have their proficiency in lasers recognized. In short, the recognized process of specialty certification cannot be expected to accommodate all of the significant new technologies that are finding their way into medical practice.

Still another concern about relying solely on board certification is that rejected applicants for privileges might sue the hospital on the grounds that their applications were not fairly treated. In *Armstrong v. Board of Directors of Fayette County General Hospital*, for example, a Tennessee appeals court found that the denial of surgical privileges to an applicant by a public hospital on the sole grounds that the practitioner lacked board certification was "arbitrary, capricious, discriminatory, and beyond the jurisdiction of the hospital."[14] [Other courts, however, have held that requiring board certification is, in fact, reasonable.]

The Medicare Conditions of Participation also specifically forbid *sole* reliance on specialty certification: "Under no circumstances is the accor-

---

*Four of the boards (Pathology, Preventive Medicine, Psychiatry and Neurology, and Radiology) offer more than one "general certificate."

dance of staff membership or professional privileges in the hospital dependent solely upon certification, fellowship, or membership in a specialty body or society."[15]

Thus, while board certification is, per the JCAH, an "excellent benchmark," hospitals would be well-advised to supplement it with other criteria, especially demonstrated competence and technology-specific training. In addition, because privilege delineation involves the credentialing by one group of physicians (the medical staff) of their peers, it is important that the board of trustees take an active role in the process, to ensure that the actions of the medical staff are not construed to constitute an illegal "group boycott."[16] Of course, it is necessary not only to afford due process to applicants for privileges, but also to maintain records that show that due process was afforded.

## Improving the Delineation of Privileges

Hospitals can improve credentialing by (1) studying the recommendations of specialty societies on guidelines for granting privileges and using them to develop their own guidelines; (2) using certification by technology-specific specialty societies as one (but not the sole) basis for granting privileges; and (3) requiring physicians seeking privileges for new technologies to attend training courses and then to work under supervision before obtaining full privileges. Hospitals should grant privileges based on specific evidence of skill, training, and ability; this might include hours of academic study and clinical training, number of procedures performed, and outcomes expected.[17]

### Recommendations of Specialty Organizations

Some specialty organizations have published guidelines to assist hospitals with granting privileges; others may be in the process of doing so. For example, guidelines are currently available on laser use (from the American Society of Laser Medicine and Surgery, Inc., Wausau, WI; this organization has no relationship to the American Board of Laser Surgery) and on gastrointestinal endoscopy (from the American Society of Gastrointestinal Endoscopy, Manchester, MA).

The "Statement on granting hospital privileges to perform gastrointestinal endoscopy"[18] (approved by the American College of Gastroenterology and the American Gastroenterological Association) might serve as a useful model for the granting of clinical privileges in new technologies. This statement suggests that privileges for each major category of endoscopy be granted separately. It recommends the establishment of a multidisciplinary endoscopic procedure committee that would advise the credentialing body on the initial granting of privileges, monitor performance and outcome, and assist in renewal of privileges.

This statement on gastrointestinal endoscopy specifies the volume of cases that trainees should have performed personally in order to be considered competent. For esophagogastroduodenoscopy, for example, 50-75 cases are specified, while 50 cases are recommended for colonoscopy. The guidelines recognize that competency can be established outside of a formal fellowship or residency program, but insist that this competency be shown to be equal to that obtained in a formal program, and suggest that it be very carefully documented. They also recognize that new procedures are being developed for which privileges will be requested and make recommendations for how competency could be demonstrated.

The American Society for Laser Medicine and Surgery, Inc., issued suggested guidelines in 1984.[19] Among their recommendations are that "The applicant shall do only those procedures which he is capable of doing by conventional means and initially do simple procedures," and that "The applicant shall establish a means to work closely with biomedical engineering personnel."

Hospitals might also wish to study the guidelines being developed by the Committee on Clinical Privileges of the American College of Physicians (ACP) for assessment of physician competence in selected procedures in nephrology and gastroenterology.[20] For development of guidelines, the ACP has selected hemodialysis, continuous arteriovenous hemofiltration, acute peritoneal dialysis, percutaneous renal biopsy, colonoscopy, endoscopic retrograde cholangiopancreatography (ERCP), flexible fiberoptic sigmoidoscopy for screening, and diagnostic esophagogastroduodenoscopy. Significantly, according to the project's chairman, Dr. Eugene Hildreth, the subcommittees will be seeking to develop generic definitions of competence, rather than emphasizing specialty certification.[21] Approved guidelines should be published in the spring of 1987.

The Inter-Society Commission for Heart Disease Resources, in 1982, published guidelines specifying the knowledge, skills, and training a physician should have in order to obtain and interpret echocardiograms.[22] These guidelines are quite detailed and specific, and may serve hospitals well as a model for the development of criteria on which to grant clinical privileges.


## Fellowship Training

Although board certification, as noted, is insufficient to demonstrate technological proficiency, an applicant for clinical privileges may have completed a post-residency fellowship in a specific area, such as interventional radiology or neuroradiology, that might be cited as evidence of technological competence. [Unfortunately, these post-residency training programs in radiology vary widely in quality, and they are not followed by a formal examination that could assess competence.[11]]

It should also be noted that there appears to be increased recognition of the importance of certification in the delivery of *levels* of care. This is reflected not only in the creation in the last two decades of boards in family medicine and in emergency medicine, but also in the fact that six specialties now offer subspecialty certification in critical care medicine (anesthesiology, internal medicine, neurological surgery, obstetrics and gynecology, pediatrics, and surgery).

## Training for Practicing Physicians

Given that practicing physicians are unlikely to undertake a formal residency or fellowship program solely to become proficient in a new technology, the best approach may be for physicians to attend organized training courses, where they can obtain "hands-on" experience, to be followed by work in the hospital under supervision. The American Society for Laser Medicine and Surgery, Inc., for example, approves courses of laser instruction.

The American Society for Gastrointestinal Endoscopy has developed a pilot program to teach flexible fiberoptic sigmoidoscopy to interested physicians. The Society is reported to be planning a nationwide effort to provide preceptor-type training in this procedure. However, no readily available program has yet been developed for more sophisticated techniques such as gastroscopy, ERCP, or colonoscopy.[7]

Informal apprenticeship under the direction of a skilled endoscopist may also be a useful approach. For example, Frakes describes learning endoscopic retrograde sphincterotomy in an informal program that included observation of an expert's practice and performance of cases under direct supervision in the expert's hospital.[22]

Short-term training programs are available in some areas of medicine. For example, one-week training programs for radiologists in magnetic resonance imaging (MRI) are being offered at numerous sites. Many other continuing education programs are available, with the approval of the Accreditation Council for Continuing Medical Education being a good indicator of quality. Unfortunately, continuing education programs are generally too brief, and lacking in "hands-on" experience, to be considered as an adequate sole means for attaining technological proficiency.

## New Approaches

Structural changes might also be implemented as a means of seeking to guarantee a higher level of proficiency. For example, at Johns Hopkins Hospital (Baltimore, MD), a cardiovascular radiology admitting service was established that permitted radiologists to serve as attending physicians, rather than as consultants.[23] Such an approach might give radiologists an added incentive to be highly proficient in the relevant invasive technologies, not only to be able to attract referrals, but also to meet the added requirements of being an attending, as opposed to a consulting, physician.

A similar method that has been employed at some community hospitals is to make physicians who wish to practice interventional radiology join the surgical department.[6] Whether this is truly a reasonable alternative remains to be seen.

Finally, and perhaps most importantly, hospitals may simply wish to become more stringent in the credentialing process. The approach that is taken in aviation, where log books are used and varying qualifying levels are required to fly different kinds of aircraft, may be a desirable model. Requiring detailed, written documentation of the experience of a medical staff applicant with a new technology may be a good policy. As long as the process of granting privileges is applied consistently and fairly to all applicants, a hospital should normally not be concerned that it is being *overly* stringent.

## Benefits of Improved Credentialing and Privileging

Improving the process of delineating clinical privileges has many benefits. It will reduce the hospital's risk of being found corporately liable for negligently screening members of its medical staff or negligently granting privileges. It will also help in accreditation, as the JCAH will, in the future, evaluate clinical outcomes as part of the accreditation process. Most importantly, it will improve the quality of patient care.

A good privileging process will also facilitate the incorporation of new procedures that promise to improve patient care and conserve resources. For example, surgical palliation has long been the standard treatment for biliary obstruction associated with cancer of the pancreas. A newer treatment, endoscopic placement of a prosthesis, which can be done by a gastroenterologist, will, in general, result in a shorter stay than would be necessitated by surgery.[24] A good process for granting privileges will recognize that many such procedures are potentially very beneficial for both patients and society and will set forth standards that allow these procedures to be safely performed in the hospital.

## Conclusion

The rapid introduction of new technologies and procedures into medicine makes it more important than ever to delineate clinical privileges carefully. The mechanism of specialty and subspecialty certification, while a good criterion, is not sufficient in itself to serve as the basis for privilege delineation. Hospitals must supplement board certification status with other information about a physician's ability to use new technologies effectively.

In order to ensure that the medical staff will not be seen as arbitrarily "freezing out" physicians who seek privileges for new procedures, it is important that the board of trustees take an active role in overseeing the credentialing process. In addition, hospital administration could facilitate the process by establishing a vice president for clinical or medical affairs in the hospital, where such a position does not yet exist. Supporting this office with up-to-date information about the recommendations of various specialty societies, and keeping current with the evolution of practice in the various specialties and subspecialties, will strengthen the credentialing process. But whatever the mechanism, the final result must be that only those who are actually proficient in a new technology should be given privileges to use it.

## References


1. Peters JD, Peraino JC. Malpractice in hospitals: Ten theories for direct liability. Law Med Health Care 1986; 12:254-9.
2. Elam v. College Park Hospital, 182 Cal. App. 3d 332, 183 Cal. Rep. 156 (1982).
3. Joint Commission on Accreditation of Hospitals. 1987 Accreditation Manual for Hospitals. Chicago: JCAH, 1987:117.
4. JCAH, see note 3, p. 118.
5. Design tougher credentialing procedures, experts advise. Hosp Risk Manage 1985; 7:57-9.
6. Becker GJ. Interventional radiology: Challenges and initiatives. Radiology 1986; 161:562-4.
7. Davidson AJ. Technological volatility and the aging radiologist. AJR 1986; 147:1322-3.
8. Waye JD. How to become trained in an endoscopic procedure after the fellowship program. Am J Gastroenterol 1986; 81:611-2.
9. Howell JD. The changing face of twentieth-century American cardiology. Ann Intern Med 1986; 105:772-82.

10. American Medical Association. 1986-7 directory of residency training programs accredited by the Accreditation Council for Graduate Medical Education. Chicago: AMA, 1986.

11. Rogers LF. The American Board of Radiology to consider *Added Qualifications*. AJR 1986; 147:1324-6.

12. American Board of Medical Specialties. Annual Report & Reference Handbook—1986. Evanston, IL: ABMS, 1986.

13. Havighurst CC, King NMP. Private credentialing of health care personnel: An antitrust perspective. Am J Law Med 1983; 9:131-201.

14. Armstrong v. Board of Directors of Fayette County General Hospital, 553 S.W. 2d 77 (Tenn. App., 1976).

15. 42 C.F.R. 405.1023(e)(4).

16. Kopit WG, Barnes CE, Latorre L. A practical guide to health care antitrust issues. Trustee 1986; 39(May): 16-8.

17. Chenen AR. Privileges system deters disputes among medical staff specialists. Trustee 1985; 38(Jan):28-9,35.

18. American Society for Gastrointestinal Endoscopy. Methods of granting hospital privileges to perform gastrointestinal endoscopy. Manchester, MA: Author, 1986.

19. American Society for Laser Medicine and Surgery, Inc. Standards of practice for the use of lasers in medicine and surgery. Wausau, WI: Author, 1984.

20. Committee on Clinical Privileges, American College of Physicians. Draft guidelines. Philadelphia: Author, 1986.

21. Thomas P. Procedures: Who will do them? Med World News 1986; 27(Aug 11):12-3.

22. Frakes JT. An evaluation of performance after informal training in endoscopic retrograde sphincterotomy. Am J Gastroenterol 1986; 81:512-5.

23. Kinnison ML, White RI, Auster M, et al. Inpatient admissions for interventional radiology: Philosophy of patient management. Radiology 1985; 154:349-51.

24. Siegel JH, Snady H. The significance of endoscopically placed prosthesis in the management of biliary obstruction due to carcinoma of the pancreas: Results of nonoperative decompression in 277 patients. Am J Gastroenterol 1986; 81:634-41.

# Index

## Q

## R

ISBN: 0-934277-17-6